Deutsches Krebsforschungszentrum

Current Cancer Research

1992

Springer-Verlag Berlin Heidelberg GmbH

Cover photo:
Laboratory still life
Photograph: Josef Wiegand

Additional material to this book can be downloaded from http://extras.springer.com.

ISBN 978-3-7985-0898-9 ISBN 978-3-662-11384-4 (eBook)
DOI 10.1007/978-3-662-11384-4
ISSN 0940-0745

Publisher:
Deutsches Krebsforschungszentrum
Im Neuenheimer Feld 280
D-6900 Heidelberg 1
Tel.: + 62 21/42-0
Telex: 4 61 562 dkfz d
Telefax: + 6221/40 12 71

Editorial responsibility:
Presse- und Öffentlichkeitsarbeit
Hilke Stamatiadis-Smidt, M. A.

Coordination:
Elisabeth Hohensee, M. A.

Co-workers:
Dipl.-Biol. Susanne Glasmacher
Dipl.-Biol. Eva Holtmannspötter
Andrea Oder
Dipl.-Biol. Renate Ries
Dr. phil. nat. Birgitt Sickenberger
Stefanie von Kalckreuth, akad. gepr. Übers.
Prof. Dr. med. Gustav Wagner
Dipl.-Biol. Frauke Werner

Translation:
Dipl.-Phys. Dirk Meenenga, B. Sc.

Lay-out:
Heidi Hnatek

Photos:
Josef Wiegand

Photos in the research reports by the authors or by members of the staff. Figs. 2, 3, 55 Prof. Dr. Neidhard Paweletz, Division of Cell Growth and Division; Figs. 4, 15, 16, 133, 141, 167, 181, 182, 183 Ulrich Soeder, Leimen; Fig. 24 with kind permission of Bildarchiv Preußischer Kulturbesitz, Berlin; Fig. 46 Prof. Dr. Ernst G. Jung, Mannheim; Fig. 99 Prof. Dr. Ulrich Kück, Bochum; Fig. 107 from J. Isao et al., The Three-Dimensional Structure of Canine Parvovirus and its Functional Implications, SCIENCE 251, 03/22/91, S. 1456 ff.,

Originally published by Steinkopff Darmstadt in 1992

New Approaches in Cancer Research

by Harald zur Hausen

For decades, the improvement and refinement of surgical techniques and the purposeful use of radiotherapy have met with considerable success. The concerted application of surgery and radiotherapy has especially contributed to the fact that many types of cancer are no longer considered incurable. Especially in the case of common cancer types, however, it is obvious that these successes are limited; the treatment results for cancers of the lung, the intestinal tract, the efferent urinary passages, and the breast are stagnating. Significant improvements only appear possible through early detection. The development of methods for early detection of lung cancer, for example, should thus be promoted.

The past decades have seen the advent of chemotherapy in cancer treatment. Dramatic successes in the treatment of childhood leukemias, lymphogranulomatosis (Hodgkin's disease), and testicular cancer have raised hopes that eventually we might be able to identify chemical substances that would fight the "big killers," i.e., today's most frequent cancer types. However, the results achieved so far have not been very satisfactory, despite some initial success. Life-saving and life-prolonging effects are offset by the high toxicity of many of the substances – which sometimes even leads to severe general defunctionalization symptoms and thus to a significant reduction of the patient's quality of life. Concentrated efforts are being made worldwide to improve this situation by carefully selected protocols for comprehensive field trials. The relatively unspecific effect of the cytotoxins, however, casts doubt on whether significant treatment breakthroughs can be expected beyond a moderate improvement of today's statistics.

Present expectations in cancer therapy are dominated by developments in other fields: advances in molecular biology and immunology and the resultant understanding of the causes of cancer. Today, two basic approaches with very different backgrounds can be defined, which, however, are growing close: one defines cancer as a result of the failure of defense mechanisms, the other as a result of the failure of intracellular regulative processes. In the following, I will compare the "immunological concept" to the "molecular concept".

The starting point was the observation that in the case of genetic or acquired immune deficiencies – the latter are now mostly due to AIDS infections – certain types of cancer, in particular all tumors of the hematopoietic system (lymphoma), occur more frequently than others. We thus had reason to assume that at least these types of cancer are kept at bay by a functioning defense system that identifies the altered cells as "foreign". Today we know that in the case of lasting immunodeficiencies, the incidence not only of lymphomas, but also of several types of papillomas of the skin and of the mucosa, of skin cancer and, for example, of cervical cancer prestages is significantly increased

At first sight, these observations support the "integral" view, which never defined cancer as a focal disease but as a disorder of the entire organism. The contradiction to the slowly accumulated understanding of cancer as a focal disease is beginning to break up: At present, about 15% of all cancers worldwide can be associated with virus infections, and 70% of these with

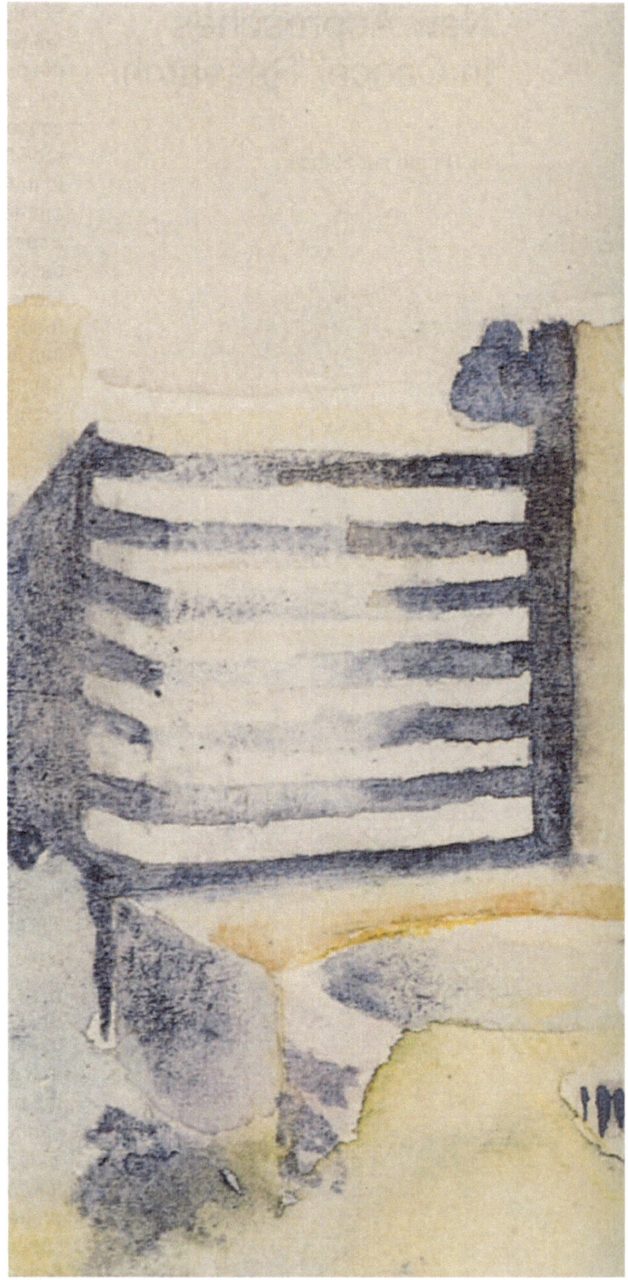

Fig. 1
The Deutsches Krebsforschungszentrum.

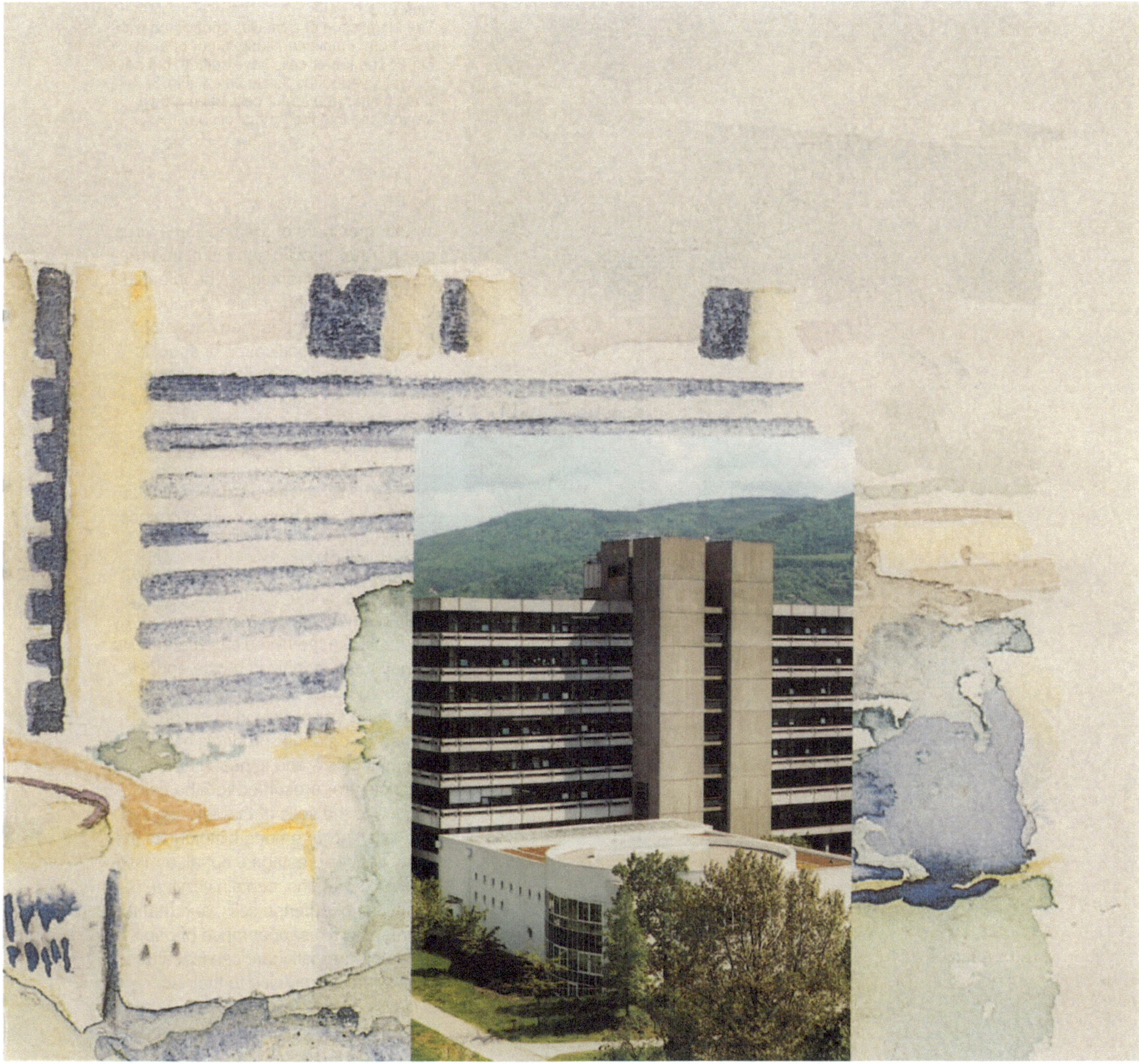

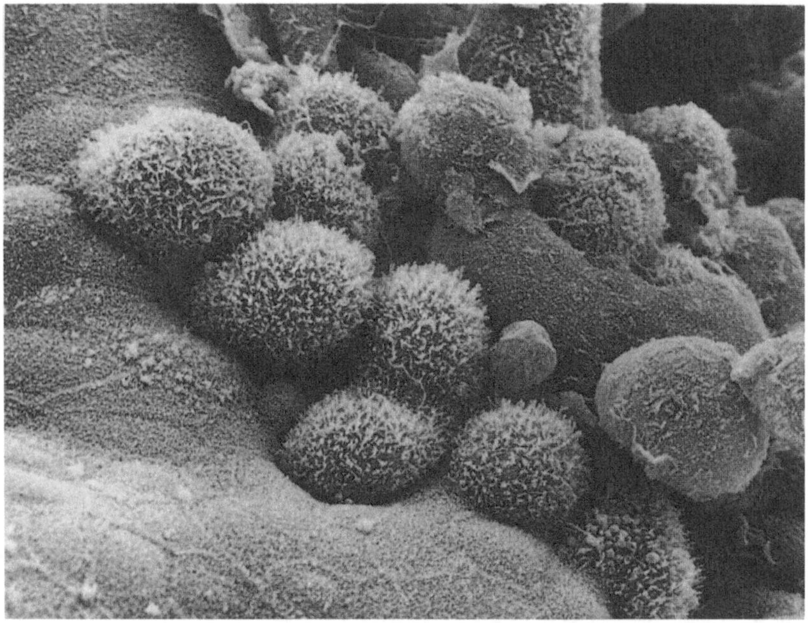

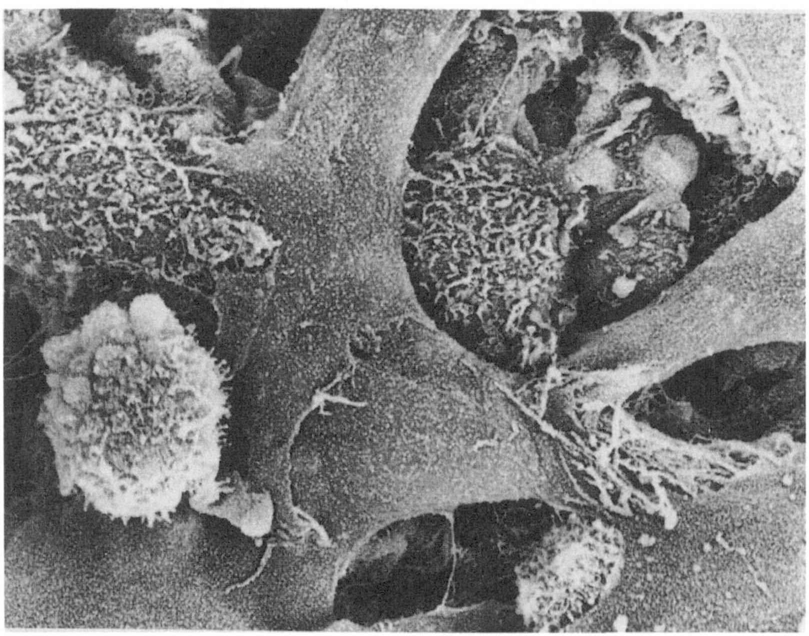

Figs. 2, 3
The lung tissue of a rat was confronted with cells from a malignant lung tumor of a rat. Fig. 2: The tumor cells have settled, but have not yet invaded the tissue below. Fig. 3: Shortly after, the tumor cells have grown around and into the normal tissue.

certain members of the papilloma virus group. After infection, the viral information remains "inherited" in the infected cells without doing visible damage. The actual "derailment" is then caused by an additional modification of specific cellular genes that obviously control these viruses. Such modifications activate specific virus genes, whose "heterologous" genetic products contribute to altering the cell's characteristics. This is where the organism's defense system has a realistic chance to intervene.

It was also observed that an alteration of only one single amino acid within a protein molecule, as may be caused by a mutation in the hereditary material, is sometimes recognized by the endogenous defense system. This is the case if the amino acid in question is carried by catabolic products of the protein molecules, and if these catabolic products are "presented" on the cell surface to the cells of the defense system. It is known among histologists that many cancer prestages, but also malignant proliferations, contain varying quantities of defense cells, and that the spontaneous disappearance of papilloma and premalignant cervical alterations is most likely due to their activities.

These findings have led to a number of treatment concepts on the basis of the identification of cancer cells by the endogenous defense system. In the following, I will briefly describe four main aspects: "monoclonal antibodies," "active immunization," "promotion of antigen presentation," and "extracorporal proliferation of tumor-infiltrating lymphozytes."

The possibility of producing specific antibodies against an almost infinite number of biologically effective molecules and their active elements led almost immediately to the question of whether they could be used in the fight against cancer. Especially cancer types that carry large numbers of certain molecules on their surface, such as melanomas, cancer of the colon, and carcinomas of the liver, seemed to present a suitable basis. However, the expectation that antibodies would have a cell-destroying effect proved to be only partly realized: Problems of concentration and distribution as well as immune reactions against these antibodies make it debatable whether this approach will lead to a breakthrough in cancer treatment. As opposed to this, the use of antibodies in diagnostics has shown better results. Radioactively marked antibodies can be used to localize certain tumors by scintigraphic imaging.

Another broadly discussed approach is the coupling of cytotoxins to monoclonal antibodies which act against tumor surface molecules in order to use this affinity as a carrier system. These approaches, however, have not proven successful yet.

During recent years, experimental approaches on the use of endogenous cancer cells to stimulate the defense system have been revived. The development of specific cell processing techniques and of the extracorporeal infection of cancer cells with viruses have aroused the expectation and hope that, after the appropriate re-introduction of the treated cells into the patient, the tumor cells' heterologous antigens or modified proteins would be presented to the body's cell-mediated defense mechanisms and would thus cause their activation. These approaches are presently being clinically tested; their prospects are difficult to evaluate. Preliminary results indicate that some activity against tumor extracts can be obtained, without, however, having an unambiguous effect on tumor growth.

A particularly interesting concept has developed from animal experiments which show that cancer types which lack certain cell surface molecules (histocompatibility antigens) grow in laboratory animals. Histocompatibility antigens are needed to present the modified tumor cell proteins to the defense system. Due to a lack of stimulation by antigens there is no defense response. The tumor cell thus uses the deactivation of the responsible genes as a "trick" to achieve inhibited growth.

Certain types of human cancers are also accompanied by a deactivation of these presentation molecules. Considerations on the treatment of such diseases are based on two questions: Is it possible to activate these "sleeping" genes with biologically active substances and thus allow the defense system to identify the cancer cell? In fact, some members of a group of molecules, called interferons, cause the reactivation of such genes. However, it is not yet known if their effect on a rare type of human leukemia, hairy cell leukemia, and the limited success in the treatment of renal carcinoma can be traced back to such a mechanism. Another approach is the use of gene therapy to introduce active surface protein genes into cancer cells in order to "force" the cells to present antigens.

The aforementioned observation of the infiltration of tumors by defense cells gave rise to the hope that a particularly successful approach to cancer treatment might be the isolation of defense cells, their intensive proliferation under optimum tissue culture conditions, and their subsequent re-introduction into the patient's circulatory system. It could be shown that the activated lymphocytes do indeed travel back to the tumor; interesting preliminary results indicate that in some cases they were even able to inhibit further tumor growth.

Insertion of genes of the tumor necrosis factor (TNF) into the activated lymphocytes by genetic engineering seems to improve their effectiveness considerably. Tumor cells are particularly sensitive to this factor. Under this therapy, some melanoma patients could be cured completely, whereas others showed no response at all.

This is undoubtedly a very remarkable development deserving special attention. While most other immunological approaches were not very successful, the combination of the immunological and genetic therapy concepts gives rise to considerable hope, even though not enough tumor types have been analyzed so far to serve as a basis for a comprehensive evaluation of this technique.

Apparently in opposition to these developments – influenced by experiences in surgery and radiotherapy, and, in particular, by concentrated experimental cancer research initiated after the turn of the century – are therapeutic concepts in which cancer is considered a focal disease. These models consider the development of cancer as a dysregulation of one single cell and are based on the understanding of molecular alterations within specific cancer cells.

There is ample proof of the fact that individual tumors originate from single cells, i. e., that they are monoclonal. Chromosome alterations, enzyme patterns, and patterns of integration of viral genome are, in general, unambiguous criteria. In the past years, the finding that the development of cancer generally – if not always – requires that the hereditary information of single cells be altered has been confirmed many times and has made the analysis of causal relationships possible. Specific rearrangements of hereditary information have been detected, for instance, for Burkitt's lymphoma, chronic myeloid leukemia, and other cancers of the hematopoietic system. Functional losses of genes play an important role in specific tumors of the eye (retinoblastomas) and of the kidneys (Wilms' tumors) and, undoubtedly, in many other tumors as well. Gene alteration by point mutation changes specific gene functions and obviously contributes to the development of cancers of the colon, the bladder, and the breast. Finally, the introduction of heterogeneous genes by virus infections and their subsequent integration into the hereditary material of the infected cell open up new functional chains and regulative defects that depend on the pattern of integration.

At present, our knowledge about molecular alterations of certain types of human cancers is very limited and speculative, despite the fact that research in this field is developing very quickly. All findings indicate that a single specific gene alteration does not suffice to trigger cancer. Rather, chains of several specific events within one and the same cell seem to be necessary to make it grow invasively and eventually to metastasize. In the case of cervical cancer, the necessary viral gene function seems to be activated only by the destruction of cellular "control genes." Activation alone results in surface changes ("carcinoma in situ"); only further changes, probably in cellular genes, make possible an invasive growth and, eventually, metastatic spread. This sequence of events plausibly explains the usually very slow transition from early tissue alterations to clinically detectable cancer, which might take several decades.

Our ability to increase our knowledge about the individual elements of the causality chains, and from there to develop a comprehensive model that can be verified experimentally, has given etiological cancerresearch a strong boost. Furthermore, this understanding is the basis of new therapeutic considerations to rationally interrupt the causality chain that leads to the development of cancer. The following description of some current developments and concepts in molecular biology, which are presently being considered for use in cancer therapy, will elucidate the vast potential of this approach.

The technique of cloning genes of biologically active substances makes their industrial production possible. Among these are the human insulin, interferons, tumor necrosis factor, erythropoietin, epidermal growth factor, and other substances which are increasingly being used in clinical therapy. Beside the interferons and the tumor necrosis factor mentioned above, colony-stimulating factors play an important role in cancer therapy. Some of these factors stimulate the growth of various components of the hematopoietic system. An important advance is the stimulation of surviving endogenous stem cells after bone marrow transplantation, which may save the lives of many patients.

The availability of various biomodulators and their clinical use constitute a first visible success of the development of genetic engineering for therapy. The growing understanding of the biological role of such factors and the continuously increasing number of newly identified biomodulators allow us to assume that one more field of therapy will change decisively in the future.

The specific information of each of our genes is coded in the sequence of specific elements of our hereditary information, the double-stranded deoxyribonucleic acid. The information is read from the information-carrying strand. In this process, complementary ribonucleic acid (RNA) is produced, which, after transcription, determines the sequence of amino acids which compose the proteins of our cells. Genetic engineering has made it possible to read the second strand (the so-called antisense RNA which does not carry information) of identified genes under the control of strong promotions. Presumably, the complementary antisense RNA and sense RNA then combine to form a double helix which inhibits the transcription of proteins. This method allows us to selectively inactivate specific gene functions.

This principle has proven of particular importance for basic cancer research and makes it possible to specifically study genes involved in cancer development. It is also becoming increasingly important in the diagnostics of gene activities which can be studied microscopically, using antisense probes and certain hybridization techniques (in situ hybridization).

The hope that we will be able to use antisense probes for the treatment of cancer or infections, however, will not be realized in the near future. First, numerous problems must be solved experimentally. How can it be ensured that such probes really find all the defective cells in the organism? How can the probes be introduced into each and all of the defective cells in an active form? Is it possible to maintain their activity over a long period of time? These cardinal questions still remain to be answered. In some cases, even short antisense oligonucleotides of specific gene transcripts have proven effective. Thus, unexpected turns of developments cannot be ruled out.

The ability of certain short RNA to cut other RNA molecules at defined positions might be of importance for the diseases discussed here. Within limits, these "ribozymes" can be "tailored" for various RNA transcripts, a fact that presents a large potential for new findings inbasic cancer research and, in the

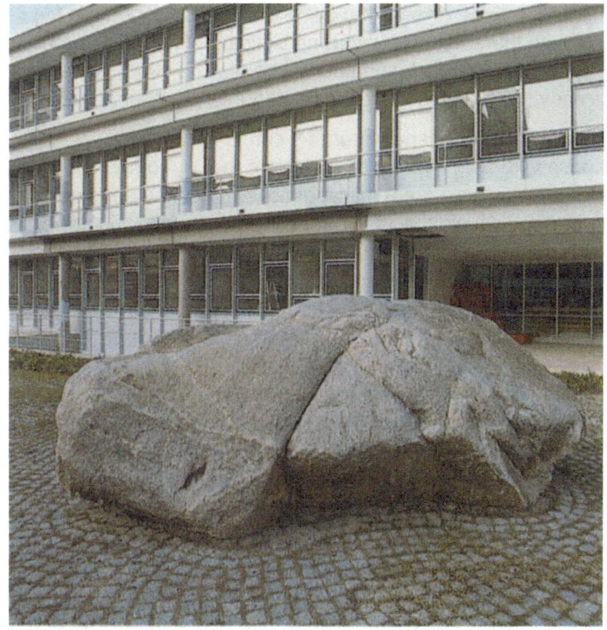

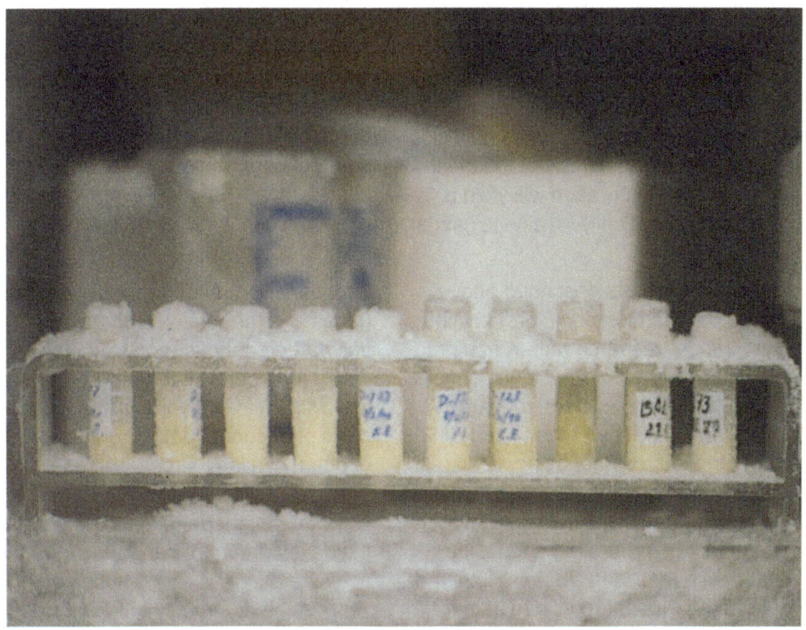

Fig. 4, 5
The reference center for human pathogenetic papilloma viruses. The Deutsches Krebsforschungszentrum stores countless deep-frozen strains of bacteria which contain the hereditary information of various types of viruses.

future, maybe also for the development of new therapies. However, no clinical application of this technique will be ready for use in the foreseeable future.

The concept of genetic surgery comprises working hypotheses which in the future may gain great therapeutic importance. Nucleic acid sequences, whose sequence is largely identical to that of specific genes, can be inserted into DNA strands at the position of their corresponding homologues. This "homologous recombination" might be used to specifically deactivate the functions of "cancer genes" in order to stop malignant growth. The plausibility of this method is obvious. Unfortunately, none of the problems of practical application has been tackled yet. At present, homologous recombination can be triggered in only one out of 150 cells, even under optimum laboratory conditions – a problem that adds to all the others mentioned before.

Intended integration of hereditary information may also be achieved by certain virus sequences, such as those of retroviruses and parvoviruses. It is also possible that the analysis of the mechanisms of their integration will yield a method to specifically inactivate cancer genes.

While the concepts described above (except for the biomodulators) concern basic cancer research rather than practical therapy, the introduction of specific genes, which in some patients are defective, is already being tested clinically. One such defect being studied at present is an inborn metabolic disease, the adenosine deaminase deficiency. The defect of the protein adenosine deaminase results in a severe immune deficiency. Present trials aim at introducing the intact gene into the patient's blood cells via retroviral carrier systems. Approaches on this basis are especially well-suited for the treatment of hereditary diseases that are due to the loss of one specific gene.

Today, it is increasingly realized that for the development of cancer the loss of specific genes ("tumor suppressor genes") is of particular importance. Reintroduction of such genes into cancer cells in tissue culture stops their growth. This technique would represent a true causal treatment. On the basis of these experimental findings we hope that in the future we will be able to treat cancer patients in a similar way.

To date, only a few tumor suppressor genes have been identified, although the findings indicate that they play a role in a large variety of human cancers. Suitable carrier systems for such genes – probably specific viral coats – are being developed, but will not be available very quickly. Two main problems, how to reach all tumor cells, and how to maintain the function of the introduced genes, still remain to be solved. Nevertheless, basic cancer research offers rational treatment concepts which – if they prove successful – will seize cancer at its root, namely, the genetic defects.

The identification of tumor suppressor genes and the resulting characterization of their genetic products allow us to design computer-aided models to interfere with their functions, either on the basis of oligopeptides, or on the basis of other, similarly structured molecules. These models might suggest new pathways that might be taken to influence the development of cancer beyond the actual genetic therapy. Though it is not yet possible to predict which of these pathways will be the most successful,

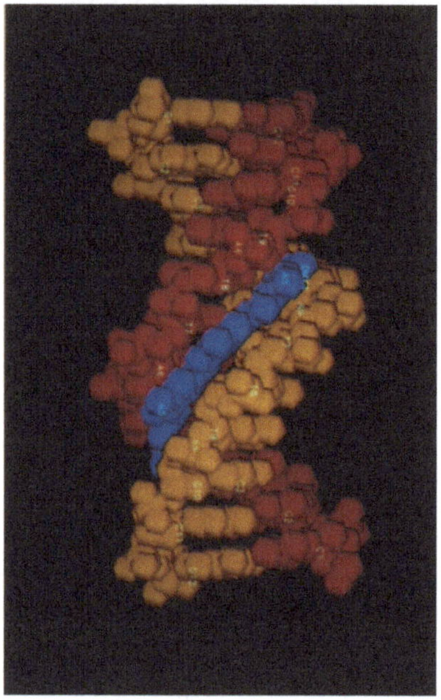

Fig. 6
Computer model of a deoxyribonucleic acid (DNA).

we would be surprised if this field of research did not yield interesting and effective new developments.

Results in the fields of molecular biology and immunology are increasingly diverting the ideas and actions of cancer researchers towards developing a rational cancer therapy, targeted at eliminating the causes. Although at present this development mainly deepens our understanding of the basic processes that lead to cancer, practical consequences for cancer diagnostics and, to a lesser extent, for therapy are now becoming apparent. We expect further developments to lead to basic changes in current treatment concepts.

Furthermore, the possible synthesis between "integral" concepts, as far as endogenous defense mechanisms are concerned, and the definition of cancer as a focal disease, is proving to be particularly advantageous to the development of new treatment approaches. Psychological factors that have an influence on hormonal regulatory processes will also gain therapeutic significance as their mechanisms are increasingly better understood.

The entry of molecular biology into medicine, which only began some years ago, will dramatically change our conception of the causes, the possible prevention, the diagnostics, and the therapy of cancer. We hope that the problems of the realization of new findings for the therapy of cancer in man will be solved as soon as possible.

Prof. Dr. Harald zur Hausen
Chairman of the Management Board of the Deutsches Krebsforschungszentrum

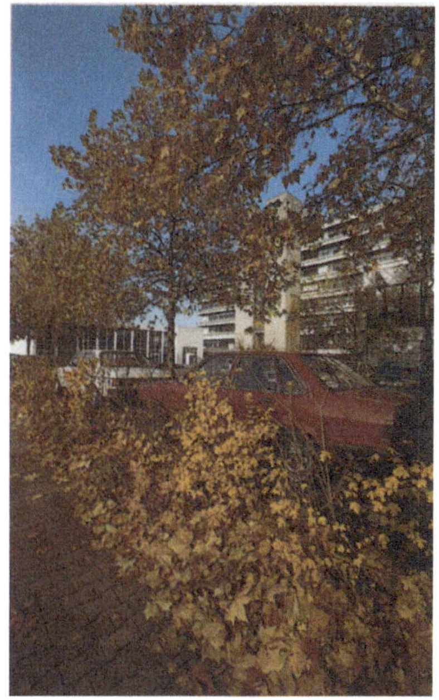

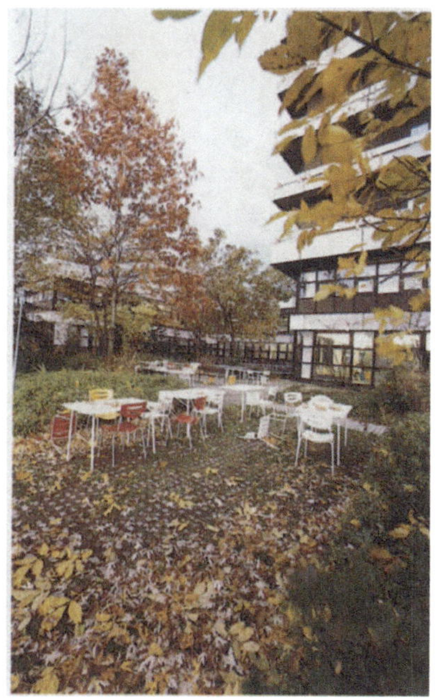

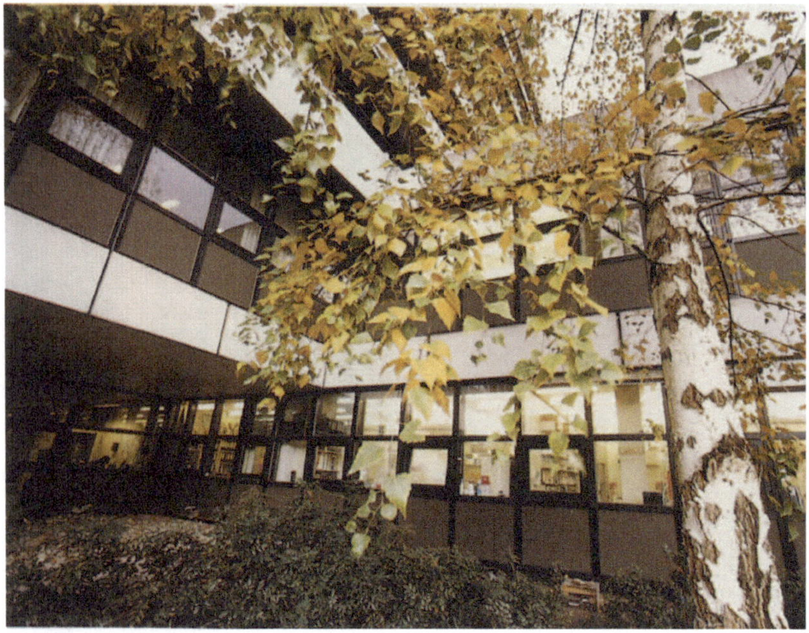

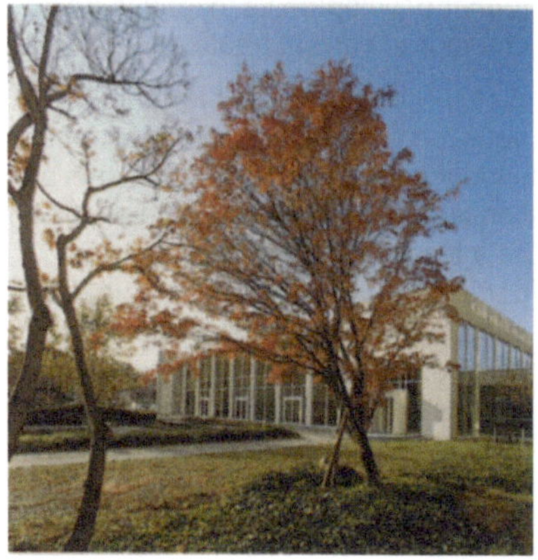

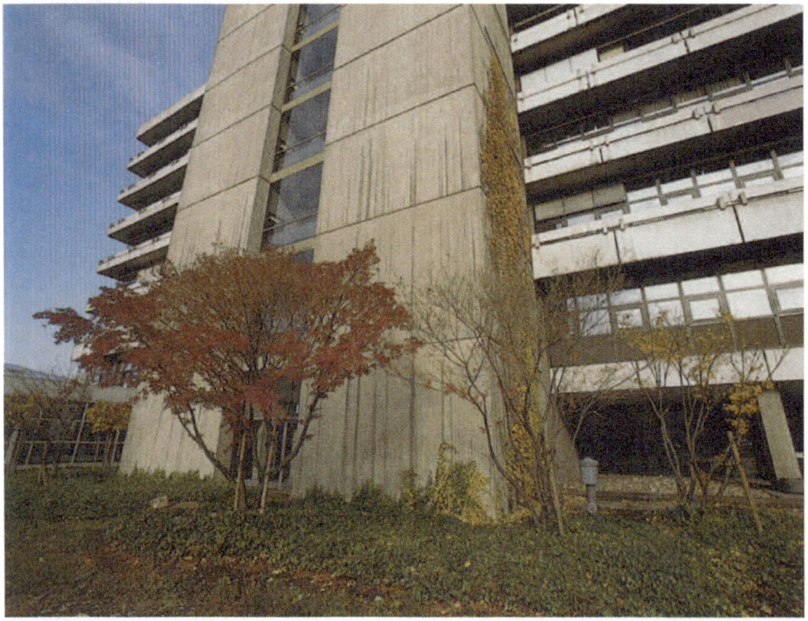

The Deutsches Krebsforschungszentrum in fall.

Mission and Structure of the Deutsches Krebsforschungszentrum

The Deutsches Krebsforschungszentrum (DKFZ) was founded in 1964 on the initiative of the Heidelberg surgeon Prof. Dr. h.c. K.H. Bauer, who died in 1978 at the age of 86. It was constituted as a foundation of public law on the decision of the Government of the State of Baden-Württemberg. Since 1975, it has been one of the major research institutions. On the basis of § 91b of the German Basic Law, it is financed by the German Federal Government (Ministry for Research and Technology: 90%) and by the State of Baden-Württemberg (Ministry for Science and Research: 10%).

In accordance with its Statutes and Articles, it is the task of the Center to engage in cancer research. As a consequence of this general formulation, the question as to whether all of the Center's research projects really entail "cancer research," a term which every discipline defines differently, is a question that must be reconsidered on occasion. In a center with a multidisciplinary structure, the discussion about the contents of the research programs never ceases, and the "equilibrium of forces" must always be re-established. This balancing process is a continuous one; it is sustained by new discoveries, the importance and weighing of which must be determined in the context of the statutory objectives. The necessary balance takes into account the interests of all the scientists, who inevitably consider the problem of cancer from different methodological approaches and assign them different priorities in competition for financial resources. On the other hand, the benefit which scientists, for the solution of their research problems, gain from consultation and collaboration with a large number of experts from all other fields relevant to cancer research is exceedingly great and cannot be provided by any other organizational form.

A new organizational structure for the Deutsches Krebsforschungszentrum was developed in 1990/91 to achieve greater flexibility, increased interdisciplinary collaboration, and rapid integration of new research approaches. All the committees of the Center agreed to these structural changes, which resulted in the Center's new Statutes and Articles (see appendix). The development of a program-oriented structure made it necessary to dissolve the Center's eight Institutes and reorganize the work in eight Research Programs, which, in general, must be concluded within 6 years. The management of the Research Programs, which consist of several of the Center's divisions working in the same field of research, or a coordinator supervises all the scientific and organizational work. The existing permanent divisions are supplemented by temporary divisions, which are planned to be concluded within 5 years. This organizational structure gives young scientists (between 30 and 35) the opportunity to assume responsibility in research. It also takes into account the rapid international development, it makes the research goal an essential element of the Center's research program, and it makes it possible to appoint the head of a Research Program – given appropriate results and qualifications – director of a permanent Division.

The fight against cancer is one of the most important tasks of contemporary science and public health policy. The complex problems of cancer research and therapy involve the biological,

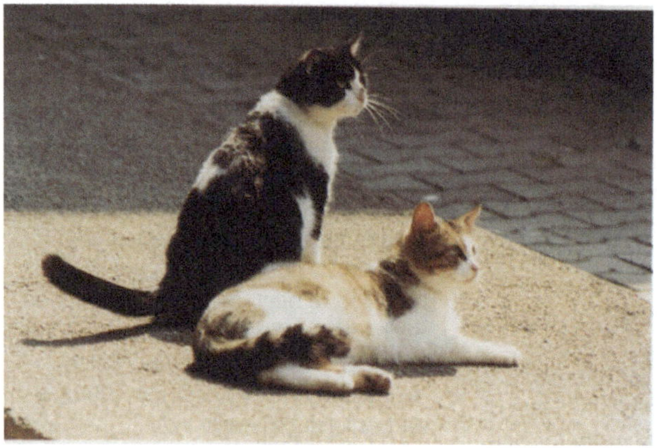

natural, and social sciences. They can only be successfully tackled in close collaboration with scientists from all these disciplines on a national and international level and by the concentration of available research capacities.

It is the objective of the Center's research program to make a tangible contribution to the understanding of carcinogenesis, to the identification of cancer risk factors, and to the prevention, diagnosis, and therapy of cancer. The multitude of human cancers is an indication of the difficulties of scientific analysis.

Taking into consideration the multitude of methods and approaches in cancer research, the Center's programs focus on eight multi-disciplinary priorities:

- Cell Differentiation and Carcinogenesis
- Tumor Cell Regulation
- Cancer Risk Factors and Prevention
- Diagnostics and Experimental Therapy
- Radiological Diagnostics and Therapy
- Applied Tumor Virology
- Tumor Immunology
- Bioinformatics.

The assignment of the existing permanent and of the future temporary divisions to Research Programs is done on the basis of their field of research. The areas of work of the Center may change continuously through the introduction of new Research Programs, the installation of new divisions, and by the alteration of the research program of an existing division. This structural organization allows the Center to implement the results of the permanent international assessment of the Center's scientific work without delay. It is expected that, in the future, more mobile working groups will evolve.

As another development emerging from the previous organizational structure of the Deutsches Krebsforschungszentrum, clinical cooperation groups, agreed to intensive talks between representatives of the University Clinic Heidelberg and scientists from the Center in 1990/91, will be created. Six such clinical working groups are planned. Each will be scientifically independent and will have an associated small clinical unit of about six to eight beds. They will make it possible to implement clinical projects in cancer research (such as the application of new therapeutic principles). It is the purpose of these research groups to implement new experimental therapies into the clinical practice for the benefit of the patient.

On June 22, 1992, the board of the Clinic of the University of Heidelberg and the Management Board of the Deutsches Krebsforschungszentrum signed an agreement on the installation of joint clinical cooperation units.

The clinical research groups will be established at the University Clinic for a period of five years. The physicians and scientists of the Deutsches Krebsforschungszentrum will provide the clinical treatment, whereas the Clinic will provide the beds and the clinical infrastructure. The Deutsches Krebsforschungszentrum will take over any costs which are not covered by the patients' health insurances.

The first two units will be established in the Pediatric University Clinic (medical director: Prof. Dr. Hans Joachim Bremer) and in the Medical University Clinic and Outpatient Clinic V (medical director: Prof. Dr. Werner Hunstein). They will be oriented to new approaches in the diagnosis and therapy of leukemias and lymphomas.

Research

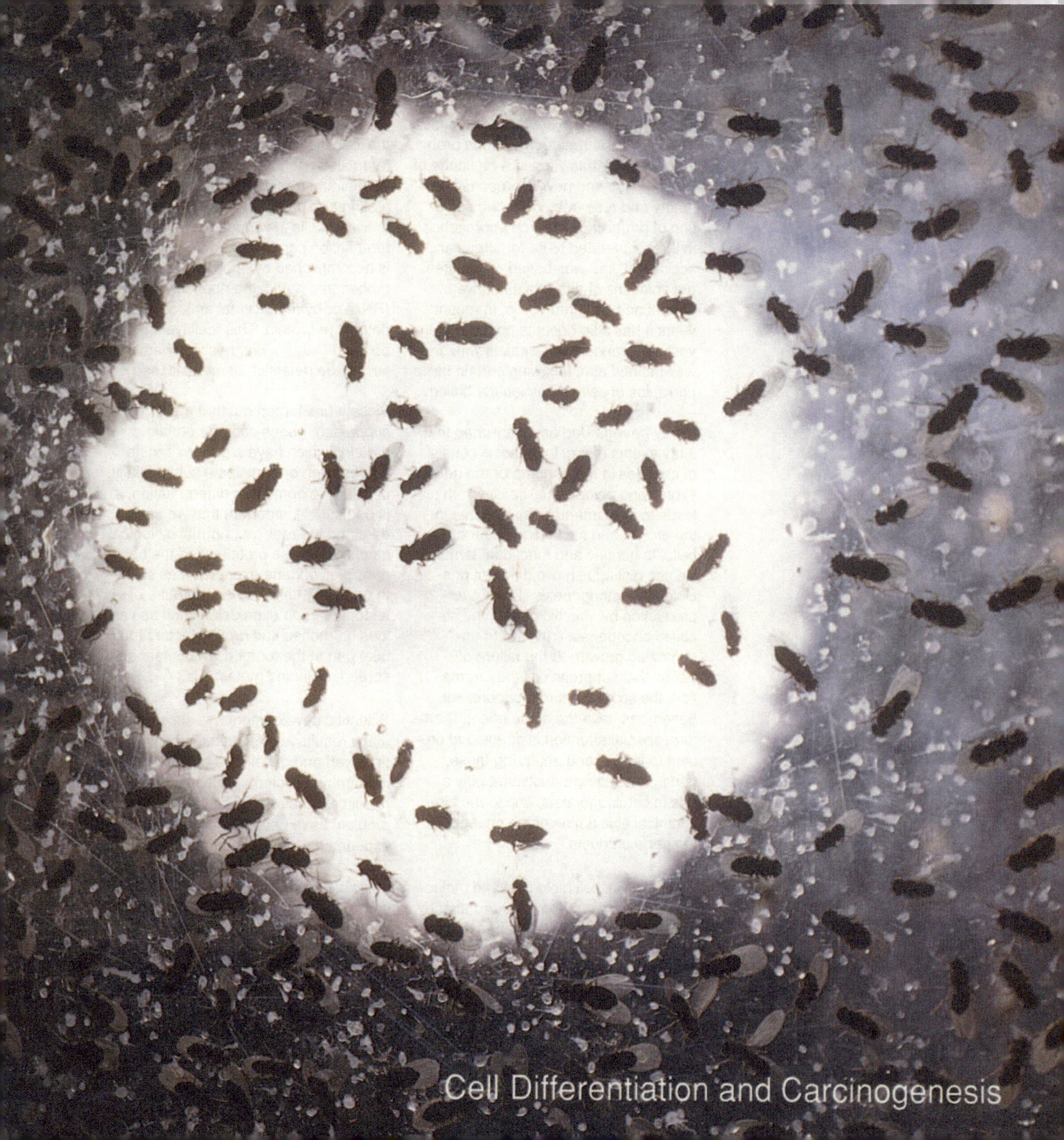

Cell Differentiation and Carcinogenesis

2

Cell Differentiation and Carcinogenesis

In recent years, the confrontation of scientists in basic research with the problem of cancer has yielded a multitude of new findings and new approaches in theory and research. While the selection of promising research approaches in the past tended to be fortuitous and accidental, i.e., was based on isolated observations of differences between normal and malignant cells, in recent years it has also become possible to investigate cancerous diseases with a well-defined aim, following certain basic principles of cell and molecular biology.

It may be regarded as established that early events of carcinogenesis consist of changes in the genome or the gene expression of individual cells, which leads to fundamental disturbances in the growth and social behaviour of cells. In genetic and functional terms, we can distinguish two different principles of tumorigenesis: 1) the overproduction by specific genes, the so-called oncogenes, can lead to uncontrolled growth; 2) the failure of genes that suppress cell transformation, the so-called tumor suppressor genes, can have the same effect. Therefore, special attention is directed at present to finding and analyzing those genes and their products that play a role in carcinogenesis, and to the biochemical elucidation of the changes in the gene products.

Furthermore, cell biological and molecular biological methods that are already available or can be established open up possibilities of practical application in diagnosis and therapy. For instance, by means of these techniques it is possible to find probes for specific chromosome changes of cancer-associated genes, including viral genes, and to use them for tumor diagnosis as well as for the identification of patients at risk . Differences in gene expression between normal and transformed cells, between resting and proliferating cells, and between cells in various states of differentiation can also be detected. This is accomplished by appropriate gene probes that detect the ribonucleic acid (RNA) or by monoclonal antibodies that detect the protein. This "cell typing" can be used in tumor diagnosis, in particular, for the detection of metastases.

Since it has turned out that many tumor suppressor genes code for certain proteins which have a general regulatory function or participate substantially in cell development or differentiation, it is particularly important that we understand the real, i.e., normal biological function of these proteins and the basic principles of gene expression as such. In particular, this also refers to the effectors of gene expression such as various hormones and growth factors that take part in the tumor development and spread, including metastasis.

Scientific development has shown that many results and techniques originally achieved and developed by pure basic research on systems which sometimes had little or no relation to the cancer problem have become trendsetting for experimental cancer research today. Thus, a further investigation of the basic biological structures and processes, of embryonic development and tissue differentiation, promises to yield more knowledge and hints for valuable new research approaches. Within the Research Program Cell Differentiation and Carcinogenesis, we will continue to pursue also fundamental questions of cell and molecular biology and to scrutinize the results for their relevance for tumor research in the narrower sense.

Coordinator of the Research Program:
Prof. Dr. Werner W. Franke

Divisions and their heads:

Cell Biology:
Prof. Dr. Werner W. Franke

Molecular Biology of the Cell I:
Prof. Dr. Günther Schütz

Molecular Biology of the Cell II:
Prof. Dr. Ingrid Grummt

Developmental Genetics:
Prof. Dr. Bernhard Mechler

Cytogenetics:
Prof. Dr. Manfred Schwab

2.1 Cancer and Genes: The Case of the Pediatric Cancer Neuroblastoma

by Manfred Schwab

The first results which indicate that cellular genes may play a central role in the development of cancer date from the end of the last century. In particular the fact that certain families are often more prone to cancers than others lead to the interpretation that hereditary factors play an important role in cancer development. Today, there is no doubt that genetic alterations play a key role in the development of cancers.

There are two levels of genetic alterations: those which occur in a somatic cell and those which affect a germinal cell. If a genetic alteration occurs in a somatic cell, only this cell possesses the altered gene and becomes a cancer cell, whereas all other cells remain normal. This type of mutation is the most common one. If, on the other hand, a genetic alteration occurs in a germinal cell, the individual remains healthy, but all cells of the offspring carry the alteration. This may result in a predisposition for a particular type of cancer.

A large number of laboratories is working worldwide to clarify the importance of various genetic alterations in the development of certain types of cancer. In principle, one single genetic alteration generally does not lead to the development of cancer. Today, the development of cancer is regarded as a multistage process, and thus it is probable that a combination of various genetic events eventually causes a normal cell to become a cancer cell. One focus of present cancer research is the search for further genetic defects in cancer cells.

In this context, the multi-disciplinary approach is increasingly gaining importance. Cytogenetics, genetics, molecular genetics, virology, and other research areas have all made specific contributions that define cancer as a genetic disease. Of particular interest is tumor cytogenetics, which has developed from a merely descriptive discipline to a field of science that has – together with molecular-genetic, virological and cytogenetical approaches – contributed significantly to the understanding of the genetic fundamentals of cancer development. The combination of classical and molecular-cytogenetic approaches is not only suited to give an insight into the genetic mechanisms of cancer development; it may also lay the foundations for the development of modern methods of early diagnosis and possibly for new therapeutic strategies.

Neuroblastoma – a Childhood Nerve Cell Cancer

Our research focuses on the elucidation of the contribution of genetic alterations to the development of a childhood nerve cell tumor, the neuroblastoma. In a more general sense, pediatric cancers have been particularly original settings that have provided the basis for developing general concepts about the role of genetic alterations in tumorigenesis. Chromosome examinations have shown that two genetic alterations are particularly common in neuroblastoma cells. The first is an increase in the number of copies of the N-myc oncogene. The second is the alteration of a certain region on chromosome 1, pointing out the role of a putative tumor suppressor gene.

The neuroblastoma model is excellently suited to demonstrate the specific interdisciplinary approach followed by our team, which includes genetics, cytogenetics, molecular genetics, protein biochemistry and clinical disciplines.

Amplification of N-myc Gene

One of the most common genetic alterations in cancer cells is the amplification of cellular oncogenes. Whereas in the genome of a normal cell only one copy of a specific oncogene can be found, selective gene amplification in the genome of tumor cells may cause the cells to have several hundred copies of that gene. Amplification is a genetic activity on the level of the DNA and results in an increased expression of genes.

Chromosome studies have drawn the researcher's attention to amplification for genetic alteration in tumor cells. In 1965, certain chromosome anomalies, which today are called "double minutes" (DMs), were discovered in neuroblastoma. In 1976, a "homogeneously staining region" (HSR) could be identified in a marker chromosome in neuroblastoma cells. However, the significance of both chromosome anomalies as well as their genetic significance remained unclarified for a long time. Although in various types of cells, DMs and HSRs were identified as sites of amplified genes causing resistance to various cytostatics such as methotrexate, this explanation could not be adequate in settings in which the tumor cells had not been exposed to cytostatics. In 1983, for the first time, evidence was found that DMs and HSRs are sites of amplified cellular oncogenes in tumor cells. Today, we assume that at least most of the chromosomal anomalies, DMs and HSRs, indicate the presence of amplified cellular oncogenes in tumor cells. Amplification seems to be a genetic alteration which mainly occurs in the cells of solid tumors. Only in rare cases has amplification been observed in the cells of hematopoietic malignancies.

Chromosome examinations showed long ago the presence of amplified DNA in neuroblastoma cells, but it was not until 1983 when it was shown that in neuroblastomas a specific gene, the N-myc, is amplified between 10- and 100-fold.

N-myc is a member of a multigene family, whose prototype is the gene myc. Amplified members of the myc gene family are present in various human tumors. The amplified N-myc gene, for example, was exclusively found in tumors that developed from cells with neural properties. N-myc amplification occurs most frequently in neuroblastomas and, to a lesser extent, in retinoblastomas, glioblastomas, astrocytomas and small-cell lung carcinomas. So far, in neuroblastomas only N-myc amplification has been observed; the amplification of other cellular oncogenes has not been reported in this tumor. This specificity points to a special function of the N-myc gene in the development of neuroectodermal tumors.

Protein Function

Amplification results in increased synthesis of the protein coded by N-myc. The N-myc protein is a phosphorylized protein located in the nucleus. Recent investigations have shown that the N-myc protein possesses properties of a transcription factor. An interesting observation is the fact that it is able to specifically associate in vivo with another protein that we were able to identify recently by immuneprecipitation. This observation opens up new possibilities of analyzing the biochemical function of a nuclear oncoprotein.

Structure of Amplified DNA

Only recently could the structural arrangement of amplified DNA be partially clarified. It was shown that the amplified DNA is much larger in size than the N-myc gene. The gene consists of only about 10 kilobase pairs (kbp), whereas in different tumor types the amplified DNA may be between several hundred kbp and 1000 kbp in length. Most surprisingly, these long DNA units are frequently arranged as head-to-tail tandem repeats which surround the N-myc gene. The well-ordered structure of the amplified DNA indicates that there may exist a specific amplification mechanism which is only partially understood.

Clinical Significance of N-myc Amplification

Important prognostic parameters for the neuroblastoma are the clinical stage and the age of the patient at the time of diagnosis. Patients with neuroblastomas of stages I and II mostly have favorable prognoses; 75 to 90% can expect to survive for at least 2 years. Patients with stage-III and stage-IV tumors have a poor prognosis. Significantly different prognoses for patient groups with tumors of stage-III have been observed in the USA and in Germany. In the USA, the prognosis for stage-III tumors is similar to that for stage-IV tumors (10 to 30%), whereas a considerably more favorable prognosis is observed in Germany. The reason for this disagreement is not yet known.

Investigations carried out independently by various working groups have shown a significant correlation between amplification of N-myc and stages III and IV. This correlation was first shown within the framework of a study on 63 neuroblastomas; amplification was not detected in 15 stage-I and stage-II tumors, but was observed in 24 of 48 (50%) stage-III and stage-IV tumors. Subsequent studies by other authors have confirmed this correlation, although the incidence of amplification was somewhat smaller (between 20 and 30%).

A significant correlation between poor prognoses and N-myc amplification was also observed when comparing patients over 1 year of age with patients under 1 year. Prognoses for patients over 1 year of age, especially for those with stage-III and stage-IV tumors, is particularly unfavorable. One study showed N-myc amplification for more than 50% of the patients older than 1 year; for younger patients, the incidence of amplification was smaller. N-myc amplification thus seems to be an independent parameter for the

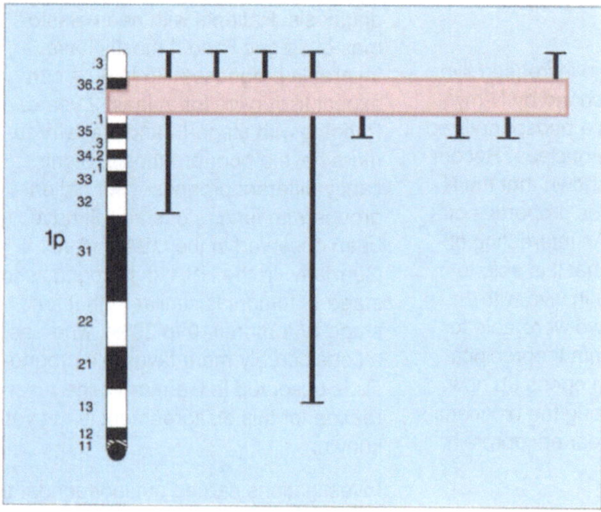

Fig. 9
In neuroblastoma cells, the short arm of chromosome 1 (1p) is frequently altered. In each patient, different sections of a specific region of this chromosome (shaded) are lost. It is not known yet whether a deletion in this region implies a loss or a failure of a specific gene.

evaluation of the prognosis of neuroblastoma.

Current therapy protocols for treatment of neuroblastoma depend on the prognosis for survival which is evaluated on the basis of the tumor stage, the degree of surgical resectability, and on an analysis of genetic alterations. The pilot study of the German Neuroblastoma Study Group recommends treatment according to protocols specific for each of four risk groups (Table 1). Risk group A includes patients with localized tumors of which at least 90% can be removed surgically (prognosis: 90 to 100%). Risk group B includes patients with localized tumors that extend beyond the organ of origin and which usually cannot be removed completely (prognosis: 65 to 80%). Risk group C includes patients with metastasizing tumors or localized tumors that do not regress after four cycles of chemotherapy (prognosis: 20 to 30%). Risk group D includes only patients with stage-IV tumors that frequently show spontaneous regression (prognosis: 75 to 80%).

Patients of risk group C receive the most intensive therapeutic treatment. Amplification of N-myc is incompatible with being included in risk groups with favorable prognoses, even if the tumor is localized. All patients with amplification are included in risk group C and are submitted to the most intensive therapy. However, this only applies to tumors of stages I-III. In the case of stage-IV tumors, neither positive nor negative differences were observed with regard to amplification when comparing the patients' prognoses. Thus, the amplification of N-myc is an independent parameter which allows us to classify a patient into a particular risk

Table 1:
Risk groups in neuroblastoma and N-myc amplification.

Risk group % of survival	Tumor
A (90–100%)	Tumor localized, almost completely resectable Stage I: microscopic residual tumor acceptable Stage IIA: small macroscopic residual tumor acceptable (<10 percent); Excluded: patients with amplification
B (65–80%)	Tumor localized; incomplete resectability Stage IIA: macroscopic residual tumor (< 10 percent); Stage IIB: ipsilateral lymph node positive Stage III: infiltration beyond median; Excluded: patients with amplification
C (20–30%)	Tumor metastazises Risk groups A and B, if amplification is positive
D (75–80%)	Stage IV

(Criteria according to the pilot protocol of the German Neuroblastoma Study Group NB90P as of August 1, 1991; head of study group: F. Berthold, Köln). Patients with N-myc amplification were always classified into risk group C, independent of other parameters.

Fig. 10
In the case of heredofamiliar cancers, the predisposition for a certain type of cancer can be proven with a simple test. The hereditary substance is isolated from a blood sample and made visible. Of 13 family members, only No. 9 is missing a section of the hereditary substance. This is the signal of a defective gene. Probably, only this child will develop that specific type of cancer.

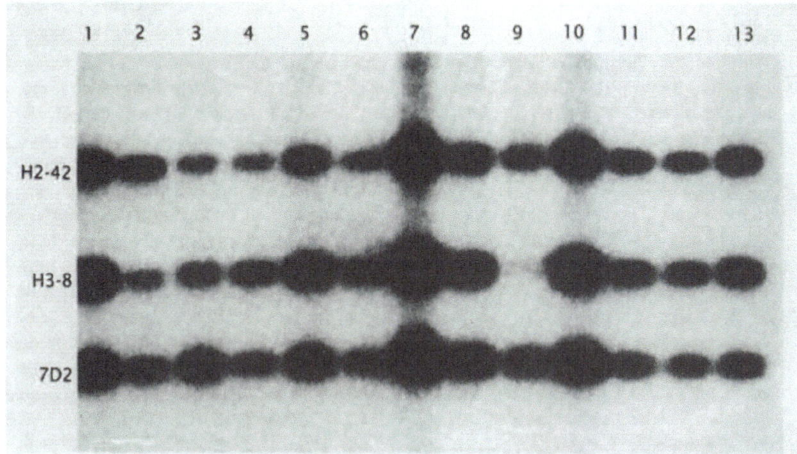

Fig. 11
Diagram of a transsection of an intestinal polyp. In the case of the familial adenomatous polyposis, the epithelium of the intestinal mucosa begins to proliferate (left). Epithelial cells invade the lower cell layer. The disintegration of the cellular order indicates the degeneration of the benign polyp into a malignant tumor (right).

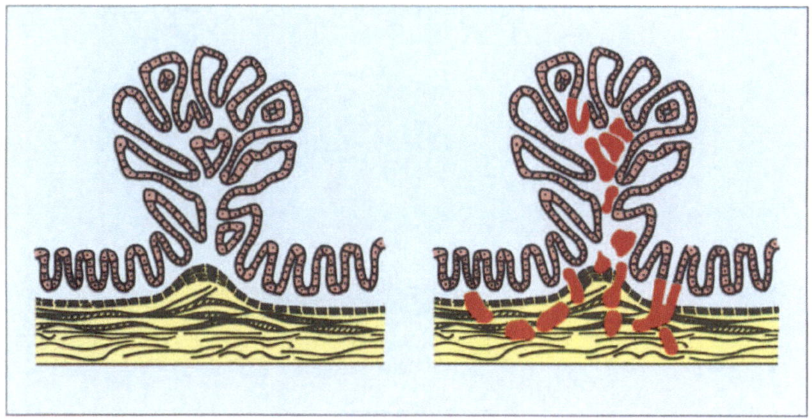

group and thus to decide on a specific treatment protocol.

Chromosome 1 Alterations

When evaluating the significance of amplification in tumorgenesis, one has to take into account that tumor cells frequently have additional genetic alterations. In the case of neuroblastomas, the deletion of genetic material from the short end of chromosome 1 seems to be of particular importance. Chromosome analyses have given evidence for 1p deletion, which was recently specified to be on bands 1p36.1-2. By using polymorphic molecular probes, 1p deletion could be detected in almost all of the neuroblastomas examined, even in cases in which a deletion was too small to be detected by chromosome analysis. However, there does not seem to exist a direct correspondence between 1p deletion and N-myc amplification. Only two out of 10 cases with deletion also showed amplification. Furthermore, N-myc is localized on another chromosome (2p23-24).

The significance of 1p deletion still has to be clarified. It remains to be seen

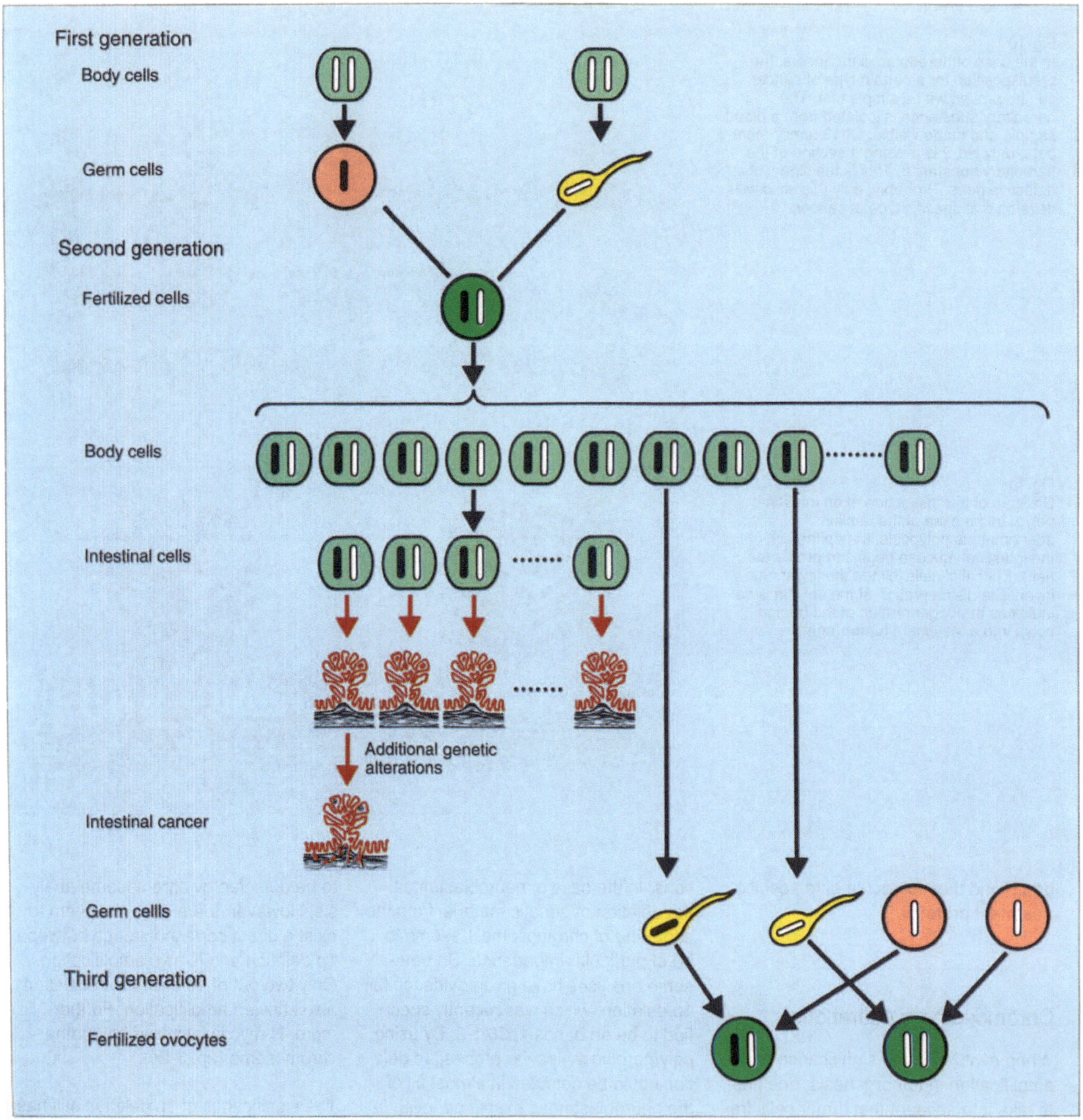
First generation
Body cells
Germ cells
Second generation
Fertilized cells
Body cells
Intestinal cells
Additional genetic alterations
Intestinal cancer
Germ cellls
Third generation
Fertilized ovocytes

Fig. 12
Transmission of the familial adenomatous polyposis (FAP). The FAP gene is situated on human chromosome 5. In the ovum (first generation), the FAP gene is altered. The child (second generation) thus inherits a deficient gene from the mother and an intact gene from the father and will eventually develop intestinal polyps. As a result of further alterations in other genes of polypous cells, almost all FAP patients develop intestinal cancer. Timely resection of the polyps prevents their degeneration into tumors.

whether a certain gene in the region is lost by deletion. Only then will we be able to tell if there is altered or deleted genetic information in the sense of a "tumor suppressor gene". Very recent progress has been made towards this goal by the identification of recurrent translocation breakpoints within bands 1p36.1-2. These breakpoints are well localized on the chromosome and are expected to provide much better access to the cloning of a particular gene than the deletions which are quite large for molecular analyses.

Gene Probes and Early Tumor Diagnosis

For neuroblastoma, the genetic alteration "amplification" is an independent parameter for the evaluation of patient prognoses. In this setting, the genetic alteration affects only the somatic cells. However, there exist a number of cancers that develop on the basis of an inherited predisposition. One typical example of this is Familial Adenomatous Polyposis (FAP), which is transmitted according to Mendelian Laws. Within the patient's large intestine, hundreds or even thousands of benign tissue anomalies (polyps) develop. This symptom is a prestage of colon cancer. If the polyposis is not detected and removed surgically at an early stage, it develops into a malignant cancer disease.

Meanwhile, the gene for FAP has been identified on the human chromosome 5. Worldwide efforts are being made to isolate this gene and to discriminate between its healthy and its abnormal form. If the gene alterations responsible for FAP are known, it will be possible to identify members of FAP families with an increased risk of developing polyposis, long before symptoms appear. It will thus be possible to concentrate on intensive clinical care and preventive measures for the patient. It will also be possible to identify family members who do not have an increased risk of developing the disease.

FAP is only one example of a possible use of gene probes in presymptomatic early diagnosis of patients with tumor risks. Genetic predisposition also seems to exist in the case of more frequent cancer diseases. For example, a form of breast cancer developing at an early age seems to be the result of genetic predisposition; in this case, too, the identification of the corresponding gene may make possible presymptomatic early diagnosis of patients with an increased risk of developing cancer.

Outlook

Currently, cancer research concentrates on three major problems. First, it seems to be important to further identify the spectrum of genetic alterations in different tumor types and to verify whether non-random genetic alterations occur in specific tumor types. Second, it is important to examine whether certain non-random alterations might be used as parameters in presymptomatic early detection of cancer diseases and whether they might be of help in deciding which of the proven therapies is to be applied. And third, it seems to be of importance to gain knowledge on the biological function of genetic alterations in cancer cells in order to obtain clues for causal therapeutic strategies.

Within the framework of these objectives, analysis of the role played by alterations of cellular oncogenes and tumor suppressor genes is of particular importance. Specific structural anomalies of both gene groups frequently occur in specific cancer diseases. On the one hand, these genetic alterations are of diagnostic significance; on the other hand, the knowledge of the consequences of these genetic alterations for multiplication and differentiation of cells may lay the foundation for approaches to causal therapeutic strategies of cancer diseases, since both cellular oncogenes as well as tumor suppressor genes obviously play a central role in the metamorphosis of a normal cell into a malignant one.

Prof. Dr. Manfred Schwab
Division of Cytogenetics

Participating scientists
Dr. Lukas Amler
Dr. Peter Barker
Dr. Ilona Becker
Dr. Kai van der Bosch
Dr. Stephan Breit

2

Raffaela Corvi
Dr. Celina Cziepluch
Susanne Dillmann
Manuela Gehring
Kerstin Reumann
Dr. Larisa Savelyeva
Jörg Schürmann
Dr. Achim Wenzel

Selected publications

Martinsson, T., Weith, A., Cziepluch, C., Schwab, M.: Chromosome 1 deletions in human neuroblastomas: Generation and fine mapping of microclones from the distal lp region. Genes, Chromosomes and Cancer 1, 67–78 (1989)

Weith, A., Martinsson, T., Cziepluch, C., Brüderlein, S., Amler, L.C., Berthold, F., Schwab, M.: Neuroblastoma consensus deltion maps to lp36. 1–2. Genes, Chromosomes and Cancer 1, 159–166 (1989)

Schwab, M.: Oncogene amplification in neoplastic development and progression of human cancers. Critical Reviews in Oncogenesis 2, 35–51 (1990)

Schwab, M.: Amplifikation von MYCN in Neuroblastomen: Paradigma für die klinische Anwendung einer Onkogenveränderung. Klin. Pädiatr. 202, 197–201 (1990)

Schwab, M.: Amplification of MYCN specifics the form of therapy for children with neuroblastoma. In: Oncogenes in Cancer Diagnosis. Eds.: C.R. Bartram, K. Munk, M. Schwab. Contrib. Oncol. vol. 39, 180–192 (1990)

2.2 Tumor Suppression in Drosophila

by Bernard M. Mechler

Cancer is not limited to humans, but occurs throughout the animal kingdom, from the most primitive metazoa to invertebrates and vertebrates, and it even affects plants. This disease is associated with the evolution of multicellularity and is generally considered a failure in the normal progression of cell differentiation. As a result, cancer cells escape the mechanism controlling normal cell growth and proliferate. When overgrowth reaches a critical threshold, complex syndromes arise and, ultimately, lead to the death of the organism.

It is now well established that cancer is primarily a disease of the genes, and numerous evidence point out that most, if not all, cancer cells contain genetic damage which appears to lie at the heart of tumorigenesis. The genetic alteration found in cancer cells is essentially of two sorts: dominant, with targets known as proto-oncogenes, and recessive, with targets known as tumor suppressor genes. Dominant mutations usually result in a gain-of-function whereas recessive mutations cause a loss-of-function.

The importance of recessive mutations in cancer formation has been genetically well documented in humans and in the fruitfly Drosophila, and current researches point out the growing importance of alterations in genes whose products negatively regulate cell proliferation as major targets in the appearance of cancer.

However, if the biochemical function of the products of tumor genes can readily be analyzed at the cell level, the relevances of these genes in terms of cancer can only be evaluated in whole organisms. It is therefore necessary to analyze these genes by studying animals which carry defined mutations or genetic alterations in these genes, and to determine under which conditions these genetic damages can induce tissue specific neoplasia during the life course of these organisms.

For analyzing genetic damages which alter the normal progression of cell proliferation and differentiation, the fruitfly Drosophila is certainly a choice subject. Our knowledge of the structure and function of the Drosophila melanogaster genome is far greater than for any other multicellular organisms. Since the first attempt to construct genetic maps made by Sturtevant in 1913, approximately 4000 different genes, perhaps a quarter of the total, have been mapped by recombination in this species. With the recent development of recombinant DNA procedures further transcription units, which were not previously recognized by classical genetics, have been precisely localized on the Drosophila genome. In this way, about 3000 transcription units have been found and mapped on polytene chromosomes by in situ hybridization. With the present maps and the available molecular genetic methods, it is now possible to clone any gene that has been identified by mutations.

Genetic and molecular analyses of Drosophila have revealed that tumorigenesis may arise from inactivation of

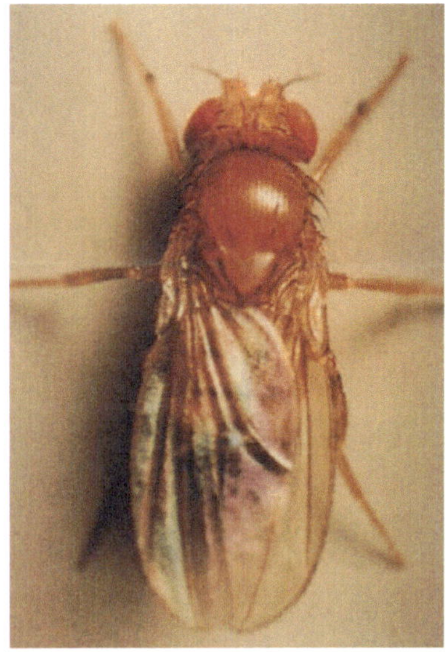

Fig. 13
Drosophila melanogaster is the geneticist's favorite laboratory animal. It is about 2 mm in size.

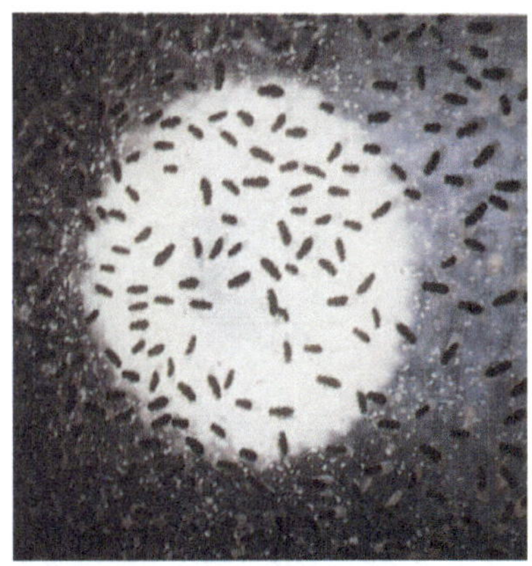

Fig. 14
Thousands of flies are bred in the Division of Developmental Genetics for the investigation of the functioning of a tumor suppressor gene.

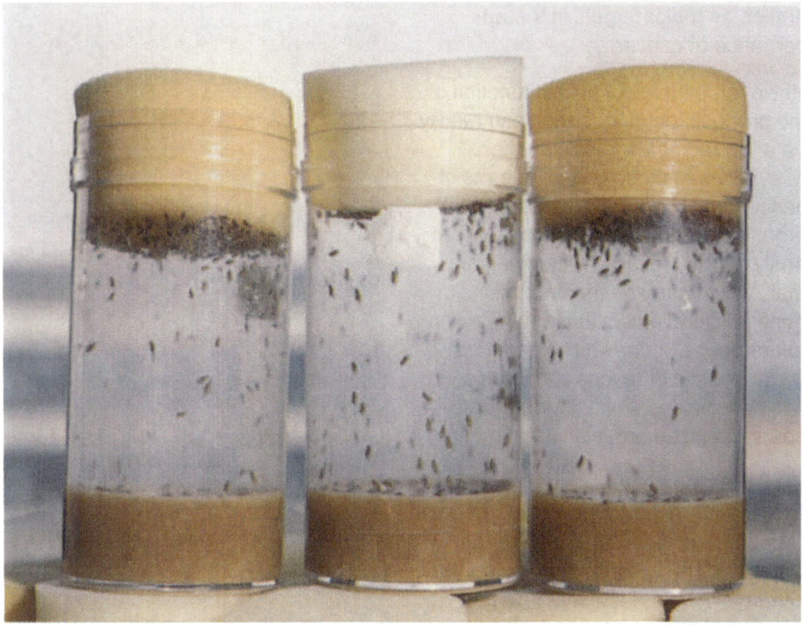

Fig. 15
The individual fly strains are kept strictly separate. Each strain has specific characteristics that allow the researcher to observe changes in the hereditary information of the phenotype.

genes controlling cell growth and differentiation. Recessive mutations in a series of genes interrupt the differentiation of primordial cells and result in uncontrolled and invasive cell proliferation. As a consequence, the mutant animals form malignant tumors in either the optic centers of the larval brain, the imaginal discs, or the hematopoietic organs. Simultaneously with the appearance and growth of the neoplasms, the development of the mutant animals becomes impaired and these animals die as larvae or pseudopupae. Among these genes, the lethal(2)giant larvae gene is the prototype of tumor suppressor genes and has been extensively studied since its discovery. Furthermore, this gene has been isolated and subjected to molecular analysis.

The Lethal(2)giant Larvae Gene

In Drosophila melanogaster the best known recessive tumor gene is the lethal(2)giant larvae (l(2)gl) gene. Homozygous l(2)gl mutations lead to neoplastic transformation of the neuroblasts and ganglion mother cells of the adult optic centers in the larval brain and neoplasia of the imaginal discs. In the mutant animals, these

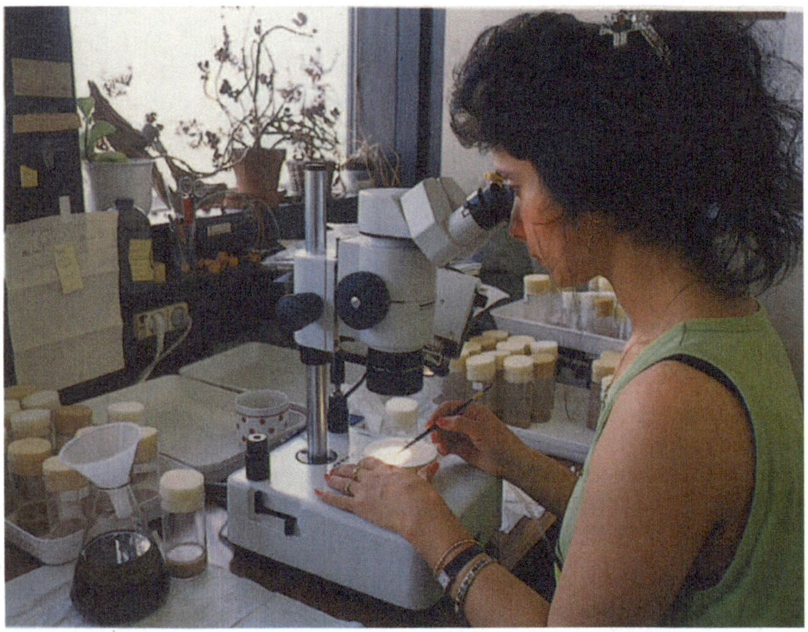

Fig. 16
The tiny insects have to be handled with kid gloves.

Fig. 17
The protein coded by the tumor suppressor gene "lethal (2) giant larvae" can be identified with the aid of an antibody in the plasma membrane of cells of the gastrointestinal tract. (The picture shows a cross section through an adult animal.) The 1(2)gl protein seems to participate in a signal transmission mechanism.

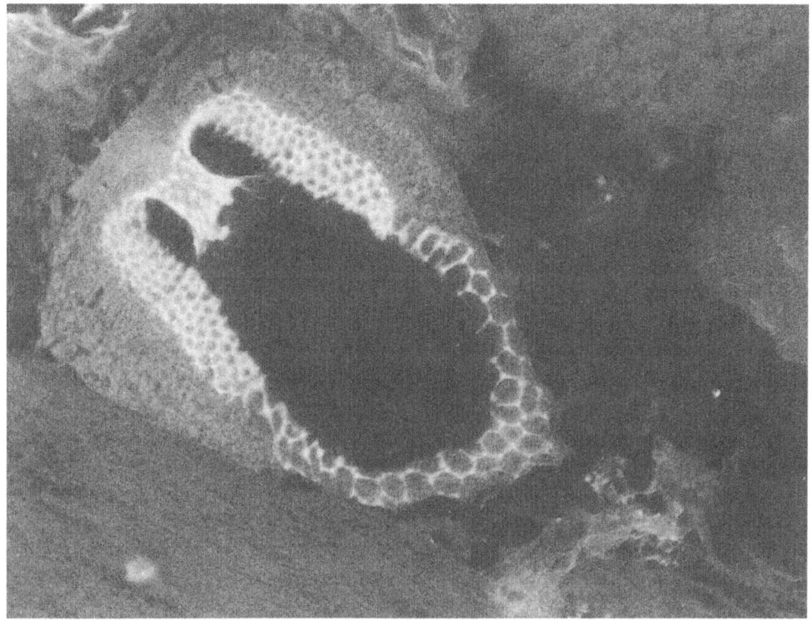

neoplasms first become visible in the third larval instar, although an abnormal pattern of growth can be detected earlier during the larval period of development. These neoplasms continue to grow during the extended life of the l(2)gl larvae and the neoplastic brain hemispheres and imaginal discs can reach several times their normal size.

The l(2)gl gene was discovered by Bridges in 1933, and intensively studied by Hadorn and his collaborators between 1937 and 1955. The l(2)gl mutation was first recognized as a lethal factor that produces pleiotropic effects with degeneration of the imaginal discs of the head, thorax, and genitalia, aplasia of the germ cells in the testes, but not of the ovaries, and underdevelopment of the salivary glands, the fat bodies, and the ring gland, which is the source of ecdysone. Lack of ecdysone leads to considerable delay in pupation, and the mutant animals die as giant larvae or pseudopupae. However, atrophy of the ring gland is apparently not the primary cause of the mutation, but appears to result from the invasive growth of the malignant neuroblasts within the brain hemispheres that disrupts essential functions required for the maturation of the ring gland. This is supported by the observations that transplantation of a normal ring gland or the injection of ecdysone can induce pupation, but cannot fully ensure the development of the mutant larvae. Furthermore, ecdysone deficiency alone is not sufficient to cause neoplastic growth. It was not until the isolation and characterization of a new allele of the l(2)gl gene by Gateff and Schneiderman in 1969 that the occurence of neoplasms was recognized in mutant l(2)gl larvae. The malignant potential of the l(2)gl brain and imaginal discs was demonstrated by transplanting these tissues in the abdomen of adult flies. Under these conditions the neoplastic cells proliferate rapidly and kill the host in 3 to 14 days, whereas normal tissues grow only moderately and exert no deleterious effect on the host.

Using techniques of molecular biology, we have cloned the l(2)gl gene and subjected it to molecular analysis. This approach has unequivocally demonstrated that the tumorous phenotype results from a lack of gene function. Furthermore, we were able to prevent tumorigenesis by introducing a normal copy of this gene into the genome of l(2)gl-deficient animals. Such successful "rescue" experiments indicate that the l(2)gl gene has characteristics of a tumor suppressor gene or anti-oncogene.

Analysis of the l(2)gl gene expression during Drosophila development has shown that the l(2)gl gene is active at the end of the two major phases of cell proliferation: during early embryogenesis and at the larval to pupal transition phase. We have further examined the requirements for l(2)gl cloning development by producing mosaic animals with clones of l(2)gl-deficient cells (l(2)gl/l-(2)gl-) in otherwise normal heterozygous animals (l(2)gl-/+) and found that the embryonic phase of l(2)gl expression is essential for preventing tumorigenesis during larval development.

The complete nucleotide sequence of the l(2)gl gene and its transcripts has been determined. This structural analysis has revealed that the l(2)gl transcript is made of 9 or 10 exons dispersed over 13 kb. The l(2)gl gene displays a relatively complex structure due to the duplication of the promoter region, as well as the first two exons. These repeats show a high degree (96 %) of homology and cover about half of the size of the l(2)gl gene. Depending on the site chosen for initiating transcription and the splicing pattern, this duplication leads to the synthesis of transcripts that differ in the 5' region. However, these variations are located upstream of the coding region, and therefore, exert no influence on the l(2)gl protein structure. Further reconstitution experiments in transgenic flies have shown that each promoter can fully govern the expression of l(2)gl.

The primary nucleotide sequence of l(2)gl transcript has allowed us to predict the structure of its protein product. With the assumption that the first ATG codon at the 5' end of the largest open reading frame found in the l(2)gl transcript is the initiation codon, the l(2)gl gene would encode a polypeptide of 1161 amino acids in length, with a predicted mass of about 127 kDa. The prediction of the mRNA and sequence analysis are confirmed by immunoglogical studies.

L(2)gl Protein

Polyclonal rabbit antibodies prepared against synthesized peptides of the N or the C terminal segments of the predicted l(2)gl protein recognize a protein of about 130 kDa. This indicates that the primary translation product of the l(2)gl gene is not post-translationally modified such to a large extent that would change its apparent molecular weight.

Amino acid sequence comparison with other known proteins is a usual way to get insights into the function of a new gene. However, computer-assisted searches have failed to detect any significant relationship between the sequence of l(2)gl and any sequence in available databanks. Searches for local relatedness of the predicted amino acid sequence of l(2)gl and motifs present in defined groups of proteins have revealed only a distant relationship between l(2)gl and ß-subunits of G-proteins.

This finding prompted us to undertake in vitro biochemical analyses of the l(2)gl protein which can be purified by immunological methods. These analyses have recently revealed that the l(2)gl protein displays an ATP-dependent kinase activity and can be autophosphorylated at serine residues. Further cell fractionation studies and microscopic examination have shown that the l(2)gl protein is predominantly found to be free in the cytoplasm, but can become associated with the inner face of the plasma membrane where it is restricted to domains facing contiguous cells.

Further examination of the spatio-temporal pattern of l(2)gl transcription and protein expression has revealed that the l(2)gl gene is intensively expressed during early embryogenesis. As it has been determined in mosaic experiments, this period of gene expression is critical for preventing tumorigenesis to take place later during larval development. During early embryogenesis, the l(2)gl transcripts and proteins are ubiquitously expressed in all cells and tissues, while during late embryogenesis expression becomes gradually restricted to tissues such as the midgut epithelium that show no phenotypic alteration in the mutant animals.

The results of the functional analysis of l(2)gl indicate that the l(2)gl protein is involved in a mechanism of signal transduction during embryogenesis which is necessary for establishing a precise program of cell proliferation and cell differentiation. Moreover, this program is set during early embryogenesis, but is implemented at a much later stage. Inactivation of the l(2)gl gene does not impair embryonic development which is completed normally, but affects developmental processes occurring during larval life. At this stage, the normal pattern of cell proliferation is altered and the cells which should form the adult tissues become committed to a pathway of continous cell proliferation and form malignant tumors. The elucidation of the function of genes like l(2)gl will contribute to our understanding of the mechanisms which control normal cell proliferation and, thus, prevent cells from becoming tumorous.

Prof. Dr. Bernard Mechler
Division of Developmental Genetics

Participating Scientists

Dr. Dennis Strand
Dr. Istvan Török

Selected publications

Mechler, B.M., McGinnis W., Gehring, W.G.: Molecular cloning of lethal(2)giant larvae a recessive oncogene of Drosophila melanogaster. EMBO 4, 1551–1557 (1985).

Jacob, L., Opper, M., Metzroth, B., Phannavong, B., Mechler, B.M.: Structure of the l(2)gl gene of Drosophila and delimitation of its tumor-suppressor domain. Cell 50, 215–225 (1987).

Opper, M., Schuler, G., Mechler, B.M.: Hereditary suppression of lethal(2)giant larvae malignant tumor development of Drosophila by gene transfer. Oncogene 1, 91–96 (1987).

Gateff, E., Mechler, B.M.: Tumor-Suppressor genes of Drosophila melanogaster. CRC Crit. Rev. in Oncogenesis 1, 221–245 (1989).

Mechler, B.M. Strand, D.: Tumor Suppression in Drosophila. In: G. Klein (ed.), Tumor Suppressor Genes, pp 123–144. Marcel Dekker, Inc. New York and Basel (1990).

Mechler, B.: The fruit fly Drosophila and the fish Xiphophorus as a model system for cancer studies. Cancer Surveys 9, 505–527 (1991)

2.3 The Role of cAMP-Dependent Signal Transduction for Cell-type-specific Gene Expression

by Michael Boshart and Günther Schütz

Differentiation and development can be described as patterns of gene expression defined in time and space. Differential gene expression largely results from regulation of transcription. Multiple regulatory processes are initiated and coordinated by extracellular signals. In multicellular organisms, signals mediated by cell-cell contacts play an important role. Furthermore, hormonal signals coordinate differentiation processes at the level of the organism. A close relation between signal transduction and cell-type-specific transcriptional control is exemplified by the tyrosine aminotransferase (TAT) gene which is expressed exclusively in liver cells and which is switched on briefly after birth. This switch is part of a terminal differentiation process by which the liver acquires gluconeogenic capacity as a response to specific metabolic requirements of the newborn organism.

Fig. 18
Shown are the regulatory elements characterized so far, which control the transcription of the tyrosine aminotransferase (TAT) gene. The TAT gene may be induced either by glycocorticoids or by cyclic adenosine monophosphate (cAMP), which activates the protein kinase A. All distances are given in kilobases (kb) and refer to the starting point of the TAT gene transcription (arrow).

The identification of cell-type-specific regulatory elements (promoters and enhancers) in a large number of genes, and cloning of cell type-specific transcriptions factors which act via these elements were prerequisites to understand cell-type-specific transcriptional control. Combination of different transcription factor binding sites in one regulatory element broadens the repertoire of regulatory specificities by synergistic interactions. Several enhancers and the promoter of a gene cooperate and determine the initiation frequency of RNA polymerase and thereby determine the transcription rate of the gene.

The role of trans-acting factors for control of cell-type-specific gene expression had been postulated in the 1960s and 1970s based on genetic experiments with somatic cell hybrids. In hybrid cells generated by fusion of different cell types the expression of cell-type-specific gene products of both fusion partners is usually repressed. This phenomenon termed "extinction" is best characterized in hepatoma X fibroblast hybrids. Killary and Fournier had shown that extinction of liver-specific genes in these hybrids has a specific genetic basis. They have identified a genetic locus on human fibroblast chromosome 17, the tissue-specific extinguisher 1 (TSE1) which repressed the expression of tyrosine aminotransferase (TAT) in hepatoma cells. The TSE1 locus maps to a chromosome distinct from the one carrying the TAT structural gene demonstrating regulation in trans. TSE1 specifically represses a group of liver genes including the TAT gene. Nothing

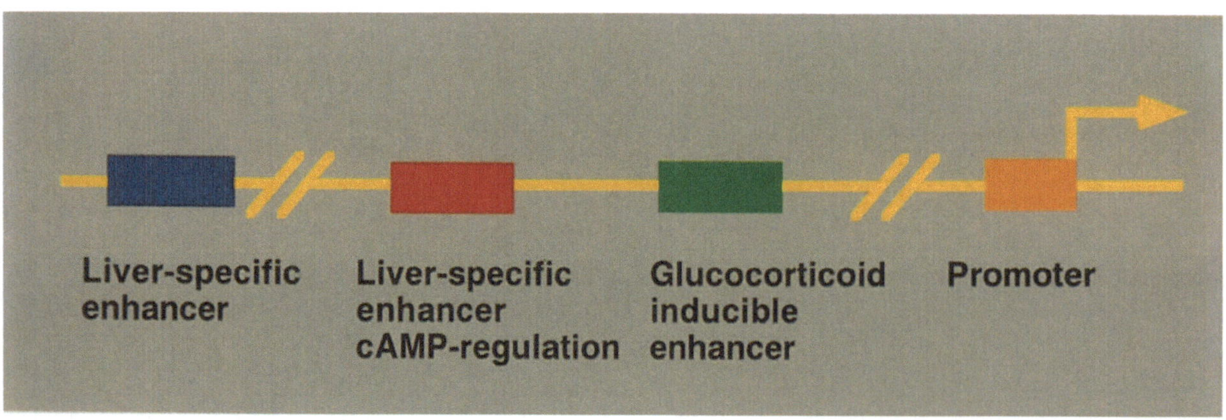

was known about the mechanisms of action of extinguisher loci when we started this project. As extinguishers are defined by genetic experiments, it was unknown whether they interact directly with DNA as repressors or whether they would indicate novel mechanisms of cell type-specific control.

The TAT gene is particularly suitable as a model to analyze the role of hormones in cell type-specific gene expression, since it is expressed exclusively in liver cells, is turned on at a defined timepoint during development, and is regulated by two signal transduction pathways. As other key enzymes of the gluconeogenesis pathway, the TAT gene is inducible by glucocorticoids as well as by glucagon acting via the second messenger cAMP. For induction via the cAMP pathway the catalytic subunit of protein kinase A is essential.

The TAT gene is only activated shortly after birth. The transcription rate is maximal 8–12 hours after birth, decreases slightly within 1–2 days, and increases again in adult liver. The postnatal hypoglycemia and the resulting release of glucagon and glucocorticoids seem to play a role for activation of the gene. Therefore, the TAT gene is suitable as a model to analyze the role of signal transduction pathways for developmental-specific transcriptional control.

Control Elements for Cell Type-Specific and cAMP-Dependent Expression of the Tyrosine Aminotransferase (TAT) Gene

The different regulatory elements which control transcription of the TAT gene are located within 10 kb upstream of the transcription start site. Specific regulatory functions could be assigned to individual elements (Fig. 18). To identify regulatory elements, parts of the TAT upstream sequence were placed in front of an indicator gene whose product can easily be determined and the transcriptional activity of these constructs was measured after gene transfer into several cell lines.

We could identify three enhancers which are important for expression of the TAT gene and localized them 11 kb, 3.6 kb, and 2.5 kb upstream of the transcription start site. The elements at –11 and –3.6 are liver-specific enhancers, the latter mediating cAMP induction in addition. The region at –2.5 kb is crucial for glucocorticoid response.

A detailed functional analysis by gene transfer experiments of the enhancer at –3.6 kb upstream of the transcription start site has defined a minimal fragment of 80 bp which mediates all properties of the enhancer. Using a series of point mutations, we found that two short sequence motifs within these 80 bp are absolutely essential, since their mutation leads to total loss of function of the enhancer. The mutual dependence of these elements indicates that they cooperate. The sequence of one of these elements is similar to cAMP-regulated elements (CREs) in other cAMP-inducible genes and mediates a strong response to increased intracellular concentrations of cAMP in highly differentiated hepatoma cells. The second essential element of the enhancer is constitutive and liver-specific and its activity correlates with the degree of differentiation of the respective hepatoma cell line. The high degree of specificity of the enhancer –3.6 kb therefore relies on cooperation of two essential elements with overlapping specificity. Therefore, the activity is restricted to highly differentiated hepatoma cells and in vivo to adult hepatocytes.

Analysis of the enhancer at –3.6 kb demonstrates that the modular structure of regulatory elements provides a safe and economical way to generate specificities. A large number of regulatory patterns can be generated by combinatorial use of a much smaller number of regulatory proteins which interact synergistically. Cooperation of several essential elements allows regulation of the activity of the enhancer over several orders of magnitude in response to much smaller changes in activity of individual regulatory factors.

Cell-specific Repression by the Tissue-specific Extinguisher Locus TSE1: Antagonism between TSE1 and cAMP Signal Transduction

Genetic analysis of extinction in somatic cell hybrids allows identification of trans-acting factors which are most likely part of mechanisms which usually control cell type-specific gene expression. Therefore, we analyzed the mechanism of action of the TSE1 locus to understand the control of cell-type-specific transcription in the liver.

A first hint to the mechanism by which TSE1 represses TAT transcription in somatic cell hybrids came from the identification of a group of liver-specific genes which are coordinately regulated by TSE1. All seven genes are expressed in hepatoma cells and show a

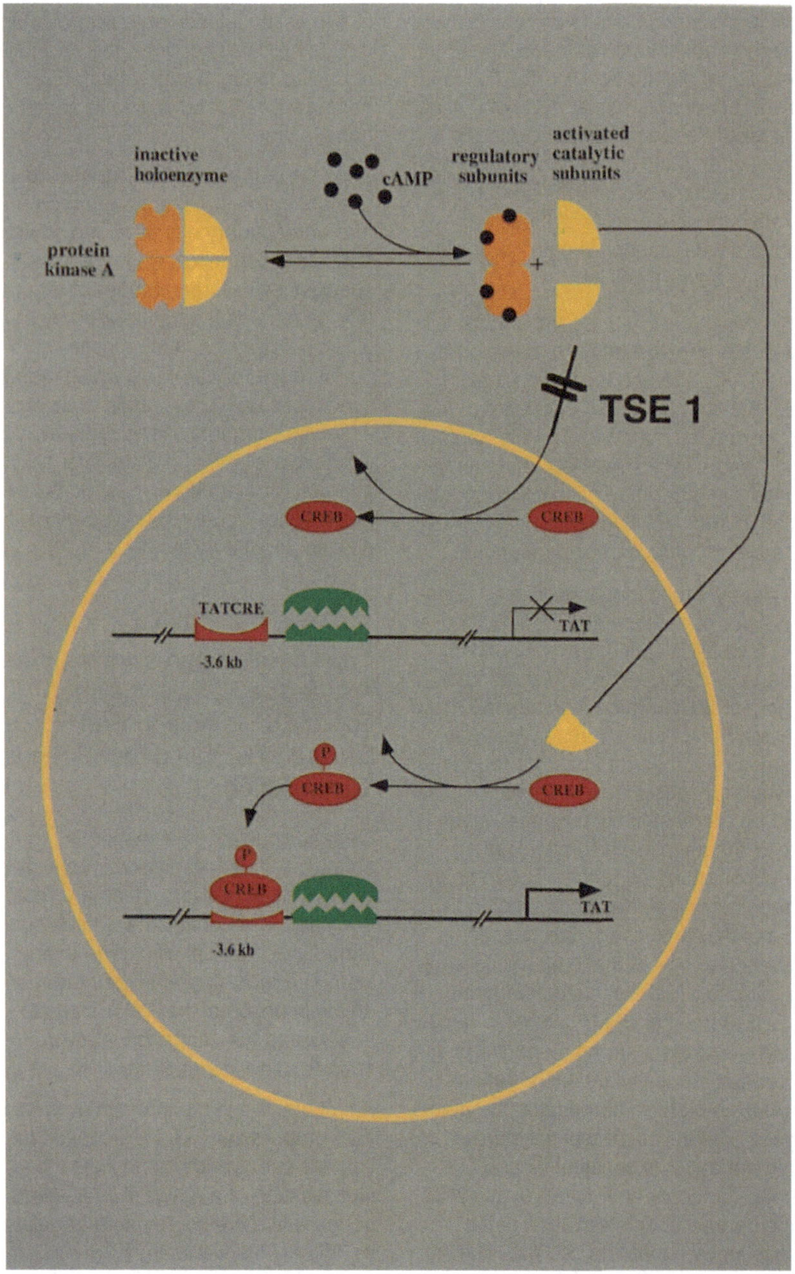

dramatically reduced repression in microcell hybrids generated by fusion of a hepatoma cell with a fragment of human chromosome 17 derived from a fibroblast which carries the TSE1 locus. We found that all TSE1 regulated genes are inducible by cAMP and that in microcell hybrids, cAMP is able to antagonize TSE1-mediated repression.

a) The Mechanism of TSE1-Mediated Extinction

By gene transfer experiments into the aforementioned microcell hybrid cell lines we could show that the cell type-specific enhancer at –3.6 kb mediates repression by TSE1. This repression of the enhancer by TSE1 can be reversed by cAMP. We could show that the cAMP-regulated element (CRE) is required and is solely sufficient for repression of the enhancer by TSE1. The functional antagonism between TSE1 and cAMP is well explained, since the CRE is the target of TSE1.

Furthermore, we found that the repression of TAT gene transcription by TSE1 results from inhibition of the cAMP/ protein kinase A signal transduction path-

Fig. 19
Suppression mechanism of the TAT transcription by the cell-specific extinction factor 1 (TSE1). This increase of cAMP concentration in the cell causes an activation of the protein kinase A. The activated subunit of the enzyme then changes the transcription factor CREB so that it can bind to the cAMP-regulated region of the TAT gene (TATCRE). CREB now causes, together with a cell-specific regulator, the transcription of the TAT gene. In contrast, TSE1 suppresses the gene expression by inhibiting the activated subunit of the protein kinase A.

way. This explains why all TSE1-regulated genes are inducible by cAMP. Since the intracellular cAMP concentration is not affected by TSE1, protein kinase A or one of its substrates should be the target for TSE1. Indeed, we could find a reduction of the basal protein kinase A activity in cells in which TSE1 is active.

b) The TSE1 Gene Product

The latter observation led to a systematic search for a protein kinase A inhibiting activity which might be identical with the TSE1 gene product. The holoenzyme of protein kinase A is a tetramer of two regulatory and two catalytic subunits which are inactive in absence of cAMP. Binding of two cAMP molecules to each regulatory subunit leads to a conformational change and subsequent release and activation of the catalytic subunit. One regulatory subunit gene (RIa) of PKA colocalizes with TSE1 on human chromosome 17. Furthermore, the expression of RIa mRNA perfectly correlates with the TSE1 phenotype in different cell lines and hybrids. High- resolution mapping of RIa and TSE1 on chromosome 17 revealed colocalization on a small segment of the chromosome within less than 500 kb. These data suggested that TSE1 and RIa were identical.

For proof of identity, an expression vector encoding the regulatory subunit was stably introduced into hepatoma cells and the resulting phenotype was analyzed. Increasing expression of the regulatory subunit led to inverse proportional changes of basal protein kinase A activity, binding of CRE binding protein to its cognate element, and finally, expression of the TAT gene. Expression of the regulatory subunit leads to a perfect phenocopy of the TSE1 phenotype. Thus, we could identify the regulatory subunit RIa as the product of the TSE1 locus. This is the first molecular characterization of an extinguisher factor. Figure 19 illustrates the action of TSE1 on TAT gene expression.

Long before cell-type-specific transcription factors had been identified, the analysis of extinction in somatic cell hybrids has already shaped the concept that cell-type-specific gene expression is controlled in trans. TSE1 is the first example of such a genetically defined factor whose mechanism of action has been elucidated. Since regulatory mutants cannot easily be obtained in mammalian cells, somatic cell hybrids are valuable tools to analyze cell-type-specific gene expression.

Perinatal Activation of the TAT Gene

A number of independent observations concerning the increase of TAT expression within the first hours after birth can be combined into a mechanistic concept with our knowledge of the role of cAMP signal transduction for cell-type-specific control of TAT expression:
a) The raise in TAT transcription parallels a raise of gluconeogenic hormones due to the postnatal hypoclycemia. b) In utero administration of cAMP leads to premature activation of fetal TAT expression. c) TSE1 activity and RIa mRNA are high in hepatoma cells which express fetal liver markers, but are low in adult hepatocytes.

The model derived from these observations postulates a dominant role of glucagon and other gluconeogenic hormones acting via the cAMP pathway for the properly timed activation of the TAT gene. RIa/TSE1 could repress basal TAT expression in fetal liver. Activation by cAMP shortly after birth is mediated by the cell-type-specific enhancer at –3.6 kb and is mechanistically equivalent to reversal of extinction by cAMP in hepatoma microcell hybrids. In any case, perinatal activation seems to be due to activation of protein kinase A and to be mediated by the cAMP response element (CRE) of the TAT gene.

Dr. Michael Boshart
Prof. Dr. Günther Schütz
Division of Molecular Biology of the Cell I

Participating scientists
Dr. Falk Weih
Dr. Mark Nichols
Dr. Doris Nitsch

In collaboration with
Dr. Keith Fournier
Fred Hutchinson Cancer Research Center,
Seattle, Washington, USA

Selected publications

Killary, A. M., Fournier, R. E. K.: A genetic analysis of extinction: trans-dominant loci regulate expression of liver-specific traits in hepatoma hybrid cells. Cell 38, 523-534 (1984)

Boshart, M., Weih, F., Schmidt, A., Fournier, R.E.K., Schütz, G.: A cyclic AMP response element mediates repression of tyrosine aminotransferase gene transcription by the tissue-specific extinguisher locus Tse- 1. Cell 61, 905–916 (1990)

Ruppert, S., Boshart, M., Bosch, F.X., Schmid, W., Fournier, R.E.K., Schütz, G. : Two genetically defined trans-acting loci coordinately regulate overlapping sets of liver-specific genes. Cell 61, 895–904 (1990)

Weih, F., Stewart, A.F., Boshart, M., Nitsch, D., Schütz, G.: In vivo monitoring of a cAMP-stimulated DNA-binding activity. Genes & Development 4, 1437–1449 (1990)

Boshart, M., Weih, F., Nichols, M., Schütz, G.: The tissue-specific extinguisher locus TSE1 encodes a regulatory subunit of cAMP-dependent protein kinase. Cell 66, 849–859 (1991)

Nitsch, D., Ruppert, S., Kelsey, G., Schedl, A., Weih, F., Stewart, A.F., Strähle, U., Schmid, W., DeVack, C., Reik, A., Boshart, M., Schütz, G.: Hormonal and liver-specific control of expression of the tyrosine aminotransferase gene. In: Molecular Aspects of Cellular Regulation, Vol. 6: Hormonal Regulation of Transcription, Eds. P. Cohen, J.G. Foulkes, Elsevier-Biomedical, 101–133 (1991)

2.4 In Vitro Culture of Mammalian and Amphibian Embryonic Cells: Models for the Analysis of Gene Expression during Development and Differentiation

by Angel Alonso
and Michael F. Trendelenburg

The process of cell differentiation is characterized by modifications in gene expression which finally lead to the appearance of a new phenotype. With only a few exceptions, major modifications in gene expression are due to changes in the transcription of cellular chromatin.

Chromosomal proteins are among the key control elements in cell-type-specific differentiation processes. The collective term "chromosomal proteins" comprises the particularly well-studied histones as well as "non-histones" which are, in comparison to histones, far less completely characterized. While the histones H2a, H2b, H3, and H4 are directly involved in the organization of the basic chromatin structure, the nucleosome, the role of H1 histones is not yet completely understood. Numerous experimental findings, however, indicate that a fundamental prerequisite for tissue-specific differentiation is a gene-specific association of this histone class with the nucleosomal chromatin basic structure. In the following, we will present an experiment aimed at the analysis of the differentiation-specific role played by a particular subclass of histone proteins, H1°.

A particularly well-suited system for the investigation of molecular mechanisms of differentiation are the early stages of embryonic development in mice. Approximately four days after fertilization the cells begin to differentiate visibly, either into trophectoderm, or into the cells of the inner cell mass (ICM), from which, later (among) others, the various embryonic tissues and organs develop. In the second visible phase of differentiation, immediately prior to the implantation of the embryo, the primitive endoderm develops from the ICM. From the primitive endoderm two different cell lines derive: the visceral endoderm and the parietal endoderm.

These first phases of cell differentiation can be reproduced in vitro (in a culture medium). Under the influence of certain chemicals or culture conditions, embryonic carcinoma cell lines (EC cells) differentiate as described above. Within four days, after active components such as all-trans retinoic acid and chemicals that affect the endogenous cAMP concentration have been administered, the EC cell line F9 (which resembles ICM), for example, differentiates into parietal endoderm.

Cells from the ICM can also be cultured in vitro without losing their manifold development capacities. An interesting aspect is the fact that, after being transferred into blastocysts, these "embryonic stem cells" (ES) participate in the normal development of the embryo. EC and ES cells thus offer good experimental opportunities of investigating (in vitro) the phases of differentiation that take place (in vivo) during murine embryogenesis in the first few days after fertilization.

Fig. 20a
Diagram of the early embryonic development of the blastocyst of the mouse from the undifferentiated to a more differentiated stage. Parts of the inner cell mass (1) develop into a primitive endoderm (2), which later differentiates into parietal (3) and visceral (4) entoblast. It was possible to exactly duplicate this natural development in the laboratory. As a consequence, investigations on this model system no longer require animal experiments.

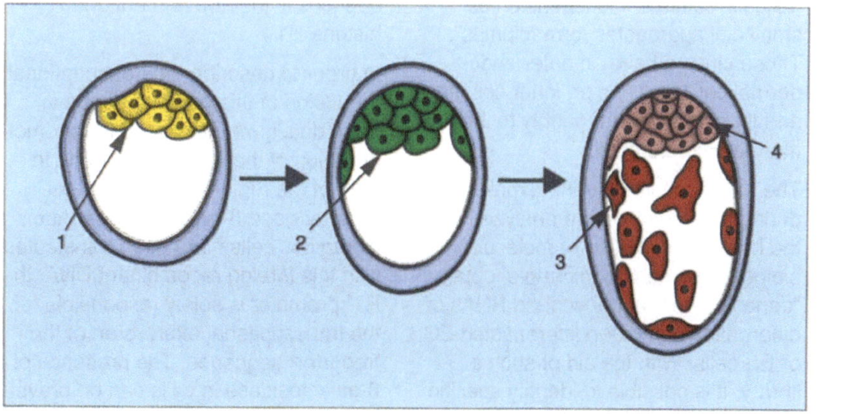

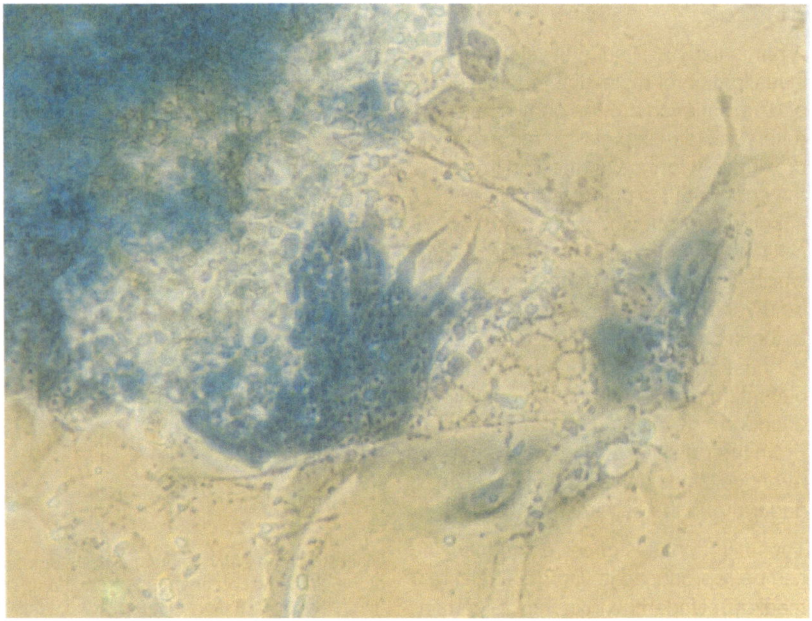

Fig. 20b
The photo shows the differentiated stage of endoderm cells of the mouse grown in a culture dish. The differentiated cells are stained in blue.

While F9 cells differentiate into parietal endoderm cells only after retinoic acid and cyclic AMP have been added to the culture medium, ES cells may differentiate spontaneously into derivatives of all three blastodermic layers. ES cells cultured in suspension as small cell aggregates form "clumps". These clumps have an outer endodermal cell layer and an inner cell mass and thus correspond roughly to the murine embroid body.

The modifications of gene expression during differentiation are analyzed with the help of techniques of molecular biology. One can, for example, obtain "gene libraries" of transcribed RNAs of differentiated and nondifferentiated EC or ES cells. With the aid of such a library, it is possible to identify specific genes that are active either only in differentiated or only in nondifferentiated cells. On the basis of such a system we isolated different cDNA clones for proteins that show different patterns of expression in nondifferentiated and differentiated F9 cells. One of these sequences is the above-mentioned histone H1°.

In order to describe the transcriptional regulation of this particular gene in more detail, we introduced the promoter region of the histone H1° gene in front of the region encoding for the reporter gene ß-galactosidase. After eukaryotic cells have been transfected with this foreign recombinant DNA, the H1° promoter is solely responsible for the transcriptional expression of the "reporter" sequence. The presence of ß-galactosidase in cells can be proven by histochemical staining. In our experiment, we transfected the recombinant DNA into nondifferentiated cells (EC and ES cell lines); then, we let these transfected cells differentiate in vitro. Such a strategy offers various options for investigating the relationship between the transcriptional control of a gene in various cell types as well as during cell differentiation.

After transfection of the recombinant DNA consisting of the histone H1° promoter region and the ß-galactosidase reporter sequence, and subsequent in vitro differentiation, the histologically stained cells with a clear activity of ß-galactosidase could readily be identified using a laser scanning microscope. It could be shown that the transcriptional activity of the H1° promoter increases in the course of differentiation, and that this transcription is tissue-specific.

We thus concentrated our efforts on the characterization of those sequences that are responsible for such a tissue-specific gene expression. For this purpose, we had to produce additional recombinants. We introduced H1° promoter sequences, which were deleted on the 5' end, in front of the sequence encoding for the enzyme chloramphenicol acetyltransferase (CAT). In this series of experiments we introduced the recombinant DNA into differentiated and nondifferentiated F9 EC cell lines. The enzymatic activity of the CAT reporter served as the measure of promoter activity. These experiments re-

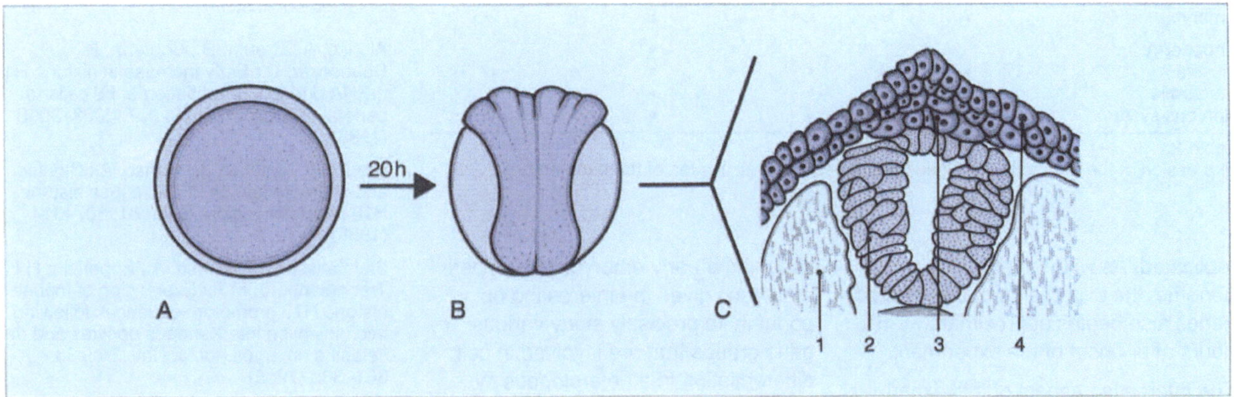

Fig. 21
After the injection of DNA into fertilized egg cells of the platanna (xenophus) (A), basic mechanisms of the control of expression during the embryonic differentiation to the neurula stage (B, C) can be investigated. (C) shows a cross section of embryonic tissues: (1) somite, (2) neural groove, (3) neural crest, (4) ectoderm.

vealed that 700 nucleotides of the histone H1° promoter are sufficient for accurate transcription as well as for the enhanced transcription after differentiation. Further experiments presently being carried out indicate that at least nine transcription factors are necessary for an optimum transcription rate.

The fact that chemical agents can be used to differentiate EC cells into various directions offers a wide range of interesting experimental options, such as analyzing the characteristics of expression of various genes in different cell types. In this respect, EC cells are an even more suitable model than ES cells, whose direction of differentiation cannot be influenced in vitro. ES cells, on the other hand, make it possible to directly participate in the murine embryogenesis. Thus, both cell types are complementary models for the in vivo analysis of the first stages of murine embryogenesis.

Another currently used in vitro system for the analysis of embryonic differentiation processes during the differentiation of larval tissues are fertilized eggs of the African clawed toad Xenopus laevis. Several properties make frog embryonic cells especially suited for the investigation of gene expression. This is why Xenopus laevis presently is the most commonly used laboratory amphibian worldwide. One can thus call upon an extraordinarily high level of knowledge that can be used in the planning of experiments. As has been shown by injection experiments, basic mechanisms of expression control of both "homologous" genes (from Xenopus) as well as "heterologous" genes (such as from mammals) can be studied with Xenopus embryonic cells. In Xenopus microinjection experiments a very much larger number of identical gene copies can be injected into the fertilized eggs than is possible in tissue cell cultures, for example. The microinjected eggs develop within only a few hours: the blastula (60 000 cells) differentiates in only 6 hours, and the embryo with differentiated tissue (neurula stage) in only 24 hours. The complete embryonic differentiation takes place separately from the maternal organism, which means that the culture of microinjected embryos only requires a simple salt medium.

As in the experiment on embryonic mammal cells described above, we again use a gene that has been coupled to a reporter gene. In this experiment, we used the mouse histone H1° gene, whose expression was investigated in various differentiating larval frog tissues. During the rapidly developing early embryonic mitosis, the injected gene copies are replicated and thus are gradually distributed into various regions of the early embryo. During this early embryonic dividing stage (approximately 6 to 8 hours after in vitro fertilization) the injected gene copies, however, are not expressed at a considerable rate, but are instead mainly

Embryo	A	B	C	D	E	F	G
Endoderm				•	•		
Muscle	•	•	•	•	•	•	•
Epidermis	•	•	•		•		
Nervous system		•	•		•	•	•

Table 2:
Expression of the mouse histone gen could be found in all tissues of the early embryo.

replicated. As with the embryonic genome, the expression of the injected genes also begins approximately 7.5 hours after onset of the experiment.

The interesting aspect of this experiment is the fact that parts of the mammalian histone gene are simultaneously present in the embryonic tissues that in this stage are already differentiated, such as epidermis, central and peripheral nervous system, brain, muscle and endoderm. Our results indicate that the genes are not distributed homogeneously in all tissues; instead, each individual embryo of an injection batch shows a proper distribution "mosaic" of the injected mouse histone genes. Table 2 shows a typical result of such an injection experiment. Each of the embryos displays a different arrangement of stained blue cell regions. In these whole-mounts only the positive regions within the various epidermal regions can be readily discerned. Only the investigation of sections yields a complete image of the histone gene distribution. Expression of the mouse histone gene could be proven in all tissues of the early embryo. This experiment thus gives the interesting opportunity to precisely study various gene groups that are involved in cell differentiation in a heterologous system.

The experiments described here may be used to analyze more precisely at which point in the development of the embryo and to what extent H1° histone genes are transcribed. Such investigations would require large amounts of mammalian embryos. In our studies, however, EC and ES cells as well as the amphibian system can be used as model systems for cell differentiation, thus avoiding the use of a large number of experimental animals.

Prof. Dr. Angel Alonso
Research Program Applied Tumor Virology
Prof. Dr. Michael F. Trendelenburg
Project Structural Gene Analysis

Participating scientists
Dr. Beate Breuer
Research Program Applied Tumor Virology

Dr. Herbert Spring
Dr. Herbert Steinbeißer
Project Structural Gene Analysis

Selected publications

Alonso, A., Breuer, B., Bouterfa, H., Doenecker, D.: Early increase in histone H10 mRNA during differentiation of F9 cells to parietal endoderm. Embo J. 7, 3003–3008 (1988)

Breuer, B., Fischer, J., Alonso, A.: Cloning and characterization of the mouse histone H10 promotor region. Gene 81, 307–314 (1989)

Steinbeisser, H., Alonso, A., Epperlein, H.H., Trendelenburg, M.F.: Expression of mouse histone H10 promotor sequences following microinjection into Xenopus oocytes and developing embryos. Int. J. Dev. Biol. 33, 361–368 (1989)

Hofman, A., Montag, M., Steinbeisser, H., Trendelenburg, M.F.: Plasmid and bacteriophage lambda DNA show differential replication characteristics following injection into fertilized eggs of Xenopus laevis: Dependence on period and site of injection. Cell Diff. Development 30, 77–85 (1990)

Schmid, M., Steinbeisser, H., Trendelenburg, M.F., Lipps, H.J.: A bovine papilloma virus type I (BPV-1) containing plasmid replicates extrachromosomally in Xenopus embryos. Nucleic Acids Res. 18, 2196 (1990)

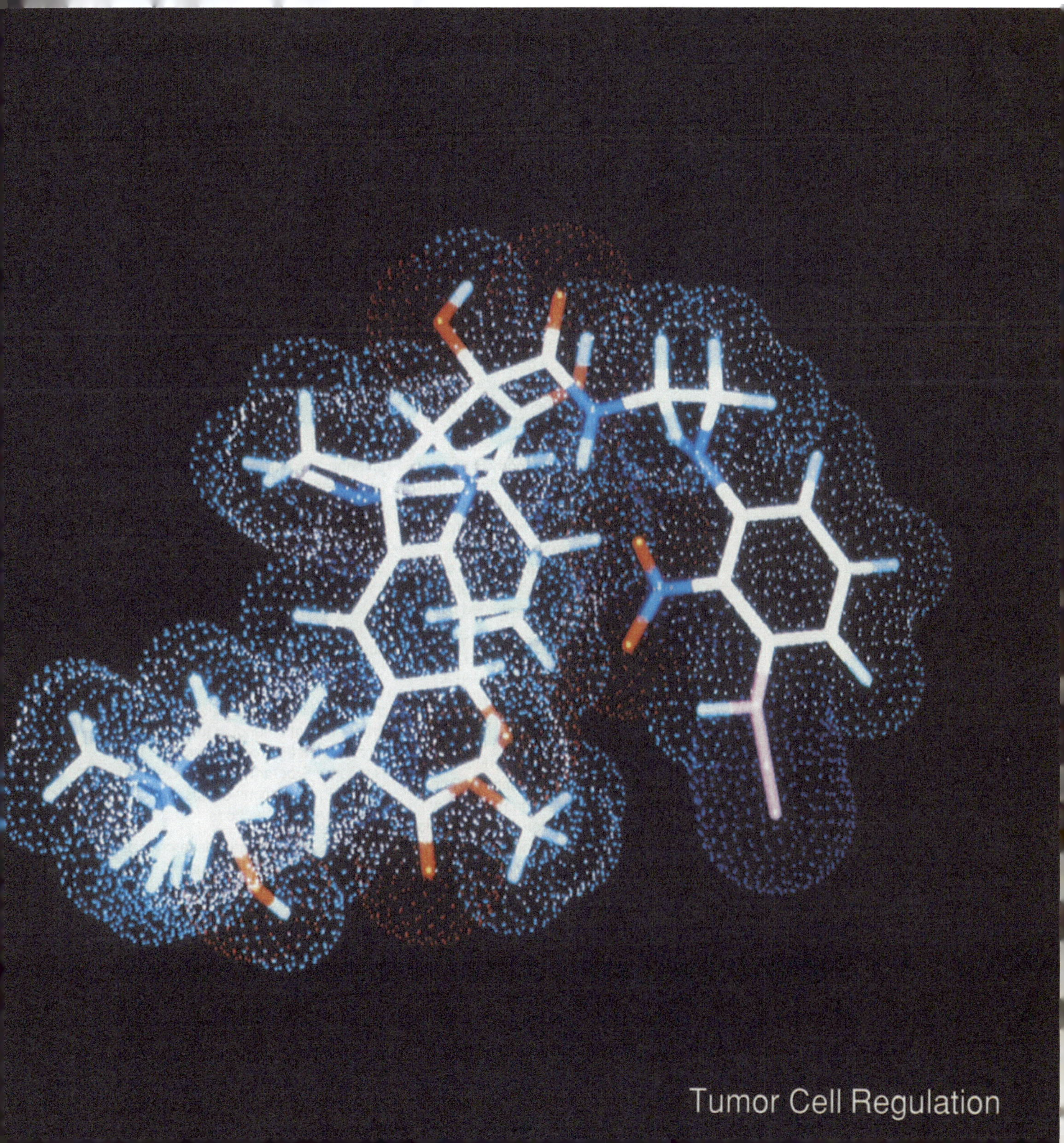

Tumor Cell Regulation

3

Tumor Cell Regulation

Today, cancer is thought of as resulting from the accumulation of genetic damages that occur accidentally or are due to external factors. The result is a permanently disturbed communication among the cells and between the tumor tissue and the organism, becoming evident by chaotic and destructive growth and senseless functioning.

Communication between cells and body tissues is mainly based upon the continuous exchange of chemical signals: Depending on their place of origin of effect, these can be characterized as hormones, neurotransmitters, cytokines, mediators, or growth factors. Each cell of the human body is able to emit and receive such signals and thus is in permanent contact with all other cells of the organism. This extremely complex system of communication ensures that all parts of the body behave coherently and cooperatively as if they were following a predefined plan.

Signals are emitted, received and interpreted. The recipient gives each received signal a meaning, which, in general, is a prompt to act. For this purpose, the cells have several complex chains of chemical reactions by which signals can be detected, modulated, modified, and passed on into the interior of the cell or even the nucleus. At their point of destination, they affect, for example, the activities of enzymes and genes, the structure of the cellular skeleton, the permeability of the cellular membrane, and thus the entire behavior of the cell. The intracellular signal transmission channels are retroactive and interlinked and thus constitute an extraordinarily complex "cellular nervous system". Presently, cellular signal transmission is, apart from the action of the genes, one of the most intensively studied areas in biomedical research, especially because it is now known that the majority of all genetic defects resulting in cancer or other diseases manifest themselves as a disturbed signal transmission.

Cellular signal transmission is one of the foci of the work done in the Research Program Tumor Cell Regulation. Several working groups are studying cellular signal molecules, in particular, the peptide hormones (growth factors) which promote or inhibit cell division and which have been proven to be directly and in many ways related to tumor growth. Other studies concentrate on short-lived mediators which are generated by tissues locally and only for short periods of time. Here, the work is focusing on the large group of eicosanoid-type mediators (such as prostaglandins, thromboxans, leucotriens, lipoxins). These highly active substances are involved in the regulation of almost all tissue and bodily functions. However, their role in pathological processes such as cancer is not yet understood. The detection of these short-lived signal molecules requires a great amount of funding to cover technical expenses. For this purpose, the Research Program's very efficient Division of Spectroscopy disposes of the latest analytical methods.

A second focus of the Research Program's work is the investigation of the intracellular signal transmission mechanisms, i.e., the cellular "interpretation apparatus". The key process is the biochemical protein phosphorylation and its involvement with proteinkinases and phosphatases. This reaction, comparable to electrochemical impulses in the nervous system, seems to be the standard signal of intracellular information transmission. Several working groups of the Research Program "Tumor Cell Regulation" are studying the isolation and characterization of protein kinases and their role in physiological and pathophysiological processes.

A third research project is investigating one of the central problems of experimental cancer research, the regulation of cell division. The complexity of the research requires the combined use of microscopic, cell-biologic, biochemical and molecular-biological methods and thus calls for an intensive collaboration, both among the Research Program's divisions, as well as with other Research Programs of the Deutsches Krebsforschungszentrum. Since the aforementioned intracellular signals and the cellular signal transmission mechanisms assigned to them (such as protein phosphorylation) directly or indirectly (by altering cell differentiation) affect the regulation of cell division, the Research Program's main projects are closely collaborated.

All these studies aim at deepening our knowledge of molecular processes whose disturbance results in the development and growth of tumors. It is hoped and expected that, on this basis, new therapeutic approaches can be developed and that the search for risk factors can be improved. It is conceivable that the development of a tumor can be stopped or even reversed by purposely changing intracellular communication processes at specific stages, such as growth, supply with nutrients, or formation of metastases. This concept has already been realized successfully in other fields of medicine, such as in psychopharmaceutical and cardiovascular medicine. Many of the cytostatics used in clinical practice today have been developed in a similar way. Their applicability is limited, however, since the carcinogenic mechanisms are not yet known and since they have serious side-effects. New methods may make it possible to better control these side-effects by purposely altering the intracellular signal transmission, and thus broadening the range of application and the success of existing cancer drugs.

Coordinator of the Research Program:
Prof. Dr. Friedrich Marks

Divisions and their heads:

Pathochemistry:
Prof. Dr. Volker Kinzel

Biochemistry of Tissue-Specific Regulation:
Prof. Dr. Friedrich Marks

Differentiation and Carcinogenesis in vitro:
Prof. Dr. Norbert Fusenig

Biochemistry of Tumors:
Prof. Dr. Dietrich Keppler

Project groups and their heads:

Biochemical Cell Physiology:
Priv.-Doz. Dr. Walter Pyerin

Molecular Biology of Mitosis:
Prof. Dr. Herwig Ponstingl

3

3.1 Development of Substitute Methods for Animal Experiments

by Friedrich Marks

Living creatures provide, to an impressive extent, evidence that the whole is more than the sum of its parts. This is why biological and medical research, despite the remarkable successes of molecular and cellular biology, cannot progress without observing, and doing experiments on intact organisms (e.g., on animals), unless one adopts an extreme ethical point of view and absolutely refuses to gain knowledge from animal experiments. Many people, therefore, consider such experiments as acceptable, even though they may be a necessary evil. The situation is quite different, though, when animals are used as test objects for the assessment of the potential hazards to man of products such as drugs, cosmetics, household and industrial chemicals. In recent years not only have the ethical considerations increased considerably – after all, such tests are usually particularly painful for the animals – but it is also uncertain to what extent, if at all, the resultant findings are applicable to man. In the following, the problematic nature of animal experiments will be illustrated by means of an example: the assessment of tumor promoting environmental factors.

Tumor promotion means the acceleration of tumor growth by factors that on their own are not carcinogenic or, in scientific terms, have no initiating effect. One thus has to distinguish between carcinogenic "initiators" of the disease and accelerating "promoters," both of which are present, in a variety of forms, in the human environment. In animal experiments, the effects of initiators and promoters may dramatically enhance each other: If the dose of the initiator is sufficiently low, only latent tumor cells develop, which by themselves (unless treated with a promoter) do not grow into tumors. Only upon promotion do they develop benign tumors, some of which will subsequently become malignant. This might be the situation humans are exposed to, since in our environment carcinogenic factors are usually present in low concentrations. It may well be possible that in the course of our lives more and more latent tumor cells accumulate, remaining unidentified and harmless as long as they do not come into contact with tumor promoters. Thus, tumor promoters are potentially extremely serious environmental risk factors, and this makes the need for suitable methods of detection all the more urgent.

Many initiators can be detected by their mutagenic effect, which can be measured in cell cultures (though Bruce Ames, one of the fathers of this "mutation test," recently doubted the value of this method). Tumor promoters, on the other hand, do not have similar characteristics, as a consequence of which they can only be detected in animal experiments. Very soon, however, scientists realized that there is an extreme variability in sensitivity not only among the organs of one organism, but also among the different species of laboratory animals. For example, a substance that is highly tumor promoting in mice may have no effect at all in rats or hamsters, or vice versa; the same may even be observed between different mice strains. In view of this, how is one supposed to transfer any findings to the human?

The precariousness of the situation may be illustrated by means of the evaluation of the carcinogenic effects of dioxine. This commonly known superpoison is one of the most effective tumor promoters in rats, while there is no definite indication yet for an increased cancer risk for humans who have been contaminated with dioxine in their work environment or as a consequence of accidents. (Considering the other toxic effects of dioxine, this, however, is a poor consolation!) A large number of similar examples illustrates the fact that, for the assessment of environmental risk factors, animal experiments (though for the investigation of basic biological relationships there is no replacement yet) are highly disputable, not only from the ethical, but also from the scientific point of view; in many cases they may even be unsuitable.

Epidemiology gives a way out of this dilemma by trying to relate the frequency of diseases to certain environmental factors or to characteristics of lifestyle. Of course, this can only be done retrospectively, whereas society and legislation demand, with good reason, that the innocuity of a new product be proven before it is introduced onto the market. Basically, toxic effects of substances such as environmental factors are due to chemical interactions with our body's biomolecules or with its cells. With the help of cell cultures or isolated cell constituents, it is possible to identify such reactions, to observe the molecular processes taking place, and to exactly assess the consequences for the life of the cell.

However, vital functions are never monocausal; instead, they are always based on a confusing multitude of interlinked molecular processes. In addition, cells in a culture dish usually react differently than in their natural environment, which is the body tissue. It is therefore still extremely difficult to infer the reactions of the organism from cell culture observations.

This – and not an occasionally insinuated sadism of the scientist – is one of the reasons for the slow development of methods that might be able to replace animal experiments. The fast development of the biological sciences, however, gives reason to hope that this problem will be solved. In fact, there are already methods for the cultivation of cells and for the molecular analysis of cellular processes that allow us to gain fundamental medical knowledge by experiments on human cells and surgical materials rather than by animal experiments. This trend will considerably intensify in future years. The development will also make it possible to reliably assess environmental risk factors, provided that the relevant cellular "key reactions" can be identified.

A project of the Division of Biochemistry of Tissue-Specific Regulation, which was initiated at the end of 1989, will illustrate how this might be achieved. In this project, we are attempting to develop a substitute for the "Draize test". Named after its inventor, this test has been used for many years throughout the world to test the mucodermal tolerance to newly developed substances, which is a common problem in the chemical, pharmaceutical, cosmetic, and food industries. Among animal protectionists, the Draize test has a particularly bad reputation, since the irritant effect is measured by way of the reaction that a test substance causes when instilled into a living rabbit's eye. The reaction may be common conjunctivitis, or, more severely, corneal clouding, or even the partial or total destruction of the eye.

Unfortunately, the biological processes involved in such inflammatory processes are extremely complex and can in no way be modeled yet in detail by cell and tissue cultures. In the cascade of events more and more new cell types are recruited and batteries of molecular processes are activated to combat the environmental poison. The recording of all events appears to be doomed to failure. Thus, the presently available substitute methods only measure the inflammatory reactions in

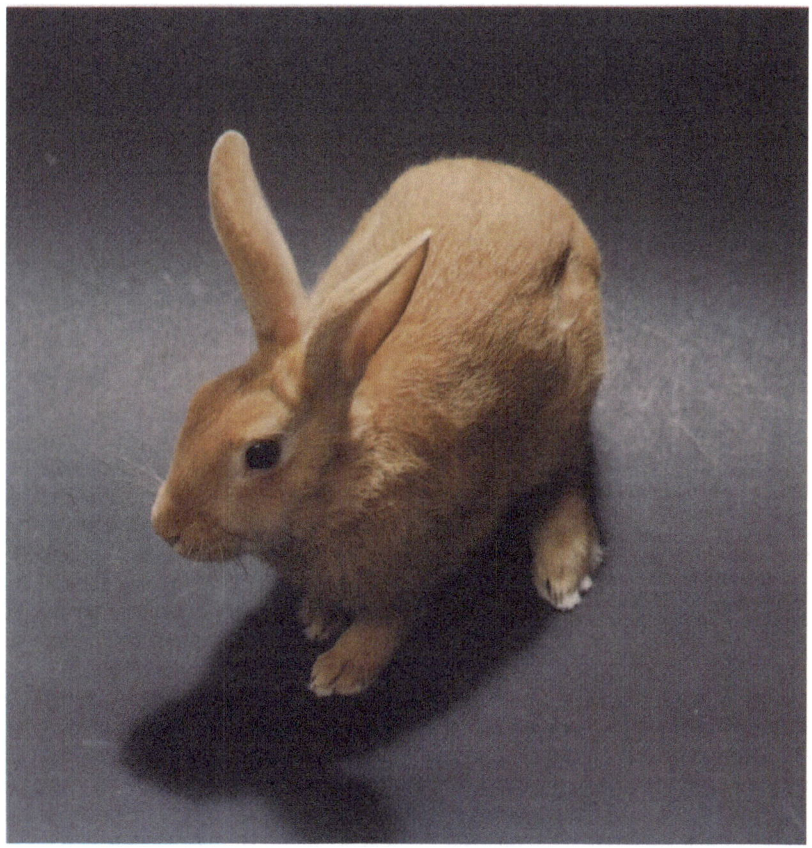

Fig. 22
Substitute methods on the basis of cell cultures are developed in order to minimize the number of animal experiments.

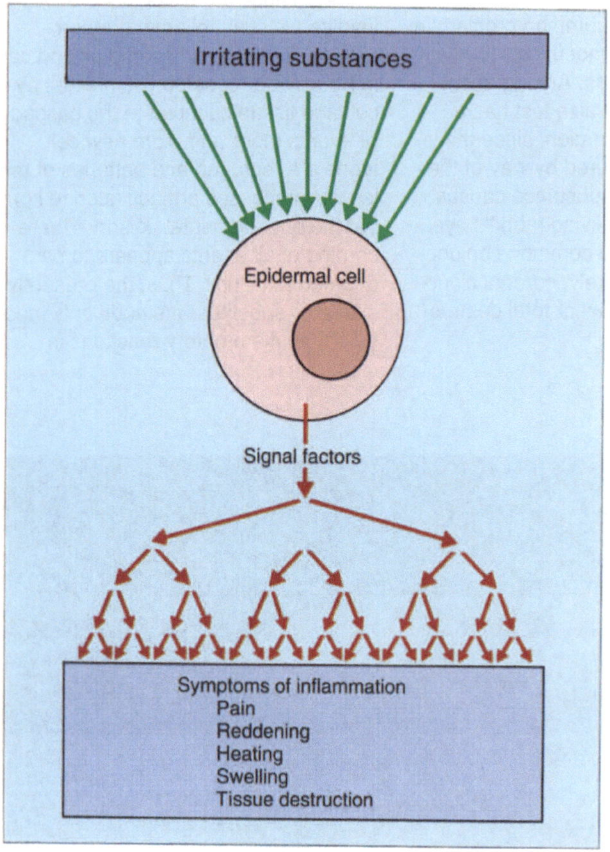

Fig. 23
Environmental factors that irritate the skin and the mucous membrane, among which are tumor promoters, cause the skin cells to release certain signal factors. These induce reactions within the organism which lead to symptoms of an inflammation. These are observed, for example, in the Draize test.

organ preparations such as isolated animal eyes, incubated chicken eggs or placenta (chorio-allantoic membrane). The disadvantages are obvious: in order to remove the organs, the animals still have to be killed; in addition, it is not at all clear yet to what extent the results can be extrapolated to the human. On the other hand, the resistance of cell cultures to toxic substances (the ability of cells to survive) is only a rough assessment and correlates very little with the conditions in living tissue. Alternative test methods are limited to certain classes of irritating substances. The Eyetex test, for example, which is based on a mixture of eye proteins, can only be used for protein denaturing substances such as acids, lyes, and detergents. There are, however, many other irritating substances.

In view of this situation, can one reasonably hope to develop a substitute for the Draize test? After all, one would have to assume that cells always react, no matter what the nature of an outside stimulus, with the same stereotyped biochemical responses. If, in addition, such a reaction were the common trigger of the cascade of cellular and molecular processes mentioned above, we would have found an ideal measure of irritation, especially if it could be observed in human cell cultures.

Prompted by the Berlin Association of Anti-Vivisectionists and supported by Schering, Inc., we are trying to track down such a common biochemical denominator of skin irritation. As a model, we use human epithelial cells (keratinocytes). These are the body's foremost line of defense against environmental factors and they initiate the inflammatory reaction by sending out biochemical signals to other tissues. Among these signals are certain tissue hormones (growth factors, cytokines), as well as the eicosanoids. The latter is a collective term for a group of biologically extremely potent agents, such as prostaglandins and leucotrienes, which are released by the irritated cell. Cytokines and eicosanoids act as "mediators" and activate the body's defense mechanisms. As a consequence, the characteristic symptoms of an inflammation, such as pain, reddening, sensation of heat, swelling, and influx of leucocytes develop. In our project, we want to examine whether the release of such mediators by skin cells is the desired stereotyped molecular response to chemical irritation, and whether identifying and measuring it in cell cultures might at least partially replace the controversial Draize test. It should be emphasized, however, that such investigations have only become possible through basic observations on living animals and the latest methodological developments. Thus, in fundamental research, animal experiments now can help to make future animal experiments unnecessary.

Why does the Deutsches Krebsforschungszentrum carry out this project, though at first glance it seems to be of little importance for cancer research? The answer is related to the tumor promoters already mentioned: it has been shown that virtually all tumor-promoters – at least those that are effective on skin and mucosa – are also serious irritant poisons that trigger massive inflammatory reactions. In fact, it has been shown that there is a direct link between irritant effect and tumor promoting effect. In our quest for biochemical symptoms of tissue irritation, we can fall back upon considerable resources of knowledge; after all, we have many years of experience in looking into the molecular mechanism of tumor promotion. Thus, by trying to replace the Draize test, we hope at the same time to set up the basis for reliably detecting and assessing the potentially extremely dangerous environmental tumor promoters.

Prof. Dr. Friedrich Marks
Division of Biochemistry of Tissue-Specific Regulation

Participating scientists

Dr. Karin Müller-Decker
Dr. Gerhard Fürstenberger

3.2 Sensitizing Multidrug Resistant Tumor Cells by Anchoring a Drug with Laser Light

by Herwig Ponstingl, Christof Granzow and Georgios Nasioulas

Knowledge of the precise nature of a malignant tumor and of its spread is the basis for therapeutic decisions. Many localized tumors can be eliminated by surgery or radiotherapy, whereas other malignancies, such as leukemias, spread throughout the whole organism. Therefore, they are treated by chemotherapy. Even in some localized organ tumors, due to their particular biological characteristics, primary chemotherapy yields better results than radiotherapy or surgery. One target for this application of chemotherapy is the small-cell lung cancer.

Even though for these diseases chemotherapy is superior to other treatments or is the only effective treatment, it is applied only as a last resort in late stages of certain organ tumors, thereby playing a rather problematical role. The extremely effective cytotoxins used as cytostatics not only inhibit the growth of the tumor cells, but also affect normal tissues with a high rate of cell proliferation, such as the bone marrow, the immune system, and the mucous membranes, which all have vital functions in the organism.

An important group of cytostatic agents are the Vinca alkaloids that are isolated from plants. They are clinically relevant as components of many established chemotherapy protocols. In the cells, the closely related substances vinblastine, vincristine, and vindesin bind reversibly to tubulin. This protein assembles into small tubes (microtubules), which are the main component of the mitotic spindle, which distributes the genetic material to the two daughter cells during division. Vinca alkaloids inhibit the assembly of microtubules and, as a consequence, cell division. However, since microtubules are also found in the axons of neurites, anti-tubulin cytostatic agents have a neurotoxic effect. Vinblastine is applied for treating acute leukemias, Hodgkin's lymphomas, testicular tumors, melanomas, and neuroblastomas; vincristine for metastatic breast cancers, chorion carcinomas, colon carcinomas, small-cell lung tumors, and squamous cell carcinomas of the head and neck; and vindesin for Kaposi sarcomas.

The spectrum of tumors amenable to treatment with antitubulin cytostatics would be considerably larger if it were possible to maintain a high drug concentration locally, which, otherwise, tends to decrease because of outward transport and diffusion. Breast cancer and small-cell lung cancer, for instance, often respond to chemotherapy with a significant prolongation of the patients' survival without, however, achieving permanent recovery. Attempts have been made to achieve higher drug concentrations by implanting a pump under the patients' skin for continuous infusion.

Chemotherapy of tumors faces yet another problem, that of chemoresistance. Some tumors, such as adenocarcinomas of the colon or the kidney, are inherently resistant to cytostatics (intrinsic or primary resistance). In the case of other cancers, such as small-cell lung carcinomas, breast carcinomas, childhood leukemias, or neuroblastomas, chemotherapy may be effective in the beginning. However, in the course of the treatment the tumors often become resistant (acquired or secondary chemoresistance), sometimes even to substances that were not used in the therapy (multidrug resistance). In experiments with cell cultures, a single cytostatic agent often is sufficient to induce resistance to a multitude of drugs.

Victor Ling of the Ontario Cancer Institute in Toronto, Canada, has identified a protein in the outer membrane of cells that develops resistance, the concentration of which frequently corresponds to the degree of chemoresistance. The protein's structure is similar to that of transport proteins which can be found in the cell walls of bacteria. It is particularly abundant in the membranes of cells in the kidney, adrenal gland, liver, colon, small intestine, the pancreas, and the uterus during pregnancy. This corresponds well to its proposed functioning as a pump for the secretion of toxic substances. This fact might also explain the inherent multidrug resistance of tumors in these organs.

Fig. 24
During cell division, microtubules direct the distribution of the chromosomes to two poles; Vinca alkaloids disturb this process. Under their influence, the distribution apparatus, which is made up of microtubules (upper right: stained in an untreated cell), cannot form (lower right). As a consequence, the chromosomes are distributed randomly inside the cell (lower left). Untreated control cells with stained chromosomes (left).

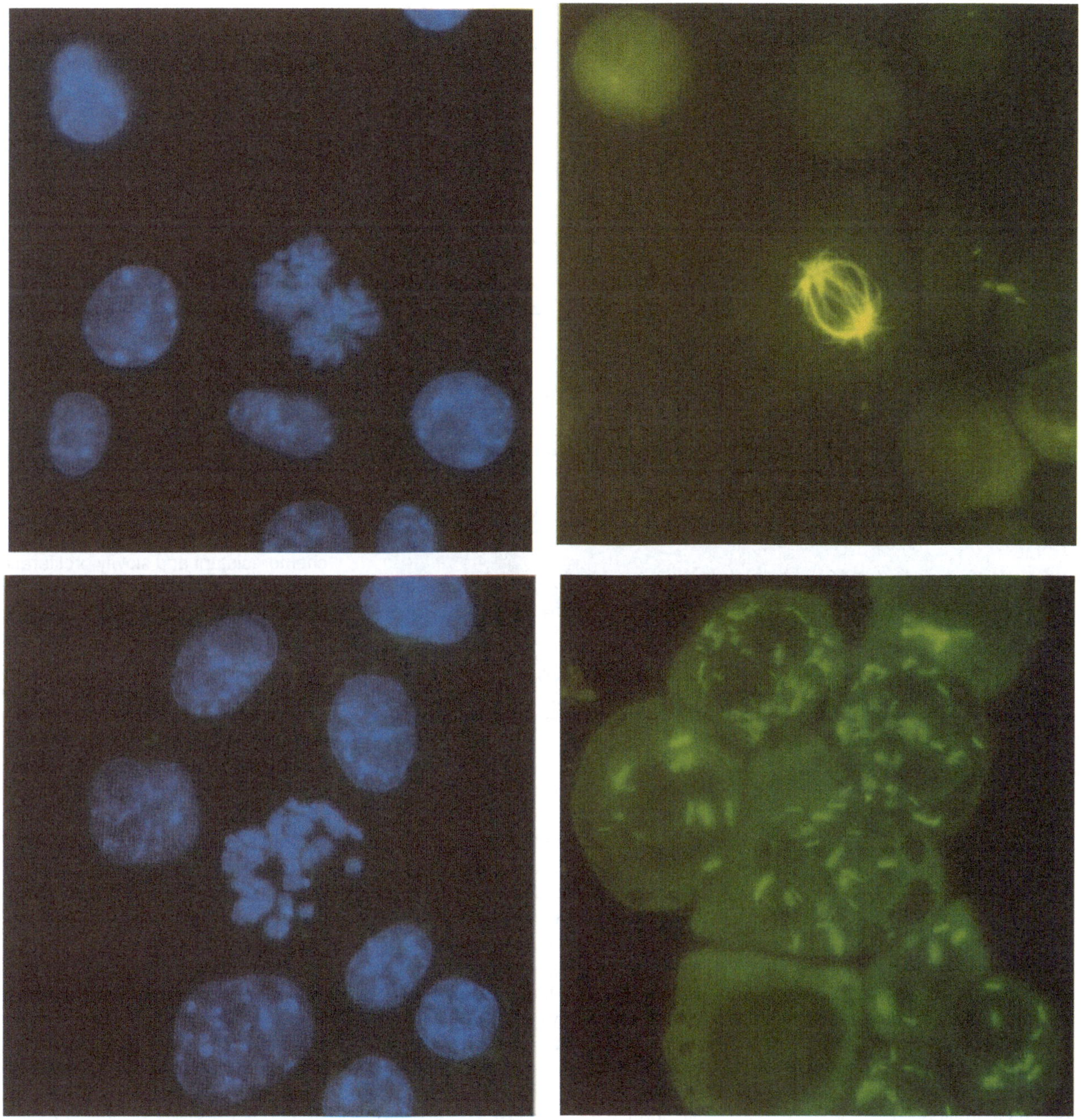

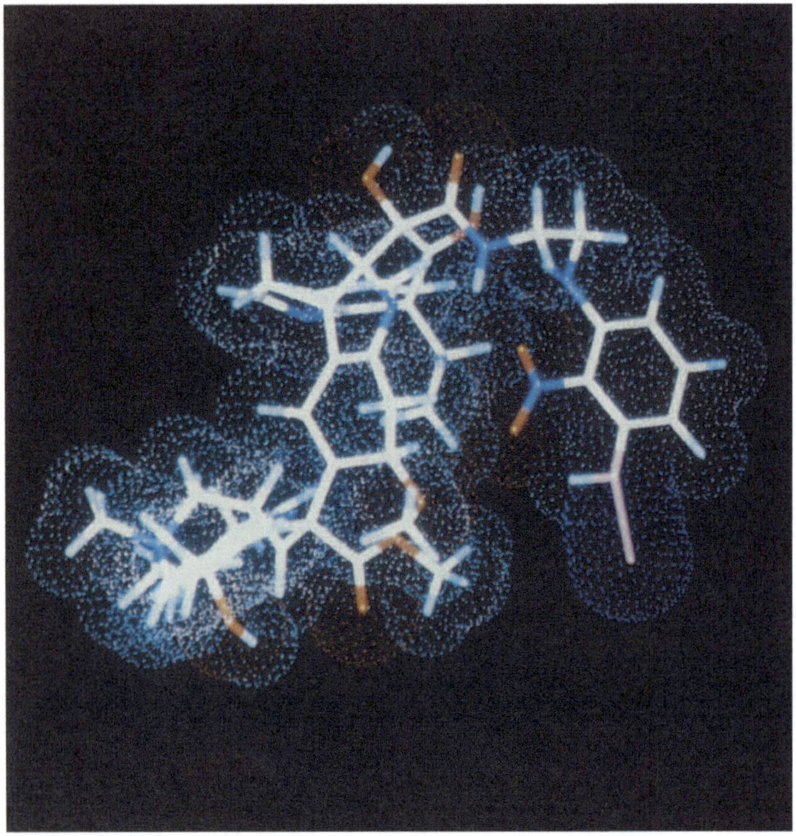

Fig. 25
Spatial structure of napavin. The arm protruding from the compact molecule absorbs the incident light; after irradiation, it serves as the anchor. (Computed by Martina Kieninger and Dr. Sandor Suhai.)

In other chemoresistant tumors, different resistance mechanisms have been identified. In some cases, mutations in the gene coding for the target protein tubulin lead to changes in the binding site and thus weaken the drug's binding to the tubulin.

If it were possible to bind a drug irreversibly to its target proteins in the cell, the binding would be stabilized and the pump of the multidrug resistance protein would become ineffective. This would be achieved by a chemically stable bond to tubulin, or, alternatively, by directly blocking the membrane pump. However, a drug that is intrinsically chemically reactive would be stalled many times before reaching the tumor cell. Thus, it was our goal to bring a cytostatically active, yet chemically inactive form of the drug into the cells and then anchor it by means of light. Therefore, we synthesized a new, light-sensitive derivative of the cytostatic drug vinblastine, which we call napavin (Fig. 25). With respect to all properties investigated so far (solubility, toxicity, inhibition of cell division, binding to tubulin, effective concentration, duration of effectiveness), unexposed napavin reacts in exactly the same way as the clinically used vinblastine. Unexposed napavin reversibly binds to its target protein tubulin and is quickly secreted from multidrug-resistant cells by the membrane pump. Upon activation by the soft laser light (about one tenth of the energy of bright sunlight for 5 minutes), a photoreactive arm forms a strong covalent bond between the substance and the tubulin molecules in the cells and thus protects napavin from diffusing or from being actively secreted. As a result, we expect chemoresistant and slowly proliferating tumors growing at light-accessible locations to become amenable to chemotherapy.

The anchoring was tested using radioactive napavin in a culture of multidrug-resistant HD33 Ehrlich-Lettré ascites cells. The medium contained napavin, which after 1 hour of incubation was exchanged for a napavin-free medium. Without being anchored by light, 70% of the napavin stored in the cells was secreted within 5 minutes. The same was true for vinblastine. Three hours later, napavin could no longer be detected in the cells. Upon activation with laser light however, the napavin concentration in the cells remained high; after 5 minutes, 83% of the originally accumulated napavin was still in the cells, after three hours 70%, and after 30 hours still 50%. Additional experiments have shown that most of the napavin was anchored to tubulin. Thus, the covalent laser light-induced binding results in a significantly higher drug level as compared to vinblastine and non-anchored napavin. As a result, the sensitivity of normally chemoresistant tumor cell lines to the cytostatic drug is improved by a factor 9 to 33.

We investigated the long-term effect of a single short napavin treatment on tumor growth in vivo in transplantable mouse tumor cells. Multidrug-resistant tumor cells were explanted from animals, incubated outside the animals with vinblastine, napavin, or the photoreactive arm alone with or without laser light, tested for their viability, and then transferred into other animals. Most of the control animals had to be killed within 15 days because of considerable tumor growth. In contrast, all mice that had received viable, multidrug-resistant tumor cells treated with napavin and laser light survived for more than 120 days without developing a tumor. Yet, the napavin concentration had been only 25 or 50% of the vinblastine concentration. In immunocompetent animals, the necessary napavin concentration is considerably lower than predicted from the cell culture experiments. We assume that in the living organism the immune system participates in the elimination of division-inhibited cells.

One problem of our anchoring procedure results from the visible blue light we need for activating the anchor in the tumor. We can penetrate into the tissue by only a few millimeters. We want the light to be exclusively absorbed by the anchor without affecting the cytostatically active part of the molecule or causing DNA alterations in tissue cells penetrated by the beam. On the one hand, light is absorbed by tissue (mainly by hemoglobin); on the other hand, a minimum amount of energy (the energy of light is inversely related to its wave length) is needed to split off a group of atoms in order to activate the anchor. These requirements are best met at the wavelengths of blue light. In this range it is possible to irradiate the skin for 10 minutes with energies equivalent to bright sunlight without causing warming. Only a small fraction of the light penetrates the skin directly; 75 to 80% of the light is diffusely scattered. Fortunately, only 1% of the energy of this scattered light is necessary to activate the napavin anchor. In some early experiments, during which we had not completely avoided daylight, the scattered sunlight led to an activation. For a high yield of uniform light we used a soft argon laser, the light of which can be guided by endoscopes with almost no loss to surfaces within the body.

At present, we are testing this procedure on solid, multidrug-resistant human tumors which only marginally respond to Vinca cytostatic drugs. The tumors are implanted under the skin of nude mice, whose immune system does not reject the foreign cells. We hope to find out whether napavin is suited for the therapy of tumors that can be reached endoscopically, such as tumors of the head and the neck, of the bladder, and colon carcinomas.

If these experiments yield satisfactory results, we plan to conduct preliminary clinical trials on tumors which are at least partially sensitive to traditional Vinca alkaloids, and which are readily accessible to laser light, such as melanomas, basaliomas, and squamous cell carcinomas of the upper respiratory and digestive tracts. In most cases, the primary tumors can be controlled by surgery or radiotherapy. Recurrent tumors, however, are often resistant to therapy. In up to 30 of the patients with squamous cell carcinomas in the oral cavity, pharynx, and larynx, secondary tumors occur at sites that are not easily accessible. In these cases the napavin laser therapy might prove to be an effective supplement to today's therapy protocols.

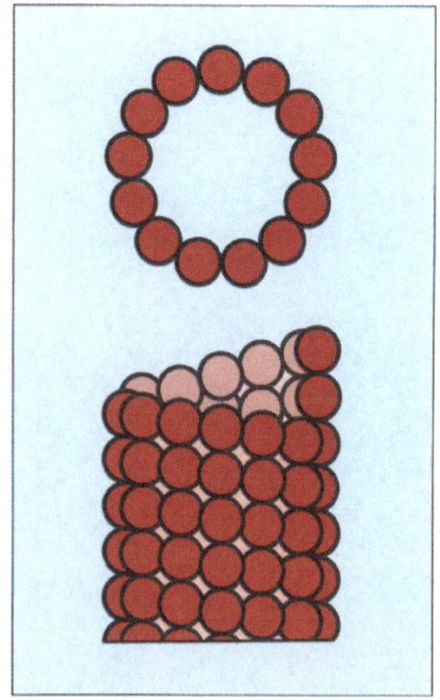

Fig. 26
Microtubules are small tubelets with a diameter of about 30 nanometers. They are composed of many tubulin molecules. They are important for the cell shape, for distributing daughter chromosomes during cell division, and in transport processes within the cell.

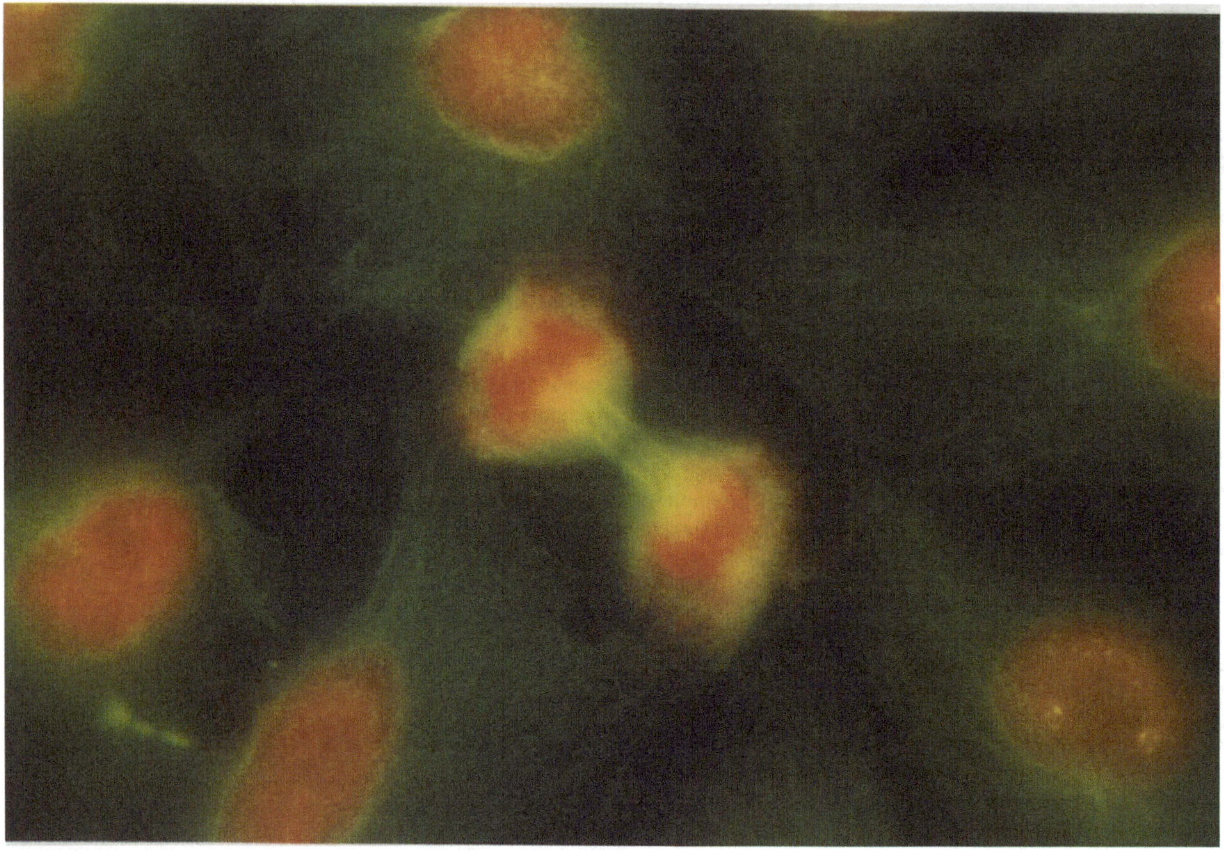

Fig. 27
The cells were stained with two different dyes. Chromosomes are stained red; microtubules are green. In the center, a dividing cell can be seen. In the non-dividing cells, the microtubules are spread all over the cell.

Our work was supported by the Wilhelm and Maria Meyenburg Foundation and by the Tumor Center Heidelberg/Mannheim.

Prof. Dr. Herwig Ponstingl
Dr. Georgios Nasioulas
Project Molecular Biology of Mitosis

Dr. Christof Granzow
Division of Biochemistry of the Cell

In collaboration with

Dipl.-Phys. Michael Stöhr
Division of Applied Immunology
Deutsches Krebsforschungszentrum

Priv.-Doz. Dr. Wolfgang Tilgen
Dermatology Division, University of Heidelberg

Prof. Koert Gerzon
Department of Pharmacology and Toxicology,
Indiana University, School of Medicine,
Indianapolis, Indiana, USA

Prof. Richard Himes
Department of Biochemistry,
University of Kansas, Lawrence,
Kansas, USA

Priv.-Doz. Dr. Siegfried Matzku
E. Merck, Darmstadt

Selected publications

Tilgen, W., et al.: Heterogeneity of human malignant melanoma cells in vivo and in vitro: role of experimental systems. Pigment Cell, Biological, Molecular & Clinical Aspects of Pigmentation, University of Tokyo Press, Tokyo, pp. 435–447 (1985)

Kartner, N., Ling, V.: Vielfach-Resistenz von Krebszellen. Spektrum der Wissenschaft 5, 64–71 (1989)

Nasioulas, G., Grammbitter, K., Himes, R.H., Ponstingl, H.: Interaction of a new photosensitive derivative of vinblastine, Napavin, with tubulin and microtubules in vitro. Eur. J. Biochem. 192, 69–74 (1990)

Nasioulas, G., Granzow, C., Stöhr, M., Ponstingl, H.: Sensitization of multidrug-resistant mouse ascites HD33 and Chinese hamster ovary CHRC5S3 cells by a photoreactive vinblastine derivative, Napavin. Cancer Res. 50, 403–408 (1990)

Granzow, C., Stöhr, M., Ponstingl, H.: Photoactivated napavin suppresses tumorigenicity in wild type and mutant, multidrug-resistant Ehrlich-Lettré mouse ascites tumour cells. J. Cancer Res. Clin. Oncol. 117 (Suppl.) 45 (1991)

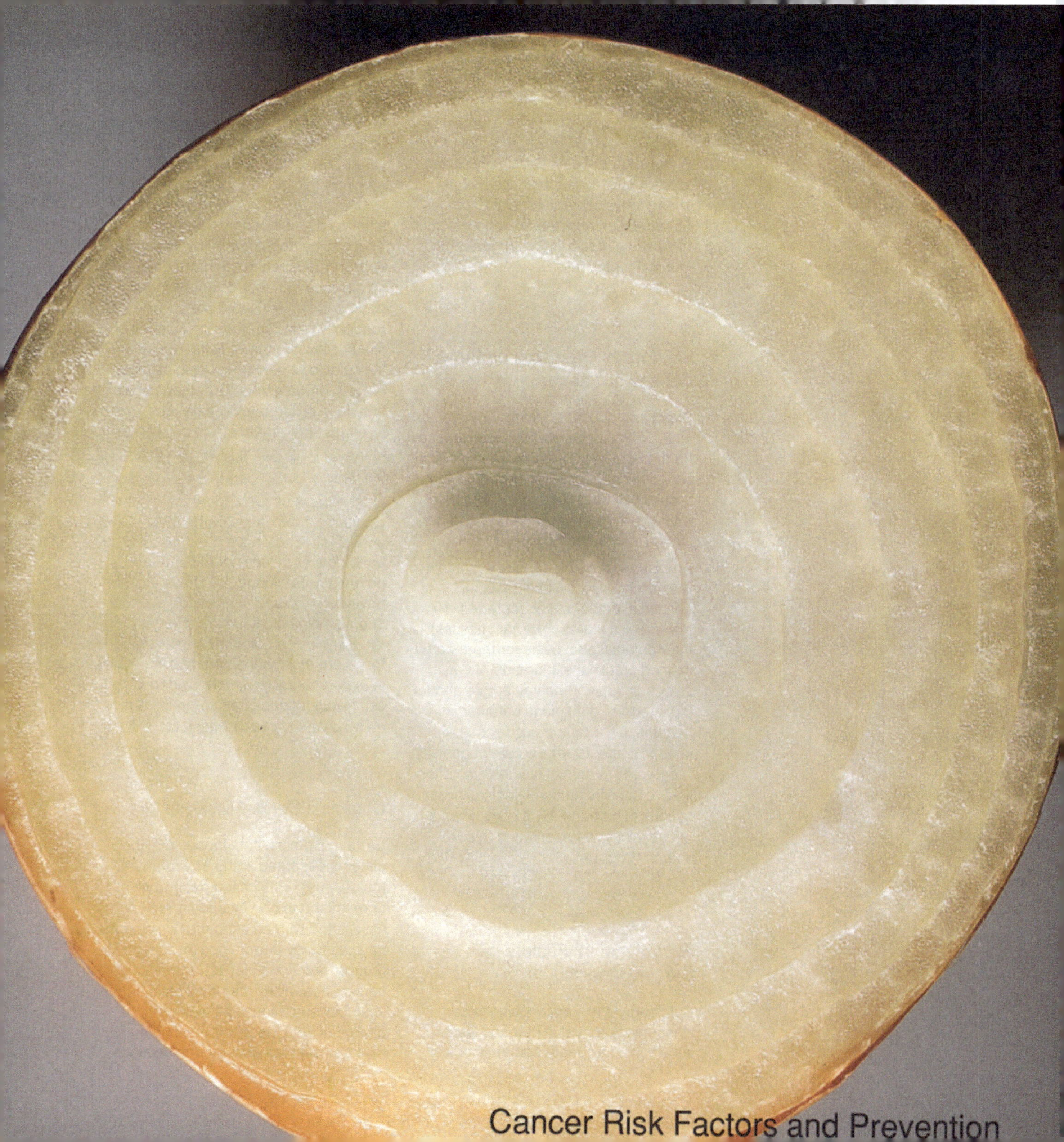

Cancer Risk Factors and Prevention

4

Cancer Risk Factors and Prevention

The assumption that human cancer is largely caused by environmental factors is undisputed today. Carcinogenic factors are chemical substances, high-energy physical radiation, and viruses. The detection and determination of such factors is a precondition for preventive medical measures.

Methods of Research on the Causes of Cancer

Direct information on environmental effects on the incidence of cancer derives from a large number of epidemiological observations showing differences in the occurrence of various forms of cancer with regard to the place, time, and person (or person group).

Animal experiments (and with some restrictions also suitable tests for genetic alterations, i.e., mutagenicity test in cell cultures of certain tissues) offer an additional basis for the theoretical and practical exploration of carcinogenic environmental factors and for the checking of findings obtained in humans. Data on the occurrence of chemical agents whose carcinogenicity is detected in animal studies also often lead to specific epidemiological investigations in humans. Both disciplines are hence jointly represented in this Research Program.

Environmental Factors in Carcinogenesis

Carcinogens are factors whose carcinogenic potential in humans was shown in appropriate epidemiological studies. Since epidemiological observations are not yet available in many situations, factors which have shown carcinogenic potential in experimental systems are also appraised as constituting a carcinogenic risk for humans. This can be documented by investigations demonstrating the more frequent occurrence of tumor diseases in experimental animals and the above-randomly more frequent conversion of tissue cells into tumor cells. Epidemiological and experimental studies must comply with a series of methodological criteria in order to allow clear inferences with regard to the causal role of the corresponding factor in carcinogenesis.

On the basis of such approaches, carcinogenic substances of the most diverse structure have been discovered up to now or at least identified as potentially carcinogenic. These include physical factors, chemical compounds and also biological factors (viruses). Whereas these categories of risk factors have mostly been studied in detail in experimental research, epidemiological investigations often comprise the entire diversity of potential factors.

Chemical Cancer Risk Factors

Certain chemical substances may be either widespread in the environment (ubiquitous) or delimited geographically or restricted to one location and hence associated with an exposure which can be specifically determined (occupational groups, nutritional habits). Appraisals on carcinogenicity may apply to single chemical substances as well as to groups of substances or to complex mixtures such as occur in the occupational environment or in consequence of cultural habits (e.g., smoking or dietary habits).

Classifications of carcinogenicity are not uncommonly made by international expert groups and have led to the current designation of 50 substances or complex mixtures as unequivocally carcinogenic for humans in the procedure of the International Agency for Research on Cancer (a cancer research institute of the WHO) practiced over many years. These include (to name only a few and without claims to completeness or to relevance appraisal): asbestos, benzene, nickel and nickel compounds, estrogens, tobacco smoke, as well as work in iron and steel foundries and the rubber industry.

Attempts have also been made to characterize and study specific exposures in individual epidemiological studies, e.g., the influence of exogenous and endogenous nitrosamine exposures on the risk of brain tumors, but as a rule more general exposures are investigated, e.g., the risk of cancer in occupations with various exposures (e.g., stainless steel welders, model builders, pesticides). Studies on the nutritional habits and risk of cancer can be evaluated with regard to the uptake of individual constituents of food (e.g., nitrate) or general nutritional patterns. Biochemical determinations of blood values (e.g., vitamins) often serve for more precise establishement of corresponding exposures.

Besides the identification of isolated factors or groups of substances, additive or synergistic actions are also of very great importance, since they probably occur much more frequently than single effects and a monocausality can only be very rarely assumed in carcinogenesis.

The occurrence and formation of already suspected carcinogens in the environment are determined by means of analytical methods. In this way it is possible to appraise the exposure of a population group to such factors. Together with the investigation of nutritional habits, this can provide important information for prevention and early diagnosis. This research (e.g., the identification of nitrosamines and their analysis) is being performed by the Deutsches Krebsforschungszentrum in an international context. Systematic animal experimental investigations with in some cases very elaborate methods (e.g., inhalation) are concerned both with relationships between chemical structures and carcinogenic action and with dose-effect relationships. Such data are necessary preconditions for appraisals of risks attributations for appraisals of risks attributable to environmental carcinogens. These studies are supplemented by investigations on synergistic and modifying effects in chemical carcinogenesis.

Co-carcinogens, which intensify the action of carcinogenic factors, can be identified by means of experiments and be isolated by biochemical methods in such a way that the structural units enable inferences with regard to the cancer-promoting action.

Viruses as Cause of Cancer

Today, four different virus types are known which are associated with certain human cancers:

- human T-cell leukemia viruses (HTLV-I) associated with a certain type of leukemia rarely occurring in adults,
- the Epstein-Barr virus, which causes certain lymphomas or tumors of the nasopharyngeal region,
- the hepatitis B virus, which is associated with liver cancer,
- the papillomaviruses, which are risk factors in cancer of the uterine cervix.

It is known how these viruses are involved in carcinogenesis. However, it is known that the viruses cannot be the unique cause for malignant cell growth. Additional factors (e.g., carcinogenic substances from cigarette smoke) must play a role in this process. The interaction of these factors with the virus genes is being investigated at present.

Epidemiological studies on cancer-associated viruses are concerned with the frequency of HPV infection in various groups of persons and the presence of other factors which are also known or suspected to be cancer risk factors and which influence this frequency.

The Effect of Radiation in Carcinogenesis

The follow-up investigation of the late fate of about 5 000 persons in whom the radioactive x-ray contrast medium Thorotrast containing thorium had been used for diagnostic reasons from 1935 to 1948 is the subject of an epidemiological study of the Deutsches Krebsforschungszentrum. In particular, this study serves to obtain more precise knowledge on the dose-effect relationships in the action of ionizing radiation on humans. The subject of this study is a comparison of the incidence of cancer cases in the exposed group of patients with that of a suitable nonexposed control group. The persons still alive are regularly being followed up.

Other epidemiological investigations are concerned with the cancer risk of persons who were exposed to radiation for occupational reasons and for whom detailed dose measurements relating to individuals are available. These may be the staff of nuclear power stations. The detailed information on doses in this group of persons, which are in a relatively low range, should in turn provide valuable information on the dose-effect relationship of ionizing radiation. An international cohort study is concerned with this topic.

The influence of diagnostic and therapeutic radiation in the region of the head and neck is one component of a case control study on brain tumors.

Descriptive Epidemiology

Besides special epidemiological studies on carcinogenesis, suitably analyzed descriptive data on the occurrence of cancer (new cases, mortalities) in West Germany and in international comparison provide an important basis for the development of specific problems and for the evaluation of cancer development in general. Theoretical models for explanation of such data are also being developed and investigated.

Coordinator of the Research Program:
Prof. Dr. Jürgen Wahrendorf

Divisions and their heads:

Cell Pathology:
Prof. Dr. Peter Bannasch

Carcinogenesis and Chemotherapy:
N. N.

Environmental Carcinogens:
Prof. Dr. Rudolf Preußmann

Metabolism of N-Nitroso-Compounds:
Prof. Dr. Manfred Wießler

Mechanism of Tumorigenesis:
Prof. Dr. Erich Hecker

Interaction of Carcinogens with Biological Macromolecules:
Priv.-Doz. Dr. Dr. Heinz W. Thielmann

Epidemiology:
Prof. Dr. Jürgen Wahrendorf

Project groups and their heads:

Tumor Promotion in the Liver:
Priv.-Doz. Dr. Michael Schwarz

4.1 Diet and Cancer

by Jürgen Wahrendorf, Heiner Boeing, Jenny Chang-Claude, and Rainer Frenzel-Beyme

The main risk factors for carcinogenesis in humans have been clearly identified as smoking, a wide range of chemicals (especially at the workplace), specific drugs (in particular, cytostatic agents), and ionizing radiation. The search for further carcinogenic conditions has thus concentrated on other complex situations in which chemical agents might, or actually do, play a part. In this context, dietary habits have received special attention, since most human tumors occur in the gastrointestinal tract. In 1980, 29.2 % of all cancer deaths among men and 35.9 % among women were due to gastrointestinal tumors.

Worldwide, the incidence of these tumors varies significantly. Stomach cancer, for example, is more common in eastern Europe, Asia, and South America than in northern and western Europe or in North America, where it has been in significant decline over recent decades. Intestinal cancer, on the other hand, is more common in industrialized countries than in underdeveloped countries. Since the lifestyles and dietary habits differ widely from country to country, and since studies have shown that in the course of time the cancer incidence among immigrants adjusts to that of their adoptive country, one can assume that one of the main causes of gastrointestinal cancers is nutrition – and thus, in principle, avoidable.

Diet is probably the most complex mixture of chemicals a human being is exposed to, and the possible influences on carcinogenesis are manifold.

To start with, all food may directly contain carcinogens or their immediate precursors (such as pesticides and additives). This fact is subject to broad discussion, though it is probably of minor significance. In addition, food components can either promote or inhibit the formation of carcinogens in the body, either from the components themselves or from their metabolic products. Examples are the formation of N-nitrosamines from nitrite and amines, and the inhibition of this reaction by ascorbic acid.

Also, food components can affect the metabolic activation or inactivation of carcinogens. Such a (protective) role is attributed to some vegetable components. Certain food components also indirectly alter the time that carcinogenic substances are in contact with a possible site of action. Dietary fiber, for example, dilutes the stool and thus reduces the transit time. In addition, food components (such as vitamin A) may directly act on the body cells and change their susceptibility to carcinogens or their growth behavior. One finally has to consider the theoretical possibility that food components may contribute to a change in the body's capability to eliminate transformed cells. This multitude of modes of action demonstrates that all epidemiological research on „diet and cancer" must stringently take account of all these subtle conditions.

The simplistic approach of comparing the average consumption of specific foods or nutrients of population groups with their cancer rates may help to generate hypotheses; however, it will not answer the question of whether, for example, the same persons who consume a lot of fat are those who develop intestinal cancer. In this respect, we need studies which demonstrate, on an individual level, a correlation between dietary habits and the occurrence or non-occurrence of cancer or other relevant changes in health.

The complexity of the dietary exposure requires careful assessment methods that provide a comprehensive picture of the normal dietary habits of an individual over a specific period of time. In order to be able to correctly analyze the manifold correlations between these figures and their interaction as risk factors, all important foods and nutrients consumed should be covered. In particular, assessment methods should be used that have been tested and validated in preliminary studies.

In the following we will present the results of three current research projects on „diet and cancer" of the Division of Epidemiology. Although all of these studies use different approaches, we will show how their results converge to form a homogeneous picture of the correlation between dietary habits and cancer.

Mortality of Vegetarians

In this prospective study, we investigated the effects of a vegetarian diet on the health status by recording all new diseases, including various types of cancer. The number of cases recorded was then compared to the number that were expected for a control group.

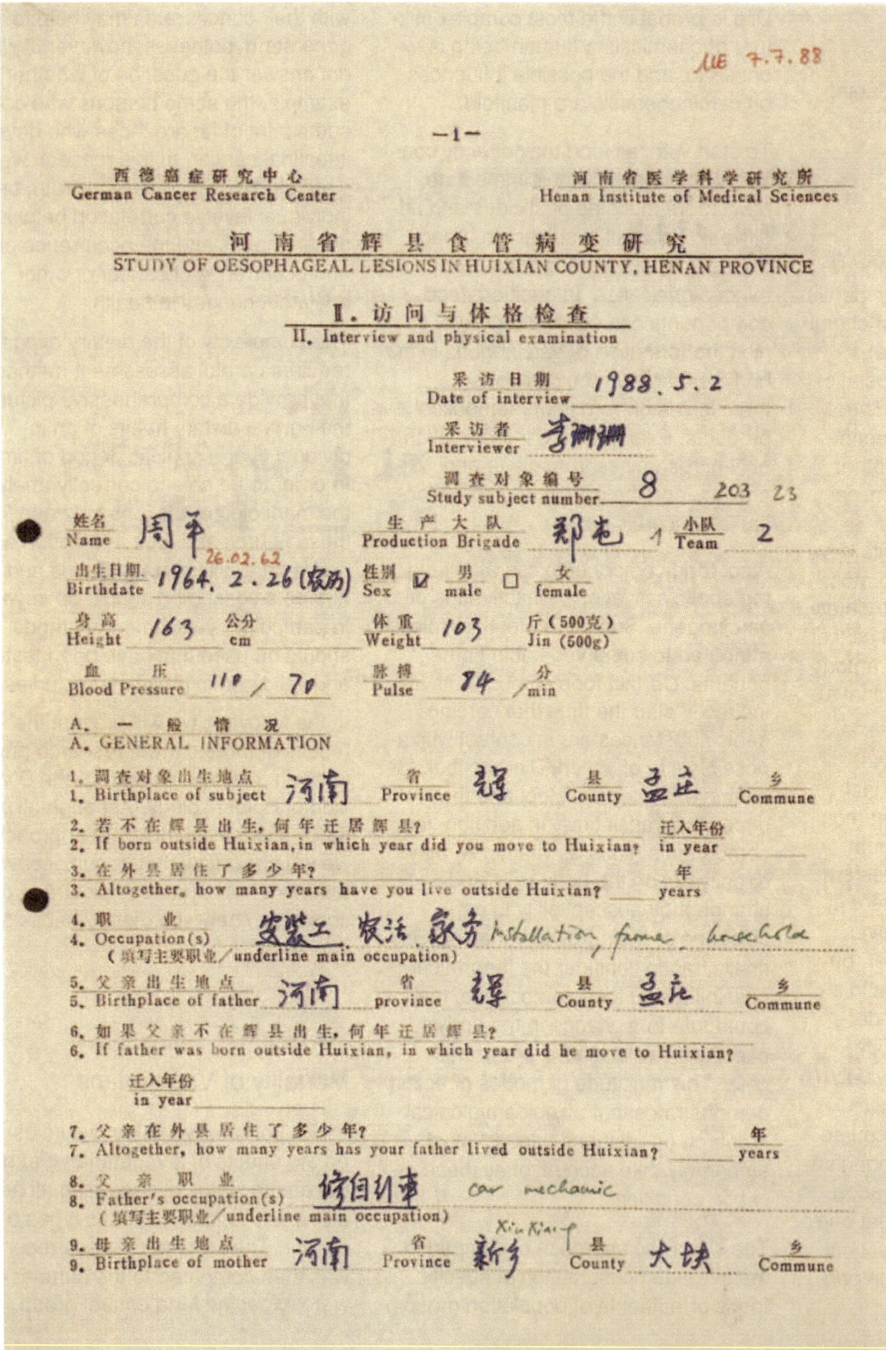

AIE 7.7.88

—1—

西德癌症研究中心
German Cancer Research Center

河南省医学科学研究所
Henan Institute of Medical Sciences

河南省辉县食管病变研究
STUDY OF OESOPHAGEAL LESIONS IN HUIXIAN COUNTY, HENAN PROVINCE

Ⅱ. 访问与体格检查
II. Interview and physical examination

采访日期 Date of interview 1988.5.2

采访者 Interviewer [illegible]

调查对象编号 Study subject number 8 203 23

姓名 Name 周平 | 生产大队 Production Brigade 郑屯 1 | 小队 Team 2

出生日期 Birthdate 1964.2.26 (农历) 26.02.62 | 性别 Sex ☑ 男 male ☐ 女 female

身高 Height 163 公分 cm | 体重 Weight 103 斤(500克) Jin (500g)

血压 Blood Pressure 110 / 70 | 脉搏 Pulse 84 分 /min

A. 一般情况
A. GENERAL INFORMATION

1. 调查对象出生地点
1. Birthplace of subject 河南 省 Province 辉 县 County 孟庄 乡 Commune

2. 若不在辉县出生，何年迁居辉县？
2. If born outside Huixian, in which year did you move to Huixian? 迁入年份 in year

3. 在外县居住了多少年？
3. Altogether, how many years have you live outside Huixian? 年 years

4. 职业
4. Occupation(s) 安装工，农活，家务 installation, farmer, household
(填写主要职业／underline main occupation)

5. 父亲出生地点
5. Birthplace of father 河南 省 province 辉 县 County 孟庄 乡 Commune

6. 如果父亲不在辉县出生，何年迁居辉县？
6. If father was born outside Huixian, in which year did he move to Huixian?
迁入年份 in year

7. 父亲在外县居住了多少年？
7. Altogether, how many years has your father lived outside Huixian? 年 years

8. 父亲职业
8. Father's occupation(s) 修自行车 car mechanic
(填写主要职业／underline main occupation)

9. 母亲出生地点
9. Birthplace of mother 河南 省 Province 新乡 Xin Xiang 县 County 大块 乡 Commune

Fig. 28
One page of the questionnaire to identify the causes of esophageal cancer in China.

Mortality as an indicator for lethal diseases is still commonly used in cancer research. Only in countries with cancer registers which contain data on all new cases is it possible to conduct studies on the basis of morbidity.

The prospective epidemiological study of the Deutsches Krebsforschungszentrum comprised 1904 individuals who followed a vegetarian or natural way of living. In 1978, we recruited participants by inserting a questionnaire in the journals of the German "Vegetarian Association". After preliminary contact, we mailed out a second questionnaire asking the participants for detailed information. In the course of the study we conducted various intermediate polls and also asked for the participants' consent that in the case of his or her death, we would be allowed to determine its cause from the death certificate. In three successive years, we toxicologically analyzed saliva samples of the participants (collected by mail) with regard to nitrite.

After an observation period of 11 years (ending in mid-1989) it became evident that the mortality in general as well as the mortality due to chronic diseases was lower for vegetarians than for the general population, which we used as the reference. Both for men and women, only half of the expected number of deaths due to cardiovascular diseases was observed. The standardized mortality ratios (SMR) (the SMR is equal to 100 if the mortality rates of cases and controls are equal) for all causes of death were 43.6 (men) and 53.1 (women), and 38.8 (men) and 46.2 (women) for deaths due to cardiovascular diseases. For malignant tumors, a similar reduction was observed only for men (SMR 47.9). For women, the mortality rate due to tumors of the gastrointestinal tract was significantly reduced (SMR 49.1); however, it was less reduced for all cancer localizations taken together (SMR 73.5). The mortality ratio due to lung cancer in men was only 7.1 and thus clearly below the expected value of 100.

These results may in part be due to the characteristics of the group of persons studied, which comprises a large number of well-educated individuals (i.e., from the academic, social, and technical professions), as well as a majority of non-smokers. The vegetarians generally had a lower relative body weight than the non-vegetarians, which is known to have a positive effect on mortality. Thus, there seems to be a general health advantage to vegetarianism, which is mainly due to a diet that contains less fat and more fibers. It was also shown that physical activity is an important factor in reducing mortality, both overall, as well as due to cardiovascular diseases. (For the latter, it was reduced by 50 %.) A similar protective effect was found for the relative body weight, even in conjunction with other risk factors. A comparison among sub-groups with different levels of adherence to a vegetarian or natural way of living showed that moderate vegetarians had a lower relative risk of death than strict vegetarians; an absolute renunciation of meat is thus less important. However, the obvious impact of a vegetarian diet on the mortality rate is emphasized by the result of our study, which indicates that vegetarianism over a period of 20 or more years has a very positive effect on both the general mortality as well as on the cancer death rate. Thus, an almost vegetarian diet with a low percentage of saturated fats and cholesterol plays a part in reducing the mortality due to cardiovascular diseases and, probably, due to cancer.

Experimental cancer research has repeatedly reported that, after the administration of carcinogens, laboratory animals with a reduced food intake developed tumors less often than those with an unlimited supply of food. In addition, certain cell-protecting characteristics were found in some vegetables, such as crucifers (Cruciferae, such as cabbage) and alliums (Alliae, such as onions and garlic). Experiments have shown that vegetarian diets lead to a better supply of protective glutathione precursors by supporting detoxication mechanisms for carcinogens. However, these relationships are neither completely understood nor reliable. In addition, they act only preventively and not therapeutically, i. e., they act only before cancer has developed. Prospective studies on other population groups, such as the Seventh Day Adventists in the USA, and a large comprehensive study in Japan, have also demonstrated the advantages of a fructovegetarian diet over a diet including meat and carbohydrates. The advantages of a natural and unprocessed diet thus outweigh its disadvantages.

Stomach Cancer in Bavaria

Descriptive epidemiological figures clearly indicate that factors related to the lifestyle or the environment have a significant influence on the etiology of gastric carcinomas. In the former West Germany, the number of stomach cancer deaths had decreased from approximately 25000 a year in the 1960s, to 14000 a year by the end of the 1980s. Adjusted for the age structure, the reduction is even more obvious: about 60% for females and, although not quite as high, significantly more than 50% for men. Aside from this clearly retrogressive trend, there is a pronounced regional variability in the occurrence of stomach cancer in the former West Germany. Observations from the 1950s until today have consistently shown that in the West German south-east, especially in the Bavarian regions of Upper Palatinate and Lower Bavaria, stomach cancer mortality rates are up to twice as high as in other regions.

Fig. 29
A study of the Division of Epidemiology has shown: vegetarians live longer.

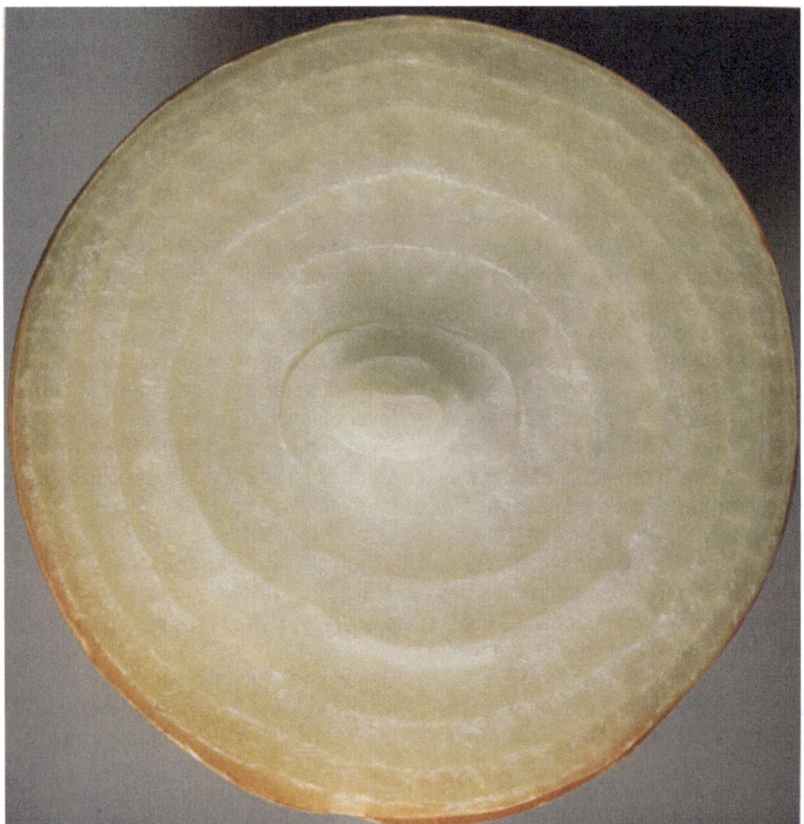

This situation is an interesting basis for etiological studies. A multi-center case-control study was conducted in regions with relatively high and low stomach cancer mortalities in order to identify the factors that are associated with stomach cancer risk. Within this study, 143 patients with a definite histological diagnosis of stomach cancer and 579 control persons were interviewed. The interviews focused on the average intake of food and nutrients before the diagnosis of the disease, various aspects of the treatment and conservation of food, questions about life style such as profession, smoking habits, and tap water quality, as well as on socio-demographic and medical information. An important result with regard to stomach cancer prevention is the fact that a high supply of vitamin C, i. e., a frequent intake of raw vegetables and fruits, reduces the stomach cancer risk by about 50 %. A high intake of processed meat increases the stomach cancer twofold, whereas a high intake of whole-meal bread and cheese was correlated with a risk reduction. In addition, it was shown that a private water supply (such as from a private well) increases the stomach cancer risk 2.5 times compared to a central water supply. Private smoke-drying of meat was not correlated to stomach cancer incidence, except when spruce wood was used. In this case, the risk was increased threefold.

A slightly increased risk was observed for drinkers of beer (average consumption between 100 and 500 grams a day); however, for a consumption in excess of this, no further increase could be proven statistically. This inconsistent trend within the categories of beer consumption, together with the inconsistent results of past studies on the correlation between alcohol consumption and stomach cancer risk, lead us to attribute little significance to this finding. However, new reports from Poland indicate that alcohol, if consumed in large quantities, might indeed play an important role in the etiology of stomach cancer. Polish studies showed a clear correlation between a high consumption of vodka and an increased stomach cancer risk.

Fig. 30
Model of the development of stomach cancer.

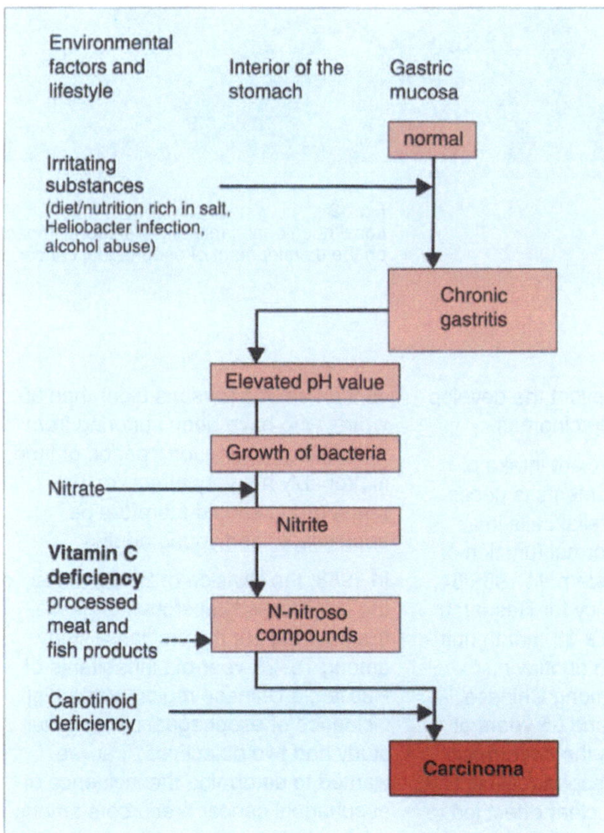

In our case-control study, we also showed that stomach cancer risk factors are more common for control persons in the high-risk area than for those in the low-risk area.

The consistency of the results of our case-control study with other known epidemiological findings from other countries, as well as the regional distribution of the risk factors within the control groups, lead us to conclude that the main etiological factors for stomach cancer in the formal West Germany were identified. 68.3 % of all stomach cancer cases could be attributed to one or several of the risk factors identified in our study.

Esophageal Cancer in China

Esophageal cancer, which is very common in northern China, in northern Iran, and in the Far Eastern republics of the CIS, is characterized by dramatic variations in its incidence, not only among different countries, but also within a geographic region, among different ethnic groups, and even between men and women. This indicates that the environment and cultural factors play an important role in the development of esophageal cancer.

Epidemiological studies in high-risk areas of China, Iran, and the CIS revealed a generally poor nutritional status of the population, which reduces the resistance to the carcinogenic effects of certain substances, and which consequently promotes the development of tumors. The frequent consumption of moldy food and certain domestic spices and foodstuffs is suspected of causing esophageal cancer in these countries. The excessive consumptions of tobacco and alcoholic beverages were shown to be the main risk factors in Europe and in the United States, but an insufficient consumption of fresh fruits and vegetables, as well as an excessive intake of carbohydrates, are also known to help the disease develop.

It is has been postulated that the first step in the development of esophageal cancer is an esophagitis. These lesions may occur at age 25 and before the development of dysplastic alterations, which are seen as precursors of malig-

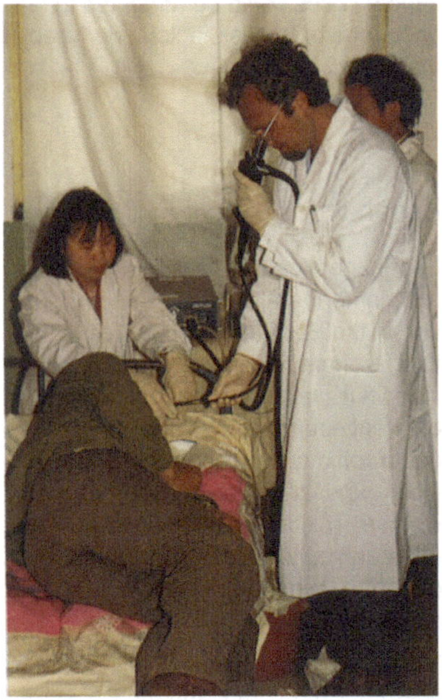

Fig. 31
In the municipality of Meng Zhuang in China, a strikingly high number of people develop esophageal cancer. The villagers, therefore, were very willing to undergo endoscopy.

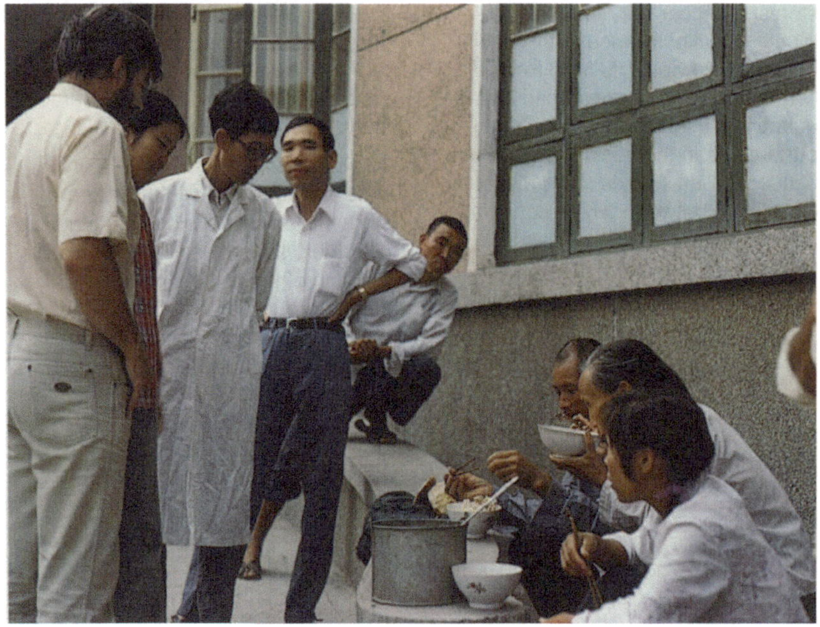

Fig. 32
Local nutritional habits have a strong impact on the development of esophageal cancer.

nant tumors. Esophagitis is an inflammatory condition, i. e., the organism's unspecific response to esophageal injuries. It is presumably caused by a coincidence of a poor nutritional status of the cells and mechanical or chemical injuries.

Since esophageal carcinomas are frequently detected in an advanced stage of the disease, and thus have an unfavorable prognosis, the early detection and treatment of dysplastic changes of the esophagus might contribute to reducing the development of carcinomas. Correspondingly, the early treatment of esophagitis might be a much more effective measure to prevent the development of esophageal carcinomas.

It is known that a sufficient intake of vitamins and trace elements is necessary to keep the epithelial cells intact and to maintain the normal function of the immunological system. In 1983/84, the International Agency for Research on Cancer conducted a 13-month nutritional intervention with riboflavin, vitamin A, and zinc among Chinese persons between 35 and 65 years of age, hoping to reduce the occurrence of precursors of the esophageal carcinoma. The lack of a clear effect led to the hypothesis that a nutritional intervention among persons older than 35 years, who have been suffering from malnutrition over a long period of time, is probably not very effective. The target group should therefore be adolescents and young adults.

In 1988, the Division of Epidemiology of the Deutsches Krebsforschungszentrum carried out the first large study among 15–25-year-old inhabitants of Huixian, a Chinese region with a high incidence of esophageal cancer. Our study had two objectives: first, we wanted to determine the incidence of esophageal cancer precursors among adolescents, and second, we wanted to

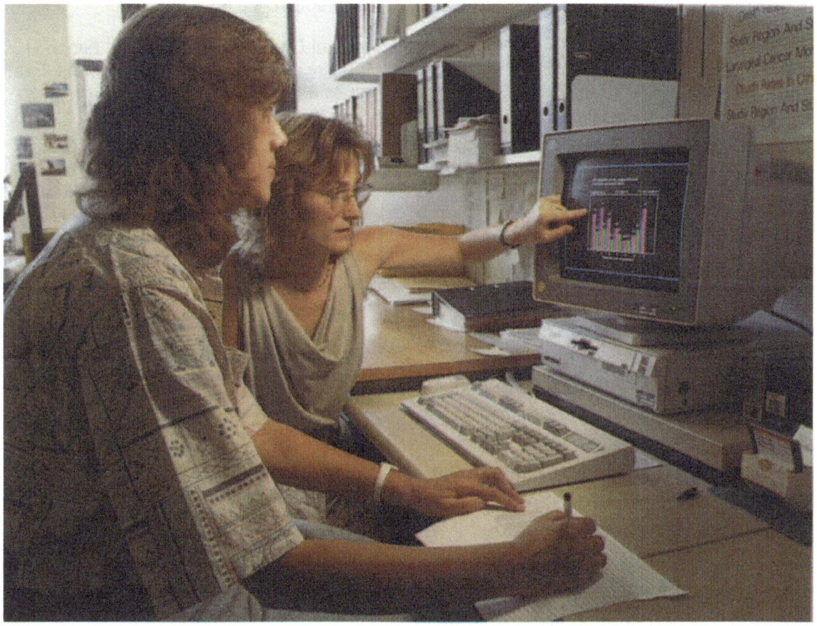

Fig. 33
The data collected by the interviewers are analyzed by the computer.

answer the question of whether certain risk factors for esophageal cancer that are known from studies on adults may also lead to esophagitis and cancer precursors in young adults.

With the aid of an international medical team and dozens of domestic assistants, a total of 545 young men and women were subjected to an endoscopic examination to identify for inflammatory alterations of the esophagus. In the course of a general medical examination, blood samples and, from some of the probands, urine specimens were taken; in addition, the participants were interviewed.

Our study showed that 43.5 % of the male and 35.9 % of the female participants showed signs of a chronic esophagitis. Among these, the majority had indicated in the questionnaire that at least one family member suffered from esophageal cancer or that they had brothers or sisters who also had chronic esophagitis. Those who primarily consume traditional foods (corn, radish, and cabbage, which during the winter is stored under the bed) fall sick more frequently. The predominant intake of corn, for example, causes a riboflavin (vitamin B2) deficiency. Signs of esophagitis were less common among participants who eat fresh fruits at least once a week, or among adolescents who consume wheat flour products at least twice daily. The biochemical analyses of the blood samples reveal, especially for the probands with esophagitis, a significant vitamin C deficiency and thus support the results derived on the basis of our questionnaire. In addition, many of the participants had a vitamin B2 deficiency; however, a correlation with the disease could not be demonstrated. Persons who frequently drink boiling hot water, tea, or soup, suffer from esophagitis four times more often than persons who do not. This seems to be due to lesions of the mucosa by excessive heat. The impact of cigarette smoking was not significant, which can be explained by the fact that, although 60 % of the young men were smokers, only 18 % consumed more than 15 cigarettes a day.

The results thus confirmed our suspicion that malnutrition and exogenous irritations may lead to inflammatory changes and to a weakening of the mucosa of the esophagus, which as a result has a lower resistance against carcinogens.

Conclusion

An epidemiological study can only contribute one tessera to the complex mosaic that describes the influence of diet on the development of cancer. Many such studies with different approaches, in different populations, and with (hopefully) similar results are needed to advance our knowledge.

The studies described above are an important contribution. They indicate that diets that are characterized by an elevated intake of fresh fruit and vegetables correlate with a lower cancer risk. This result, together with the knowledge gained in experimental research, as well as in numerous other epidemiological studies, allows us to conclude that we have found a causal connection.

In addition to the specific studies described (specific with regard to the localization of the cancer and the population studied), comprehensive prospective cohort studies are useful and necessary to obtain a complete picture of the impact of the individual dietary factors and their interplay on the cancer risk. In the beginning of such studies, information on the dietary habits of tens of thousands of individuals are carefully collected. These individuals are then observed over a long period of time in order to record all cases of newly developing chronic diseases.

Such studies are expected to answer most comprehensively the question of which dietary aspects have an influence on cancer risk.

Considering the importance of the topic „diet and cancer," it is not surprising that the public expects scientists to issue practical recommendations. Of course, recommendations on how to prevent specific diseases cannot be made for isolated conditions; instead, they should contribute to improving the general health.

An increased intake of fresh fruits and vegetables can be seen as an indisputable positive factor. It is also recommended that the intake of fat be reduced, especially with regard to cardiovascular diseases. In addition, a protective effect against intestinal cancer is attributed to an increased intake of dietary fibers, which, if handled moderately, can be recommended generally.

Dietary habits have always given reason for much speculation. In analogy to the results of the Bavarian stomach cancer study, Thomas Mann in his novel „Buddenbrooks" (1901) had Tony Buddenbrook write a letter from Munich to her mother in Lübeck and complain about the Bavarian dietary habits: „There is too little vegetables ... This makes my stomach rumble."

Prof. Dr. Jürgen Wahrendorf
Dr. Heiner Boeing
Dr. Jenny Chang-Claude
Dr. Rainer Frentzel-Beyme
Division of Epidemiology

Selected publications

Frentzel-Beyme, R., Claude, J., Eilber, U.: Mortality among German vegetarians. First results after 5 years of follow-up. Nutrition and Cancer 11, 117–126 (1988)

Wahrendorf, J., Chang-Claude, J., Qiu, S., Yang, G., Munoz, N., Crespi, M., Raedsch, R., Thurnham, D., Correa, P.: Precursor lesions of oesophageal cancer in young people in a high-risk population in China. Lancet II, 1239–1241 (1989)

Wahrendorf, J.: Dietary fat, dietary cholesterol and obesity as risk factors for colorectal cancer, kidney cancer and other tumours. In: Diet and the Aetiology of Cancer, Ed. A. B. Miller, Springer, Berlin 13–19 (1989)

Chang-Claude, J., Wahrendorf, J., Qui, S., Yang, G., Munoz, N., Crespi, M., Raedsch, R., Thurnham, D., Correa, P.: An epidemiological study of precursor lesions of oesophageal cancer among young persons in a high-risk population in Huixian, China. Cancer Res. 50, 2268–2274 (1990)

Boeing, H.: Epidemiological research in stomach cancer: progress over the last ten years. J. Cancer Res. Clin. Oncol. 117, 133–143 (1991)

Boeing, H., Frentzel-Beyme, R., Berger, M., Göres, W., Körner, M., Lohmeier, R., Menarcher, A., Männl, H.F.K., Meinhardt, M., Müller, R., Ostermeier, H., Paul, F., Schwemmle, K., Wagner, K.H., Wahrendorf, J.: Case-Control study on stomach cancer in the Federal Republic of Germany. Int. J. Cancer 47, 858–864 (1991)

4.2 Studies on Risk Factors for Brain Tumors in Adults

by Brigitte Schlehofer

Tumors of the brain have been known since ancient times. Although these tumors are among the more uncommon types of cancer, the question of the risk factors responsible for the development of brain tumors has increasingly become of interest in the past years. In cooperation with the International Agency for Research on Cancer (IARC, Lyon, France) our group is attempting to clarify this problem.

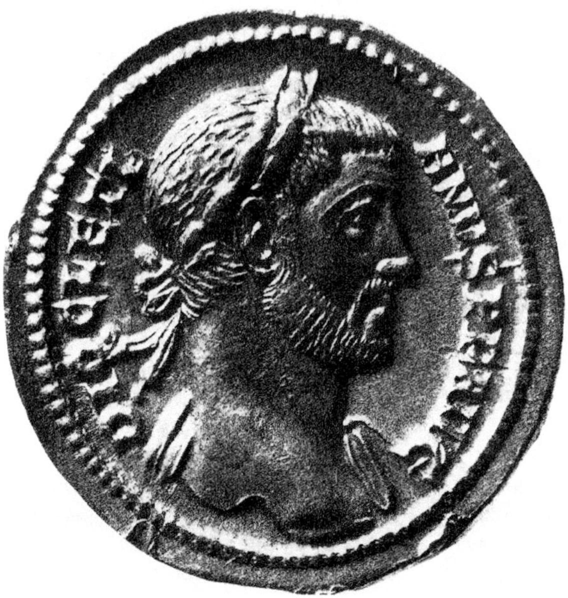

Fig. 34
In 81 A. D., the Roman emperor Titus died from a brain tumor.

Why Studies on Brain Tumors?

World-wide, the incidence of brain tumors shows significant geographical variations. It ranges from 1.0 to 15.7 (per 100 000 persons and year) for men, and from 1.0 to 9.0 for women, with the higher rates being observed in western countries. In part, this is certainly due to improved modern diagnostic methods such as x-ray examinations, computer tomography, and magnetic resonance tomography. An increased occurrence of brain tumors is also observed after a successful treatment of leukemia during childhood. Other possible reasons for the higher brain tumor rate in western countries are still unknown.

What are Brain Tumors?

It has to be emphasized that the term „brain tumor“ comprises very different tumor types, depending on the tissue it originates from. When trying to clarify the causes for the development (etiology) of a brain tumor, it is therefore essential to establish whether it originated from the proper cerebral matter, from the meninges, or from appendix cerebri (for example, from the anterior lobe of the pituitary gland), or whether it is an embryonic tumor, a vascular tumor, or even a metastasis of a tumor in some other organ.

In our study, we only considered the „primary brain tumors“, among which are the, mostly malignant, gliomas (originating in cerebral matter) and the, mostly benign, meningiomas (originating in the meninges). The most common malignant brain tumor in adults is the glioblastoma. The second most common tumor, the meningioma, occurs in women twice as frequently as in men.

Modern surgical and irradiation techniques help to improve the quality of life of many brain tumor patients and even offer a chance of recovery for many of them; the prognosis, however, largely depends on the specific nature of the tumor. The chances of recovery of patients with meningeal tumors, for example, are relatively favorable, whereas the prognosis for patients suffering from tumors of the cerebral matter is still unfavorable.

Since the therapeutical options are limited and preventive measures still unknown, the clarification of the etiology (the cause) of these tumors becomes increasingly important.

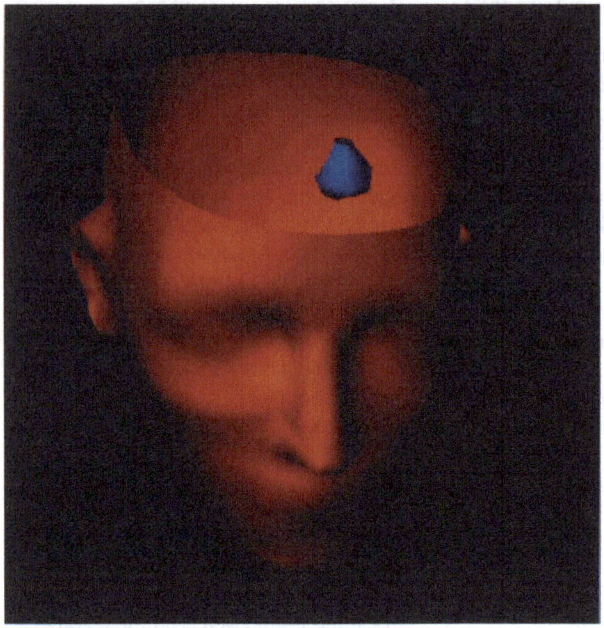

Fig. 35
The position of a brain tumor can be visualized with the help of a computer. On the basis of these images, the surgical intervention is planned.

Results from various epidemiologic studies suggest a multitude of possible causes, comprising occupational or environmental exposures, various previous diseases, individual and constitutional conditions, and nutritional factors. Due to significant differences in methodology and in the number of patients examined, however, the results of these studies are often irreproducible. This is why it is still not known which factors really control the development of brain tumors.

How Can Risk Factors be Examined?

In order to further investigate the etiology of brain tumors in western countries, Australia, Canada, the Federal Republic of Germany, France, Sweden, and the United States initiated an international „case-control study“ in 1986. On the basis of a comprehensive standardized questionnaire approximately 1500 patients ("cases") and 3000 healthy persons ("controls") were asked to answer questions on various suspected risk factors.

The study's main focus is the determination of the influence of radiation exposure, the clarification of the role of (endogenous and exogenous) exposure to N-nitroso compounds (for example, occupational or nutritional exposure), and the investigation of personal life style and environmental conditions.

In 1987 and 1988, we interviewed 226 brain tumor patients of the neurosurgical clinics of the University of Heidelberg and of the Clinical Center Mannheim, as well as 418 randomly selected control persons from the Rhine-Neckar-Odenwald region that were frequency-matched to the distribution of patients by age and gender. All persons were questioned by trained interviewers about their individual life styles.

The answers of patients and controls with respect to the different risk factors were compared. Using statistical methods, we assessed for each type of exposure the risk for inducing a brain tumor.

These data are also included in the international study. Since the questioning of the case and control groups was identical with regard to contents and methodology in all participating countries, it is possible to pool the data for analysis. The significance of our results is increased by the large number of participants from different countries.

First Results of the Rhine-Neckar-Odenwald Study

Of the 226 patients who developed brain tumors in 1987 and 1988, 115 suffered from gliomas, 81 from meningiomas, and 30 from cranial nerve tumors. For each patient, we randomly selected two control persons matched by age and gender. For each subtype of brain tumor, each set of questions regarding a possible risk factor was evaluated separately.

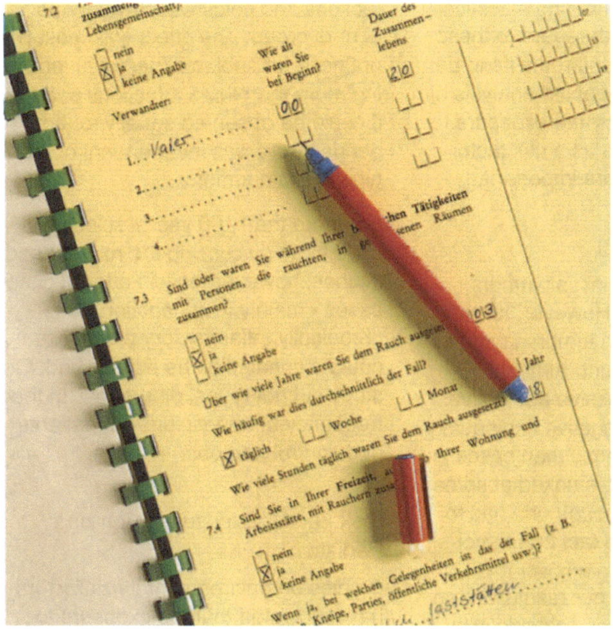
nein
ja
keine Angabe
Wie alt waren Sie bei Beginn?
Wie häufig war dies durchschnittlich der Fall?
Monat
Woche
täglich
Jahr

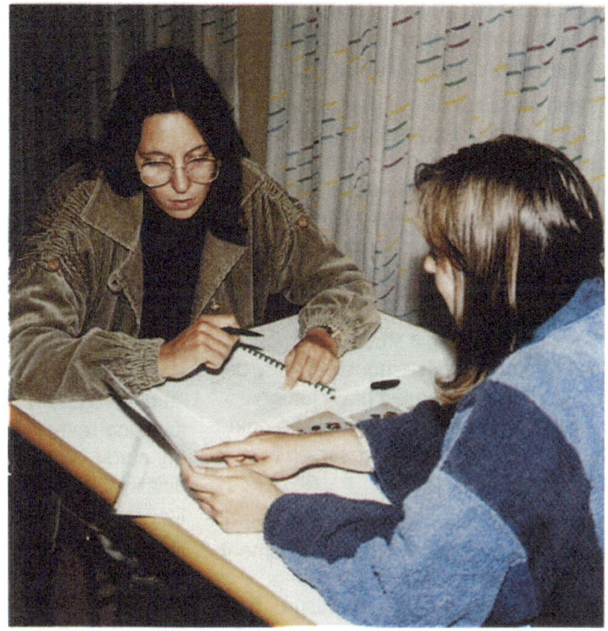

Fig. 36
A special questionnaire was developed to find out causes and risk factors associated with the development of brain tumors.

Fig. 37
An interviewer questions a female patient who has agreed to take part in the study.

Risk Factor: Occupation

An examination of the employed persons among the participants of our study showed that patients more frequently worked in the chemical and metal industries, in the agricultural sector, or as painters than the control persons. In their workplace, they were subjected to a higher exposure to solvents, tar-containing materials, dusts, pesticides, or similar substances than comparable persons in the population. However, in our study, an increased risk arising from this kind of occupation could not be established as statistically significant.

However, we did observe a remarkably increased brain tumor risk in women who had worked in the electrical or electronics industries over an extended period of time. No such increase, however, was observed in men working in this industry.

This finding, although only based on a few cases, has to be related to increasing evidence of a possible relationship between the development of brain tumors and exposure to electromagnetic fields, as can be seen in the case of people working or living near high tension lines or powerful transformers. However, it must also be taken into account that workers in the electrical and electronics industries are frequently in contact with chemical substances, such as solvents or lubricants, which might also be possible hazards.

No studies have yet been carried out to investigate the occupational risk factors for brain tumors in women. Our findings indicate that occupational epidemiology should pay more attention to female workers, also taking into account the prevention of diseases other than those related to pregnancy.

Risk Factor: Chemical Substances

In brain tumor etiology, particular importance is attributed to the above-mentioned N-nitroso compounds (mainly nitrosamines) and their prestages (nitrites and nitrates or amines that can be nitrosated). Since the 1960s it has been known that nitroso compounds may induce tumors of the nervous system in animals (IARC report).

These compounds are present in many articles of everyday life, such as in joss sticks, cigarette smoke, cosmetics, drugs, pickled meat, cheese, and sometimes even in vegetables and water. They can also be found in some industries, especially the rubber, metal, leather, and cosmetics industries.

Since epidemiologic studies showed that workers in these industries may be subject to an increased brain tumor risk, particular attention should be paid to the chemical substances used in these branches.

When evaluating the influence of N-nitroso compounds on the development of brain tumors, not only the „exogenous" (occupational) exposure, but also the „endogenous" exposure (from within the body) has to be taken into account. Under certain, not totally clarified circumstances, the stomach is able to produce N-nitroso compounds from dietary intakes of nitrate and proteins. The results of this comprehensive evaluation still remain to be seen.

During further investigations, carcinogenicity was also established for polycyclic hydrocarbons (in animal experiments) and for vinyl chloride (in animals and in humans). Results from occupational tumor epidemiology suggest that other chemical substances might also play a role in the development of brain tumors. Studies indicate an increased occurrence of such tumors in workers in the rubber and petrochemical industries, in the agricultural sector, and in the metal industry. These results, however, could not always be established.

In our study, we did not find statistically significant results with regard to these chemical substances. It remains to be seen whether in the pooled analysis of the international study the exposure to chemical substances as a risk factor will turn out to be more important.

Risk Factor: Smoking

In the etiology of almost all tumors, smoking ranks first. However, for the development of brain tumors in adults smoking is insignificant. Almost all studies regarding passive and active smoking revealed negative findings. In our study, more controls than cases indicated that they had smoked at some time in their lives. Though one has to take into account the fact that tumor patients might tend to answer this question incorrectly, our results are so unambiguous and they coincide with the trends of other studies that they can safely be regarded as established.

Risk Factor: Previous or Constitutional Diseases

Apart from suspected environmental risk factors, we also investigated endogenous reactions, such as genetic, hormonal, and infectious factors. Only such diseases were considered in the analysis that occurred at least 2 years prior to the development of the brain tumor.

In women, we observed an almost five-fold risk of developing tumors of the meninges if they had suffered from an inflammation of the meninges sometime before. It has not yet been possible to establish the factors responsible for this.

In contrast, the brain tumor risk of persons who suffered from allergies or infections and colds was lower in the control group. The effect was most pronounced for subjects (persons) indicating more than three infections per year; it could be observed equally for both genders and was independent of the type of brain tumor.

For more than 100 years, scientists have been discussing the role of head injuries; however, only in a few isolated cases - mainly in connection with chronically inflammatory processes - could a connection be established. Our study did not reveal differences in the frequency of head injuries in patients and control persons.

Risk Factor: Exposure to Ionizing Radiation

Studies on environmental risk factors have indicated that the exposure to ionizing radiation might play a part in the development of brain tumors. These studies are, for example, long-term studies on Hiroshima bomb victims or on children who had received therapeutic radiation treatment of the head.

However, whether radiation treatment of the head in adults or occasional x-ray examinations (for example, after an accident) can be regarded as risk factors is still a very controversial matter.

We did not observe an increased risk for persons who received radiation treatment or who underwent repeated x-ray examinations after an accident or for diagnostic reasons. Similarly, we did not find an increase in brain tumor risk in persons with routine dental x-ray examinations. It should be pointed out, however, that some of the patients were able to name the number of x-rays taken and the examined organ, but not the total number of radiographs taken; it is thus not always possible to calculate the radiation dose correctly.

Future Research Activities

In order to understand the etiology of brain tumors better, a number of factors from various areas of life still need to be investigated. One of these is the exposure to N-nitroso compounds, which also exists in other areas than those mentioned above.

The pooled evaluation of all the data gathered by the international group, is expected to clarify the remaining uncertainties in the etiology of brain tumors.

Dr. Brigitte Schlehofer
Division of Epidemiology

Participating scientists

Prof. Dr. Jürgen Wahrendorf
Dr. Maria Blettner
Division of Epidemiology

In collaboration with

Prof. Dr. Stefan Kunze
Neurosurgical Clinic,
University of Heidelberg

Dr. Winfried Sachsenheimer
Neurosurgical Clinic,
Clinical Center Mannheim/University of Heidelberg

Prof. Dr. Horst Schmitt
Institute of Pathology,
University of Heidelberg

Research Program:
Adult Brain Tumor Study,
International Agency for Research on Cancer, Lyon, France

Selected publications

Schoenberg, B. S.: Nervous System. In: Schottenfeld, D., Fraumeni, J. F. (eds.) Cancer Epidemiology and Prevention, 968–983 (1982).

Schlehofer, B., Kunze, S., Sachsenheimer, W., Blettner, M., Niehoff, D., Wahrendorf, J.: Occupational risk factors for brain tumors: results from a population-based case-control study in Germany. Cancer Causes & Control 1, No. 3, 475–476 (1990).

4

4.3 Air Pollution and Cancer Risk – Epidemiologic Results and Regulatory Methods

by Heiko Becher

What exactly is air pollution? Air pollution can be defined as the contamination or pollution of the air we breathe by substances produced by civilization. In fact, in urban and industrialized areas the air may be considerably polluted by a large number of substances (WHO, 1987; IARC, 1990; Tomatis, 1990); to a lesser extent, this is also true for rural areas. The total degree of pollution, as well as the concentration of individual components may considerably vary geographically, seasonally, and over the years. Which substances might be carcinogenic and what are the consequences for the assessment of cancer risk generated by a particular type of pollution?

The International Agency for Research on Cancer, IARC, in Lyon, France, evaluates agents and their compounds, as well as classes of agents, in terms of their carcinogenicity. The IARC started categorizing substances in 1972, and since then it has continued expanding and updating its assessments on the basis of scientific evaluations of the most recently published results. Particular emphasis is placed on epidemiologic results. In epidemiology (the science of the geographical and temporal distribution of disease frequencies and the factors causing and influencing them) results are obtained from studies on humans. Thus, there is a direct relevance for mankind.

A number of substances which have been classified by the IARC as “carcinogenic” or “probably carcinogenic” have been detected in the outdoor air. Some of them are listed in Table 1. The pollution of the outdoor air has different causes, the major one being the combustion of fossil fuels or the emission of pollutants in the course of various industrial processes. In the public view, the detection of carcinogenic substances in the air is considered in itself to be sufficient proof of a connection between air pollution and cancer. This then leads to a demand for an almost complete ban by law of the relevant emissions. However, it is often not realized that the measured concentrations of pollutants are frequently several orders of magnitude lower than where their carcinogenicity has been detected. For example, the level of arsenic emission in conurbations in Germany is generally below 15 ng/m^3. In an extensive epidemiologic study, in which it was shown that arsenic is a carcinogen for tumors of the respiratory tract, the concentration of arsenic in the workplace was above 10 mg/m^3, which is almost a million times more. This example illustrates the difficulties: although for quite awhile epidemiologists have been trying to scientifically bolster the simple and plausible assumption that “air pollution leads to cancer”, the results obtained so far are neither convincing nor consistent.

Ten years ago, Doll and Peto (1981) published what has become a well-known quantitative assessment of cancer risk due to air pollution. According to their estimate, air pollution accounts for 1–5% of all cancer cases, with 2% considered as the “best estimate”.

However, other factors, such as smoking or nutrition, are much more relevant; 60–80% of all cancer deaths can be attributed to these two factors. These percentages have not only been found by Doll and Peto, but have also been confirmed by more recent studies.

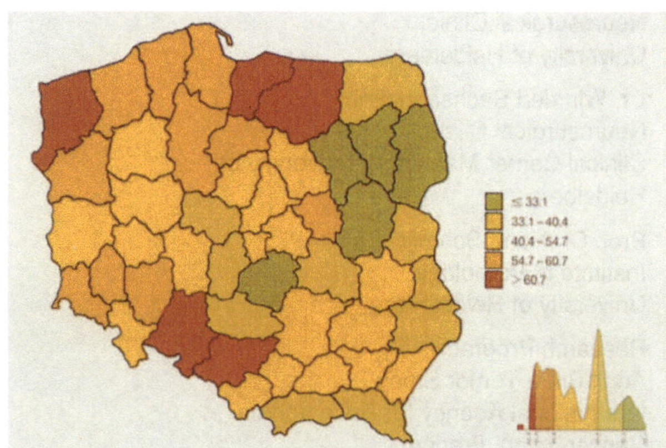

Fig. 38
Incidence of lung cancer in men in Poland (death rate per 100 000 persons per year, standardized rate).

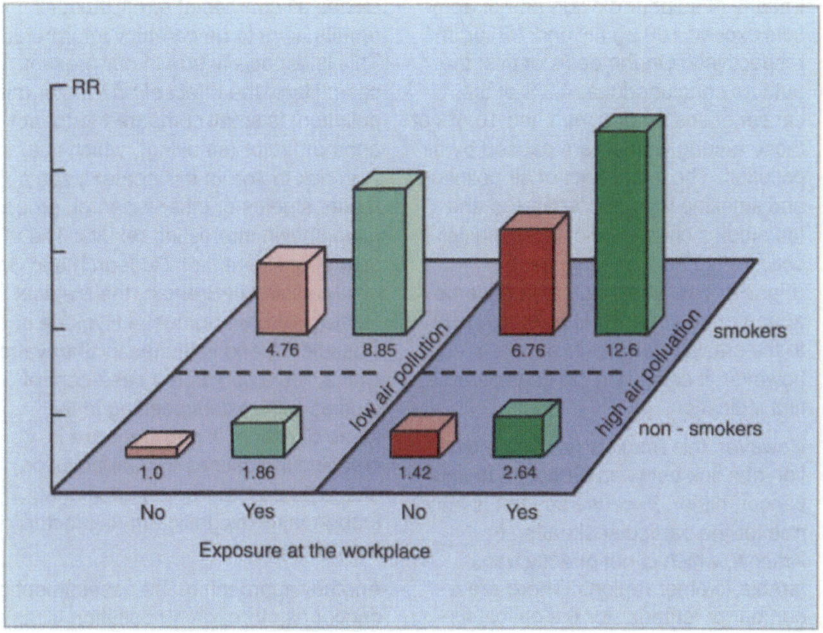

Fig. 39
Relative risks (RR) for the three main risk factors: smoking, exposure at the workplace, air pollution, as well as their combination.

Doll and Peto's assessment of the effects of air pollution has often been quoted in the past 10 years; however, a confirmation (or reliable correction of their figures either way) has not been possible. Occasionally, regional differences in cancer rates are used to bolster the hypothesis that "cancer is caused by air pollution". Certainly, there are striking differences between cancer rates in industrialized and rural areas, such as for lung cancer in the Federal Republic of Germany. However, prior to considering air pollution a potential cause for this, we have to know and to take into account the distribution of the other risk factors, since they might correlate with the factor "air pollution". For example, there is a correlation between smoking and density of population, on the basis of which many of the regional differences in cancer rates can be explained: there are more smokers in urban areas. Population density is, on the other hand, connected with air pollution. Thus, simple correlation analyses of air pollution and cancer rates involve the danger of pseudo-correlations. Though these analyses are not suited to reveal causal connections, they may indicate that a scientific problem should be tackled with the aid of other research methods.

In order to come closer to answering the question of whether cancer is caused by air pollution, a number of research projects have been carried out in the Department of Epidemiology of the Deutsches Krebsforschungszentrum in recent years. Our work is based on the following principles:

– The organ system which is directly exposed to air pollution is the respiratory tract. Within this system, lung cancer is the most frequent cause of death. For most of the substances listed in Table 1, the carcinogenic effect on the respiratory tract has been proven (exception: benzene is considered to be a risk factor for leukemia).

– A study to identify air pollution as a risk factor should be made in a region in which a high concentration of pollutants occurs. This is to ensure that the results are within an epidemiologically significant order of magnitude, since, according to results known so far, the influence of air pollution on lung cancer risk is relatively small, especially when compared to the most important risk factor, cigarette smoking.

– Parallel to this study, other approaches to describe the hazards of air pollution should be investigated: The quantitative effect of individual substances on cancer risk should be assessed on the basis of data taken from literature in order to calculate the extent of a specific risk. The advantage of this approach is that recommendations for a regulatory concept can be made.

In collaboration with a Polish group headed by Prof. Wieslaw Jedrychowski, University of Kracow, a case-control study was carried out in Kracow; the evaluation was done in Heidelberg

(Jedrychowski et al., 1990). A case-control study is an epidemiologic study in which a group of patients – here, lung cancer cases – are compared with a reference or control group. If a factor occurs more often in the case group than in the control group, e.g., smoking, it is considered a risk factor. The level of risk can then be assessed with the aid of adequate statistical methods; it is generally given as "relative risk" (RR). An RR of 10 for a certain factor means that where this factor occurs, the risk of lung cancer is 10 times greater than otherwise. In this study, a significant effect of air pollution on lung cancer risk was proven. Estimates have shown that the lung cancer risk for people living in the most polluted area of Kracow is 41% higher than for those living in the outskirts (where pollution is lower). The area of Kracow is one of the most highly polluted regions of the world; in the center of the city the average concentrations of sulphur dioxide and of aerosols exceed 100 μg/m³ and 150 μg/m³, respectively. On the basis of this, the authors concluded that 4.3% of the cancer cases among men and 10.5% of those among women are caused by air pollution. The joint effect of air pollution and smoking was also analyzed and the studies clearly indicated a multiplicative effect of these two factors (Fig. 39). This effect had also become apparent in an earlier U.S. study. Due to the smaller number of cases, however, it could only be considered a first indication.

However, this result is no clear indication of a link between air pollution and cancer, either, because so far it is only true for the particular situation in Kracow, which is not directly transferable to other regions. There are a number of "criteria" for the critical assessment of epidemiologic studies. For example, interfering factors, which may have an impact on the observed effect, have to be taken into consideration. This can be achieved by appropriate data collection and by using adequate statistical methods. However, there is no epidemiologic study which totally excludes all sources of error; thus, all results have to be carefully interpreted. This is especially true in our present case: Here, the effect of one factor (air pollution) is small compared to that of another factor (smoking), which is a high risk factor. In this context, some recent studies of other research groups have shown interesting results: The Institute for Prevention Research and Social Medicine in Bremen, the Medical Institute of Environmental Hygiene in Düsseldorf, and institutes in Shenyang, China, have conducted case-control studies with results pointing in the same direction. Thus, there are increasing indications that air pollution has to be considered an additional, though fairly insignificant, risk factor for lung cancer.

Another approach to the assessment of cancer risk through air pollution is, as mentioned above, based on an evaluation of the dose-response-relations for all major environmental carcinogens. In

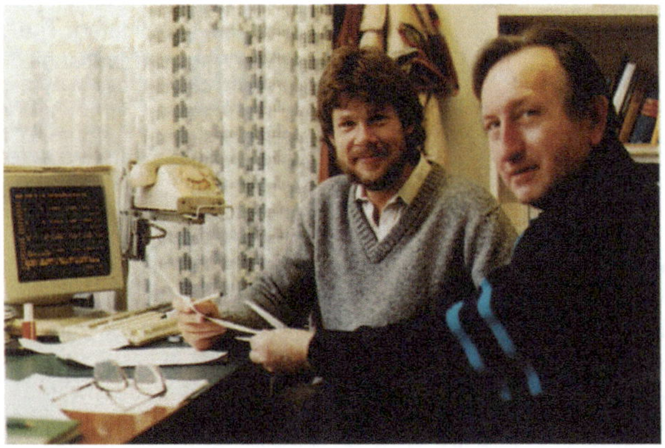

Fig. 40
The Polish epidemiologist Wieslaw Jedrychowski and the statistician Heiko Becher analyzing the data in the Deutsches Krebsforschungszentrum.

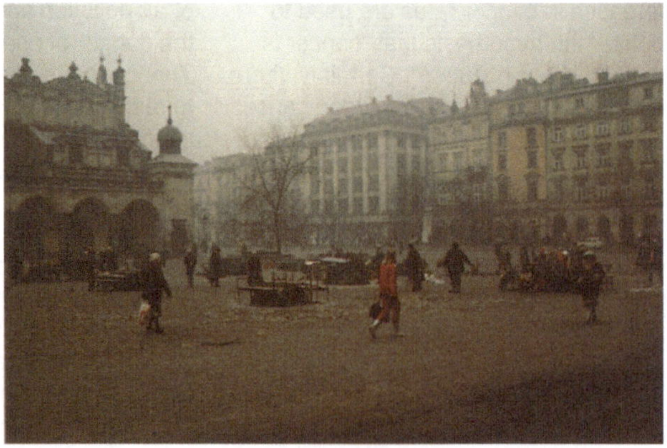

Fig. 41
Market place in Kracow.

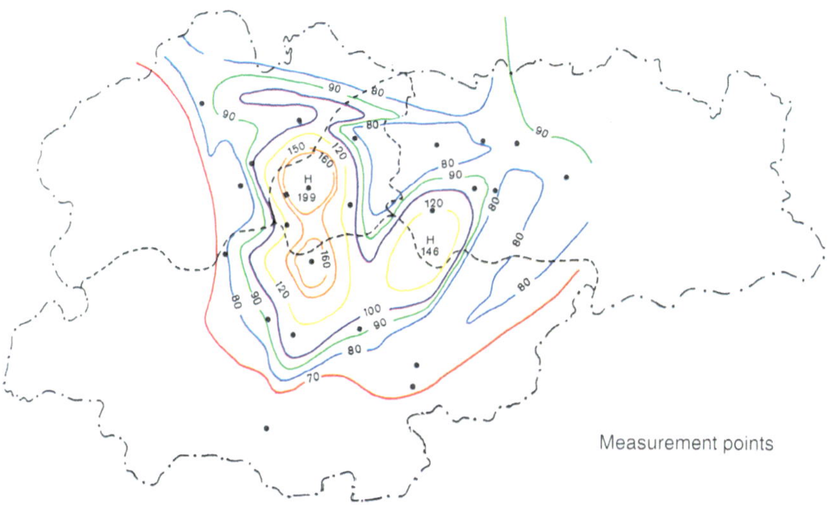

Fig. 42
Distribution of aerosols in the air (in nanograms per cubic meter) in Kracow.

theory, it should thus be possible to produce assessments for any load profile. In the framework of this research project, national and international results for a number of environmental carcinogenic agents have been studied and dose-effect-relations evaluated; where necessary, additional analyses have been made. Generally speaking, a dose-response-analysis reveals the dependence of the cancer risk on the concentration of a pollutant. Of particular interest is the shape of the dose-response-curve close to its origin, that is, for low concentrations. Dose-response-assessments are preferably done on the basis of epidemiologic data, although sufficiently reliable data are not always available.

From our studies so far, we have been able to deduce parameters for some substances, such as for arsenic and benzene, that are sufficiently validated to be used in the regulatory decision-making process. Recently, the so-called "unit risk" became a widely used parameter. The unit risk for a particular substance is the additional probability of death due to cancer if the concentration of this substance in the air is 1 µ/m^3. Making a sufficiently reliable estimate of the unit risk for a substance (from a study) is very time-consuming. Moreover, different approaches are possible, none of which is necessarily the correct one. Therefore, we also investigated whether different approaches lead to similar results. It has been shown that – irrespective of the epidemiologic study used as the basis and of the statistical methods employed – the assessment of the unit risk resulted in comparable values, which is a clear indication of the reliability of the parameter. On the basis of these findings, a national group of experts is at present developing evaluation standards to lessen the cancer risk through air pollution. On the basis of the current extent of air pollution in the Federal Republic of Germany, an efficient strategy for the reduction of the emission of carcinogenic agents is to be proposed in order to reduce harmful effects on the environment as much as possible.

Summary and prospects

In the light of a number of recently published results, it seems probable that air pollution is an independent additional contribution to cancer risk. It must be pointed out, though, that our investigations have reached the limit of what can be found by epidemiologic studies. In the future, therefore, more epidemiologic and experimental studies will be needed to provide a more accurate quantitative assessment of this effect. Molecular-biological methods are increasingly being applied in epidemiology; using them may well be a further step towards answering our question. With the aid of special techniques it is possible to detect DNA adducts in body cells. These are alterations in the genetic code, which are possibly caused by polycyclic aromatic hydrocarbons (PAH) and which may affect, for example, leucocytes. An international research group has detected a large number of such DNA alterations in population groups exposed to severe environmental pollution. The Division of Epidemiology of the Deutsches Krebsforschungszentrum now plans, in collaboration with the University of Kracow (Prof. Wieslaw Jedrychowski) and Columbia University, New York, USA (Prof. Frederica Perera), to conduct a

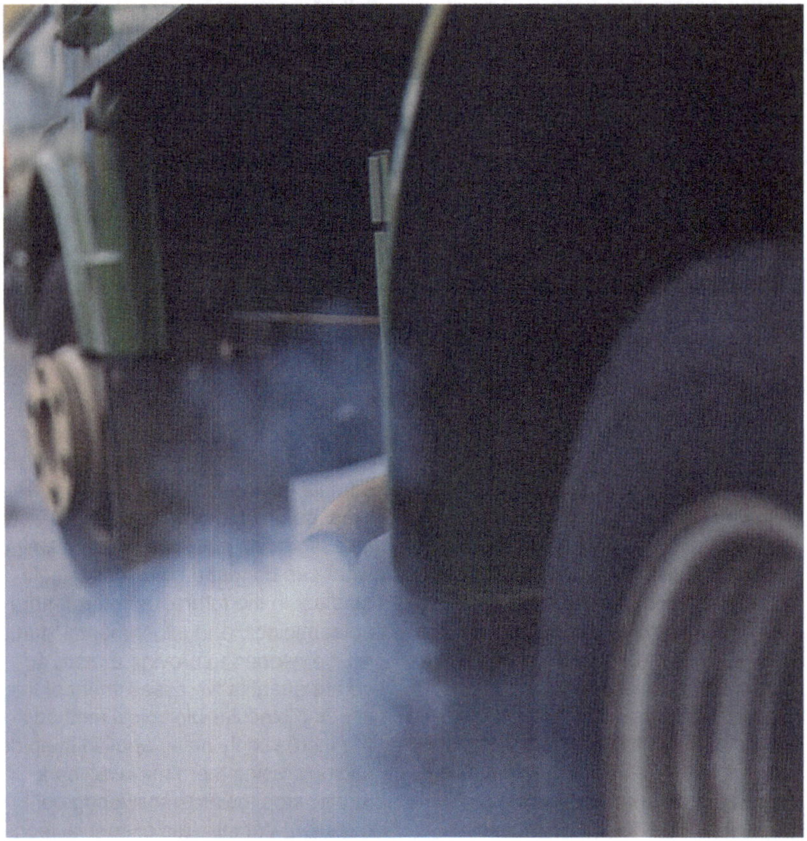

Fig. 43
The vehicular traffic, aside from the heavy industry and the use of coal for home heatings, is the main cause for air pollution in Kracow.

further study, in which the effect of air pollution on the development of DNA adducts and cancer will be examined with the aid of molecular-biological methods.

Dr. Heiko Becher
Division of Epidemiology

Participating staff
Renate Angerer
Dr. Jürgen Wahrendorf

In collaboration with

Prof. Dr. Wieslaw Jedrychowski
Department of Epidemiology
Institute of Social Medicine,
Medical School, Kracow, Poland

Priv.-Doz. Dr. Karl-Heinz Jöckel
Dipl.-Biol. Wolfgang Ahrens
Institute of Prevention Research and Social Medicine, Bremen

Prof. Dr. Jürgen Timm
University of Bremen
Department of Mathematics, Bremen

Selected publications

Doll, R., Peto, R.: The causes of cancer: Quantitative estimates of avoidable risks of cancer in the United States today. Journal of the National Cancer Institute 66, 1191–1308 (1981)

Becher, H., Wahrendorf, J.: Variability of unit risk estimates under different statistical models and between different epidemiological data sets. In: Moolgavkar, S. (Ed.): Quantitative Cancer Risk Assessment, 267–285 (1990)

Jedrychowski, W., Becher, H., Wahrendorf, J., Basa-Cierpialek, Z.: A case-control study of lung cancer with special reference to the effect of air pollution in Poland. J. Epidemiol. Community Health 44, 114–120 (1990)

Tomatis, L. (Ed.): Air Pollution and Human Cancer. ESO Monographs. Springer, Berlin (1990)

Wahrendorf, J., Becher, H.: Quantitative Risikoabschätzung für ausgewählte Umweltkanzerogene. UBA-Bericht 1/90, Hrsg. Umweltbundesamt, Erich Schmidt Verlag Berlin (1990)

Jöckel, K.H., Ahrens, W., Wichmann, H.E., Becher, H., et al.: Occupational and environmental hazards associated with lung cancer. Int. J. Epidemiol. 21, 401–412 (1992)

4.4 Exposure Studies in High-Risk Areas

Human Cancers and Their Prevention

by Maqsood Siddiqi and Rudolf Preussmann

Although considerable progress has been made towards improving diagnostic procedures and also, to some extent, in evolving new strategies for treatment of cancer, our efforts in determining causes and understanding the etiological basis of human cancers have not met with similar success in the recent past. Some of the early hopes that extrapolation of a vast amount of information generated from animal studies would provide a fair basis of understanding human carcinogenesis has not yielded the expected results. A large number of chemicals whose carcinogenic potential and dose-response information is available from experiments in different species of animals allows, at best, a basis for applying precautionary safety measures in human context rather than being an informational feed-back for investigating mechanisms of human carcinogenesis. Thus, it is being increasingly realized that assessments made from risk-exposure studies with high doses of carcinogens in animals under controlled laboratory conditions may not be truly representative of the situation(s) in man. As it is emerging now, the majority of human cancers are not inherent, but may arise from exposure to elements resulting from interactions between environmental factors and genetic, physiological, and nutritional status of susceptible individuals. This certainly makes it necessary to explore which factors positively or negatively influence the development of cancers in the context of human environment, and to give due consideration to various parameters and variables operative in human situations.

Diversity of Human Environment Influences Cancer Incidence

Cancers are known to occur with varying frequencies in different parts of the world. A comparison of incidence rates in high- and low-risk areas show differences in magnitudes ranging from a 30 times higher incidence of stomach cancer in Japan than in Uganda, a 200 times greater incidence of esophageal cancer in China compared to Holland, and a 1000 times higher occurrence of liver cancer in Mozambique than in North America. Such comparisons formed the basis of currently held opinion that human cancers are multifactorial and are largely influenced by local environment and are linked to the lifestyles of susceptible populations in these areas. An indepth study of different environmental variables and lifestyle parameters in high-risk individuals is, therefore, expected to provide valuable information on predisposing, causal and promotional elements for different cancers. Such environments could indeed be considered as model surroundings for investigating the etiological basis of human cancers.

Exposure to N-Nitroso Compounds Constitutes a Probable Risk for Human Cancers

Among the major cancers which are suspected to be associated with lifestyle of susceptible populations are those of lung, upper respiratory region, and of the gasterointestinal tract. Whereas, smoking and chewing of tobacco has been considered a high probability risk for the former, dietary N-nitroso compounds are suspected to be involved in the potential risk for the latter. A large body of epidemiological and analytical data now supports tobacco-specific N-nitroso compounds to be etiologically linked with occurrence of lung and nasopharyngal cancers in man. However, despite considerable indirect evidence for the involvement of dietary N-nitroso compounds with respect to esophageal, stomach and bladder cancers, an unequivocal proof of their causal role is still lacking.

We have directed our studies on environmental carcinogenesis at the Deutsches Krebsforschungszentrum towards investigating the causes of environmentally oriented cancers by conducting analytical field studies in several high risk areas in different countries. Our main concern through the years has been to understand the role of environmental N-nitroso compounds in human cancers. It may be noted that, on the basis of animal studies and due to widespread occurrence of N-nitrosamines in human environment, their etiological involvement, particularly in gastrointestinal cancers, has long been proposed. However, efforts to show a higher exposure of such compounds in susceptible individuals or groups of populations has not yet succeeded. This, in our opinion is mainly due to the complex nature of influences exerted by environment on the human body and also on account of the difficulties faced in quantitatively measuring biological consequences of such exposures in humans. We have tried to overcome some of these shortcomings by combining analytical and field investigations in our studies on bladder cancer in Egypt and on esophageal and gastric cancer in Kashmir. Simultaneous development of analytical techniques necessary to optimize informational output from such field studies is also an important component of our integrated approach.

In the Nile Delta area of Egypt, bilharzial infection by S. hematobium, S. mansoni or mixed infection is considered a predisposition to bladder cancer. We have recently concluded a collaborative field study in that area which provides conclusive evidence for the involvement of N-nitroso compounds in the etiology of bladder cancer. A comprehensive biomonitoring program has been organized to investigate S. hematobium-infected patients, both with and without coincidence of S.mansoni infection, prior to and after diagnosis of bladder cancer, for urinary nitrate, nitrite, and nitrosamines. All investigations were also applied to a comparative control group in Egypt. The data was compared with similar analyses from a group of normal persons in Germany. Our study has been able to establish that significant in vivo formation of nitrite and volatile N-nitroso compounds in bilharzia patients may be responsible for the high occurrence of bladder cancer. The presence of nitrate-reducing bacteria in the bilharzial bladder, many of which are known to mediate nitrosation of secondary amines, appears to be the underlying cause of high levels of nitrite and, potentially, carcinogenic nitrosamine formation, leading to increased incidence of bladder cancer. Thus, the study establishes a a close link between environmental predisposition and high occurrence of bladder cancer with possible involvement of N-nitroso compounds.

Cancer Risk Factors are Intrinsic to the Human Milieu – The Kashmir Example

In the context of geographically distributed cancers, Kashmir offers certain unique environmental features whose interaction with different facets of human life appear to be responsible for causing a high risk of esophageal cancer in the area. These unusual environmental parameters which are clearly reflected in the lifestyle of local residents, have allowed interesting observations to be made with regard to the high occurrence of this disease there. Although the study is still in progress and more data is yet to be derived, we propose to utilize some of the available results to explain how lifestyle patterns may influence cancer incidence in otherwise healthy surroundings.

Kashmir is a high altitude valley situated in the extreme north of the Indian subcontinent. It is comprised of a population distinct in their ethnic, sociocultural, and religious backgrounds. By and large, they are a traditional, nonmigratory people with stable dietary habits. Inter-marriages among close relatives is a common practice, leading to an almost pure and genetically homogenous population. These sociological parameters are of vital importance in such studies since they ensure reliablity of retrospective observations on lifestyle.

A high occurrence of esophageal cancer is now fully established in Kashmir. Although the prevalence of this disease has been known in the region for a long time, perhaps due to lack of proper diagnostic facilities in the area, it was first reported only in the early 1970s. The region still does not have a cancer registry and, therefore, in order to establish a high occurrence of the disease in the area, we had to initially depend mainly on the information provided by local doctors or from unclassified hospital records. Currently, however, good diagnostic and treatment facilities are available, at least in the main town of the province, and there is an adequate data maintenance system. The esophageal incidence rates are now being studied by epidemiologists in the area, but hospital records show that, on average, about 500–600 new cancer cases are diagnosed each year from a total population of 3.1 million in the Kashmir valley. In addition, next to esophageal, a high rate of gastric carcinoma is also found in Kashmir.

The Kashmir valley is surrounded by the geographical areas of Ladakh and Jammu, which are inhabited by people of totally different sociological and cultural backgrounds. Both these regions show low levels of incidence for esophageal and gastric cancers.

Mainly based on case-control studies, the consumption of alcohol and smoking of tobacco had been earlier shown to be major risk factors for esophageal cancer in Europe and United States.

The chewing of tobacco, use of betelnut, opium, and special dietary habits were implicated in the high occurrence of this disease in Asia and Africa. In addition, deficiencies of zinc, vitamin B1, vitamin A, lack of intake of fresh fruits, vegetables, and animal proteins were also considered to be linked to increased risk of this cancer in Iran, China, and other high risk regions.

A preliminary assessment of lifestyle pattern in Kashmir, however, revealed that none of the prominent risk factors so far associated with high risk of esophageal cancer were relevant in this area. Kashmir is devoid of alcohol consumption since the people are predominantly Muslim. Use of chewing tobacco or betelnut is practically unknown to local inhabitants, while cigarette smoking is a recent phenomenon and practiced mainly only among the younger generation. The population is entirely non-vegetarian with several traditional food dishes based on lamb meat and fish.

While the absence of normally associated risk factors for the disease became obvious, the brief survey also revealed an equally striking dietary style practiced by the local inhabitants. The Kashmiris, on account of climatic constraints and distinct sociocultural traditions use rather unusual foods and beverages. Having a temperate climate with severe winters and moderate summers, the people consume large amounts of a special kind of salted tea prepared from green tea leaves with addition of common salt and sodium bicarbonate. It is generally consumed boiling hot, several times a day. Further, due to a short growing season and long winter, locally grown vegetables are preserved by sun-drying or by pickling, and fish is either sun-dried or smoked. Most of the preserved foodstuffs are inadequately stored for long periods. Dried red chilies are most commonly used in various foods. A large consumption, in all seasons, of a Brassica vegetable locally called "Hak" together with regional varieties of spinach is an outstanding feature of the local diet.

Analytical Field Studies – Framework to Understand Human Cancers

A preliminary assessment of dietary habits was immediately followed by analytical studies on different preserved foodstuffs. Several commonly consumed food items were found to contain trace levels of preformed N-nitrosodimethylamine (NDMA) and in some cases N-nitrosopyrrolidine (NPYR). Foodstuffs were also subjected to in vitro nitrosation under simulated gastric conditions (nitrite, 25 µM). Sun-dried fish and vegetables yielded considerably high amounts of NDMA in addition to several non-volatile N-nitroso compounds. This series of experiments made it amply clear that, while consumption of preserved foods in general may cause exposure to preformed NDMA and/or NPYR, an exposure of much higher magnitude could be expected due to intragastric nitrosation of dried (and fresh) vegetables.

At this stage, the scope of study was enlarged by undertaking a multi-directional field study in the area with active collaboration of scientists and clinicians in Kashmir. There are three main components of the study, a) the assessment of dietary and other lifestyle parameters and chemical identification of probable risk factors through analysis of food and beverages, b) the biological monitoring of normal, high risk (those having chronic esophagitis), as well as cancer-affected persons for measuring nitrate/nitrite balance, and for evaluation of micronutrient status, and c) the collection of tissue and blood samples for detecting DNA adducts formed due to environmental exposure to genotoxic substances. In addition, a questionnaire has also been administered in the region for obtaining information on quantitative dietary intake and on various other lifestyle parameters relevant to the study. The questionnaire is used in the normal population in different parts of the Kashmir valley, as well as on persons attending clinics for gasterointestinal disorders in local hospitals. The information obtained from this survey has provided useful guidelines for analytical studies on foodstuffs and allows reliable estimates of food consumption and its constituents.

An initial evaluation of the field data indicated that there may exist a gradient in occurrence of esophageal cancer risk within the high-risk area of Kashmir. We have been able to tentatively mark the clusters of high- and low-risk villages within the valley on the basis of information gathered by personal interviews with residents and local medical workers. Efforts to validate our field observations with analytical and clinical evidence is in progress. An important fact which emerged from this study was that people who own large farmlands which allows them to grow more vegetables and chilies, use a good proportion of their harvest for sun-drying and for pickling. Their economic prosperity thus leads to increased availability and consumption of sun-dried vegetables,

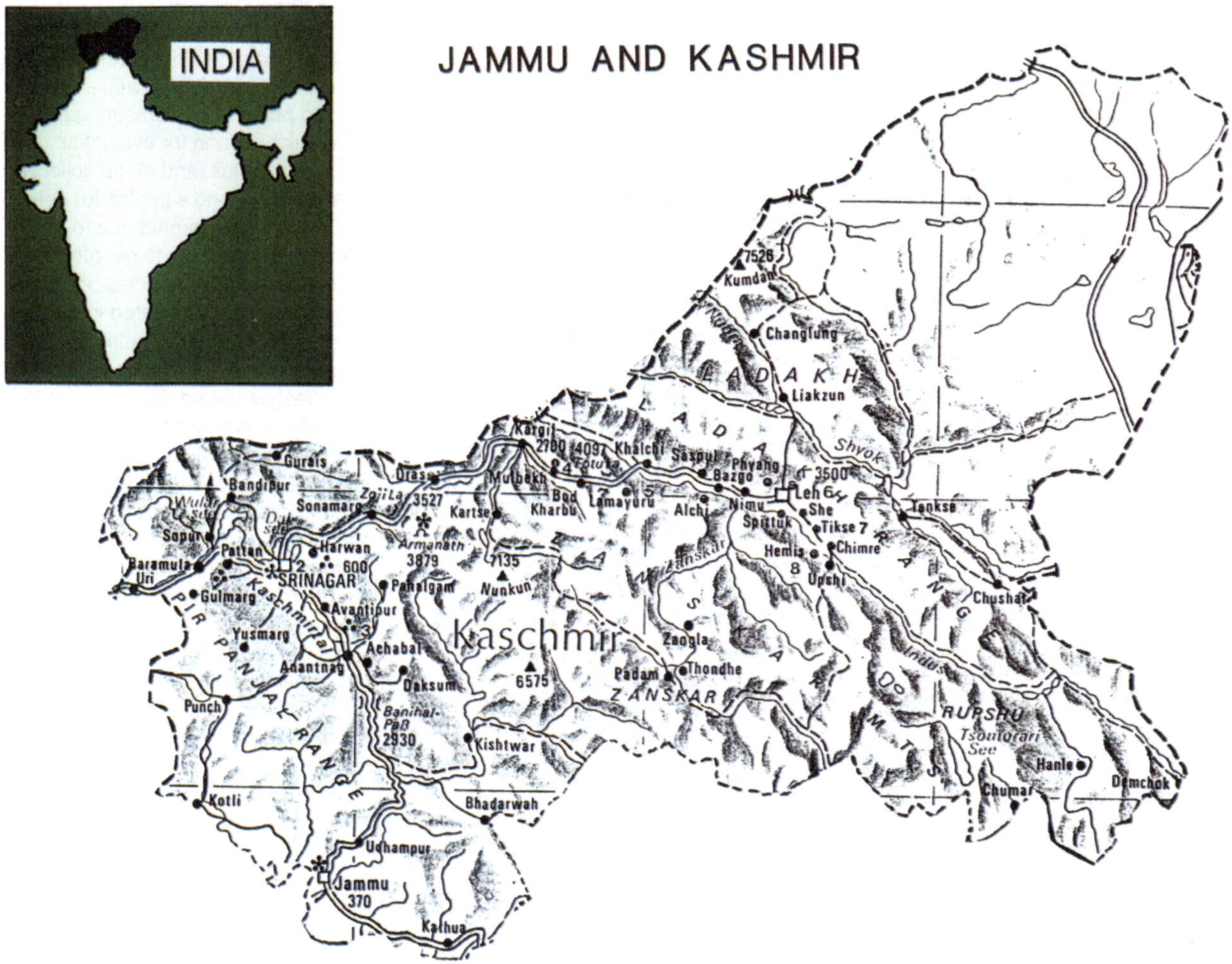

Fig. 44
A study in Kashmir investigated the causes of esophageal cancer. This cancer has a high incidence in Kashmir, but is significantly less common in neighboring Jammu.

red chilies and spices, and also to increased consumption of salted tea. Gasterointestinal diseases are found to be more prevalent in this class of people. However, economic limitations in the non-farming class, although they are practicing a similar diet, leads to restricted or no use of sun-dried vegetables. A third catagory of people identified by our survey is the fishermen who normally live around lakes and have fish and rice as their staple diet for year round. They also sun-dry a lot of fish, mainly for sale in the market. Consumption of vegetables, fresh or sun dried was found to be far less among this class, as is the occurence of gasterointestinal disorders. In our survey of several fishing villages no incidence of esophageal or gastric cancer was reported by the people.

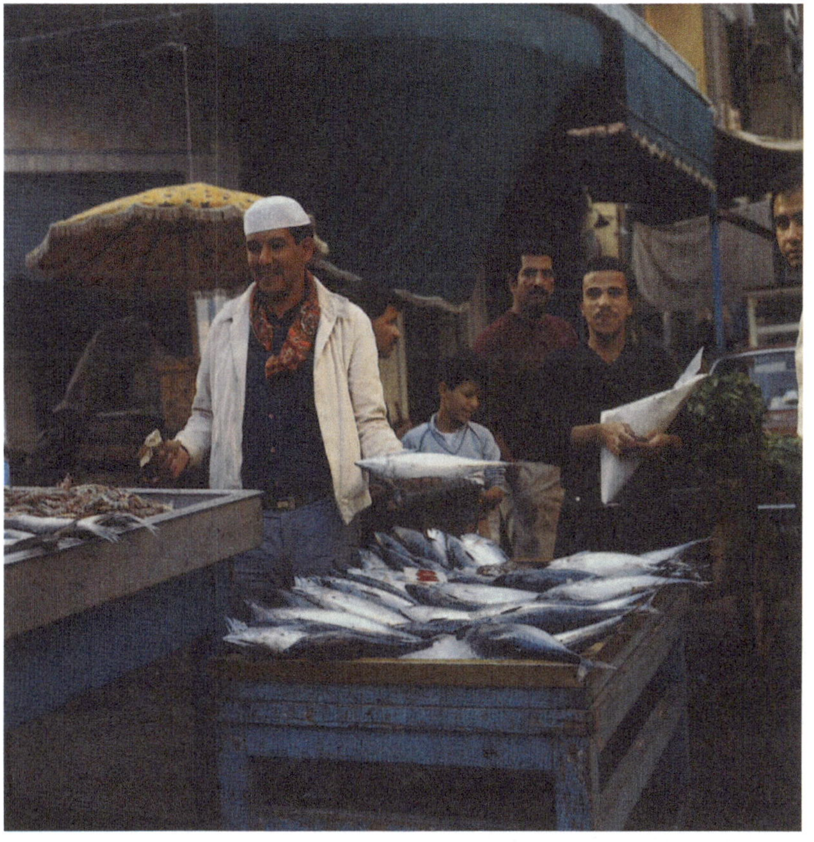

Fig. 45
Market in Egypt.

Dietary Nitrosatable Precursors may Determine Exposure to Critical N-nitroso Compounds

Once the overall scenario of local life-style and dietary habits started emerging as a definite pattern, it was considered necessary to subject the available dietary data to critical evaluation, deleting those food items whose consumption is either negligible or also quite common in areas of low incidence. A short listing of foods was thus carried out for more detailed quantitative analytical studies in order to understand the role of N-nitroso compounds as a probable risk factor for high occurrence of the disease. A large number of fresh and sun-dried vegetable samples have since been analyzed for nitrate and nitrite content and also for known and as yet unknown nitrosatable compounds which may act as precursors for an increased exposure due to endogenous formation of critical N-nitroso compounds. It is important to mention here that the development of two new techniques in our laboratory around this period facilitated precise measurements of dietary amines and alkylating potential of nitrosoamide-like compounds in food which were not possible in earlier studies with similar aims.

A high exposure to dietary nitrate and secondary amines in the general population of Kashmir appears to be evident from our studies. This is the first report to show an increased exposure to dietary secondary amines in a high risk human population. It is interesting to note that despite a higher per capita consumption of vegetables in Germany, exposure to secondary amines from vegetables alone is nearly three times higher in Kashmir. Since vegetables are the main sources of dietary amines in Kashmir, comparison of total food estimates are not likely to be different. In confirmation with our earlier observations, measurements on sun-dried vegetables have consistently shown presence of preformed N-nitrosamines. In addition, samples of locally grown "Hak", particularly from high-risk villages, are found to contain exceptionally high amounts of NDMA and NPYR (up to 91 µg/Kg). The relevance of these observation is being investigated. Sun-dried "Hak" has also been shown to contain a precursor which gives rise to a nitrosamide-like compound on in vitro nitrosation.

Red chili consumption (7 g/person/day) in Kashmir is nearly three times higher than the maximum level reported from

Bombay in India. We have good evidence now for the presence of methylbenzylamine (whose N-nitroso derivative is a specific esophageal carcinogen in animals) in chili samples analyzed from Kashmir. Thus, high consumption of red chilies in the area appears to be a potential dietary hazard. More studies are underway to evaluate its role in human gastrointestinal cancers. Thus, the analytical studies amply demonstrate a higher exposure to potential precursors of N-nitroso compounds in the local population. An increased proportion of nitrite in saliva and elevated levels of urinary nitrate in the normal population further support a higher exposure to nitrate as evidenced by food analysis.

Environmental Predisposition Facilitates Risk of Cancer

Cancer is believed to be a multifactorial disease in which host factors are suspected to play a vital role in predisposition as well as in its promotion. Our biological monitoring program is basically aimed at finding the role of such variables in the etiology of esophageal cancer. Recent results in this direction indicate prevalence of low blood vitamin A and zinc levels in the normal population. Independent from our studies, a group of clinicians has reported in a well-carried out study that nearly 88 % of the normal population in Kashmir suffers from chronic esophagitis. The regular consumption of hot salted tea could be the most likely reason for such high prevalence of this putative preneoplastic condition in the general population.

Thus, persistence of chronic esophagitis with micronutrient deficiency appears to predispose a large section of population towards high risk for the disease. Further work in collaboration with clinicians to verify this phenonmenon is in progress. It is worth investigating if susceptibility to environmental genotoxic compounds is much greater in an already predisposed group of individuals.

Sharing of Risk Factors Between Esophageal and Gastric Cancers

As briefly mentioned earlier, it is now evident that the high occurrence of esophageal cancer is closely followed by that of stomach carcinoma in Kashmir. As clinicopathological evidence for both these cancers suggests an environmental origin, and since chronic esophagitis and gastritis are observed with equal frequency, a sharing of risk factors in the etiology of these two cancers can not be ruled out. This is an outstanding feature which emerges from our study in Kashmir and needs further exploration in other high risk areas, too.

In this context, we suspect that the salted tea so commonly and frequently used in Kashmir could be a detrimental agent to esophageal and gastric mucosa due to the tea's high temperature and salt content, respectively. Thus, in conclusion, it can be stated as a working hypothesis that while indiscrimate use of hot salted tea and deficiencies of micronutrients may predispose the local population in Kashmir, increased exposure to preformed and endogenously produced N-nitroso compounds through high consumption of sun-dried and fresh vegetables (particularly that of "Hak") and red chilies could constitute the critical carcinogenic risk for high occurrence of both esophageal and gastric cancers.

Identification of Risk Factors is Necessary for Preventive Measures

The two field studies discussed here clearly suggest that identification of discreet risk factors in the human environment can be of paramount importance in recommending appropriate preventive measures to reduce the occurrence of disease. As implied in the results obtained from our study in Egypt, public health measures for controlling bilharzial infection are expected to reduce the incidence of bladder cancer in that area. Similarly, on the basis of currently available data from the Kashmir study, it can be safely recommended that reduction of consumption of hot salted tea, "Hak", and red chilies, together with adopting improved methods for drying and storing vegetables will certainly be instrumental in decreasing the rates of gasterointestinal cancers in that region.

Prof. Dr. Maqsood Siddiqi
Department of Biochemistry,
University of Kashmir,
Srinagar, Indien

Prof. Dr. Rudolf Preussmann
Division of Environmental Carcinogens

Participating scientists

Dr. Rajiv Kumar
Dr. Peter Mende
Dr. Bertold Spiegelhalder
Dr. Anthony Robert Tricker

In collaboration with

Prof. Dr. Mostafa Hassan Mostafa
Institute for Graduate Studies,
University of Alexandria,
Alexandria, Egypt

Selected publications

Siddiqi, M., Tricker, A.R., Preussmann, R.: The occurrence of preformed N-nitroso compounds in food samples from a high-risk area of esophageal cancer in Kashmir, India. Cancer Letters 39, 37–43 (1988)

Siddiqi, M., Tricker, A.R., Preussmann, R.: Formation of N-nitroso compounds under simulated gastric conditions from Kashmir foodstuffs. Cancer Letters 39, 259–265 (1988)

Tricker, A.R., Siddiqi, M., Preussmann, R.: Occurrence of volatile N-nitrosamines in dried chillies. Cancer Letters 38, 271–273 (1988)

Tricker, A.R., Mostafa, M.H., Spiegelhalder, B., Preussmann, R.: Urinary excretion of nitrate, nitrite and N-nitroso compounds in Schistosomiasis and bilharzia bladder cancer patients. Carcinogenesis 10, 547–552 (1989)

Sissiqi, M., Preussmann, R.: Esophageal cancer in Kashmir – an assessmant. J. Cancer Res. Clin. Oncol. 115, 111–117 (1989)

Kumar, R., Mende, P., Tricker, A.R., Siddiqi, M., Preussmann, R.: N-Nitroso compounds and their precursors in Brassica oleracea. Cancer Letters 54, 61–65 (1990)

Siddiqi, M., Kumar, R., Fazili, Z., Spiegelhalder, B. Preussmann, R.: Increased exposure to dietary amines and nitrate in a population at high risk of esophageal and gastric cancer in Kashmir (India). Carcinogenesis 13, 1331–1355 (1992)

4.5 Reduced Fidelity of DNA Replication – A Reason for the Development of Cancer Cells?

by Odilia Popanda and Heinz Walter Thielmann

A critical number of permanent changes in the genomic DNA, especially in some particularly important genes, is needed to transform a normal cell into a cancer cell. Such mutations occur in the process of cell multiplication and result from erroneous DNA replication. Of crucial importance in this process is a specific enzyme complex that uses the DNA as a template and copies it according to the rules of base-pairing. Normally, this complex replicates DNA with an extraordinary high fidelity of only about one error per 100 billion copied DNA elements (bases), with a human cell containing approximately 14 billion bases. It is obvious that the correct functioning of this catalytic complex is indispensable for the preservation and correct transmission of the hereditary information. All events that cause this enzyme complex to malfunction and that consequently reduce the fidelity of replication are therefore of special interest for experimental cancer research. Our research impetus thus focuses on the following two questions:

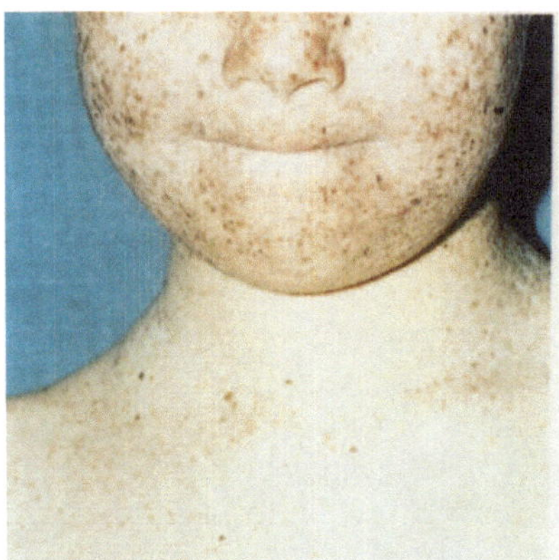

Fig. 46
Persons suffering from the rare hereditary disease Xeroderma pigmentosum react to sun light by developing irregularly colored, dark freckles. The skin becomes dry and ages prematurely. Skin cancer develops. This is caused be defects of the repair mechanisms which normally maintain the genomic integrity.

1) Does the replicative complex function less accurately if the cells are exposed to high-energy rays (such as ultraviolet light) or chemical carcinogens?

Rays and chemical carcinogens transfer energy or react with the genomic DNA of the genetic molecule and cause chemically defined damage. Ultraviolet rays, for example, may dimerize two neighboring pyrimidine bases of a DNA strand in such a way that during replication the altered elements of the template cannot be recognized and, as a consequence, no complementary base can be found. If such damage cannot be reversed by DNA repair before replication, the copying process might even fail, threatening the life of the cell.

However, cells with damaged DNA seem to be able to counteract such lethal threats. For example, cells of patients suffering from xeroderma pigmentosum (extreme heliosensitivity with dry, hyperpigmented skin) can not, due to a genetic defect, repair DNA damage caused by sunlight. Yet their cells are able to proliferate even if exposed to ultraviolet light, though with a higher rate of mutations. An early outbreak of skin cancer is the result. Does this mean that the survival of a cell damaged by carcinogens is possible only if the DNA replicating enzyme complexes work less precisely – even at the cost of permanent DNA alterations (mutations)?

Such emergency functions – collectively referred to as "SOS responses" – are known from studies on bacteria that have been exposed to chemical carcinogens or irradiation. They aim at overcoming non-repairable DNA damages or obstacles to DNA replication that pose a threat to the survival of the cell. In a bacterium, such an emergency repair involves the mobilization of about 20 different genes whose products support both the DNA repair mechanisms and, at the same time, allow DNA replication. A key aspect of such an SOS response is the fact that the bacterium tries to ensure its survival (that is, multiplication) by reducing the fidelity of replication of its DNA polymerases. Amazingly, it is the cell itself that mobilizes the instruments that transform the chemical modification of the DNA template into a permanent alteration of the hereditary information. It is obvious that the same, or a similar mechanism, if acting in mammalian cells, will have fatal effects.

2) Do DNA polymerases of cancer cells cause more errors than those of normal cells?

Frequently, cancer cells contain more than twice as much DNA (more than one set of chromosomes) as normal cells, and they reduplicate DNA more often than normal cells. At the same time, they are genetically unstable, which means that they may mutate into ever more malignant cancer cells. Does this signify that the DNA replicative complexes of cancer cells, which have to reduplicate more DNA in a shorter time, work less exactly than those of normal cells? If this were true, it could mean that the altered replicative complexes, which are similar to those appearing during treatment with carcinogens, might develop into permanent functions of cancer cells during tumor development.

Multiplication of the DNA

We shall begin with a brief description of the most important enzymes and mechanisms which normally catalyse the multiplication of the hereditary information extremely accurately.

Reduplication of DNA is performed by a multi-enzyme complex, whose various subunits catalyze different steps of the copying process. DNA helicases and helix-destabilizing proteins uncoil the DNA template strands; each of the single strands then serves as a template for the synthesis of a new DNA strand. The result is two double-stranded DNA molecules. This step is catalyzed by the most important parts of the complex, the DNA polymerases, which select and integrate the complementary DNA bases.

The new bases are selected according to the defined rules of base-pairing which determine that the new bases have to be strictly complementary to those of the template strand. This mechanism is controlled by two interacting, active centers of the enzyme,

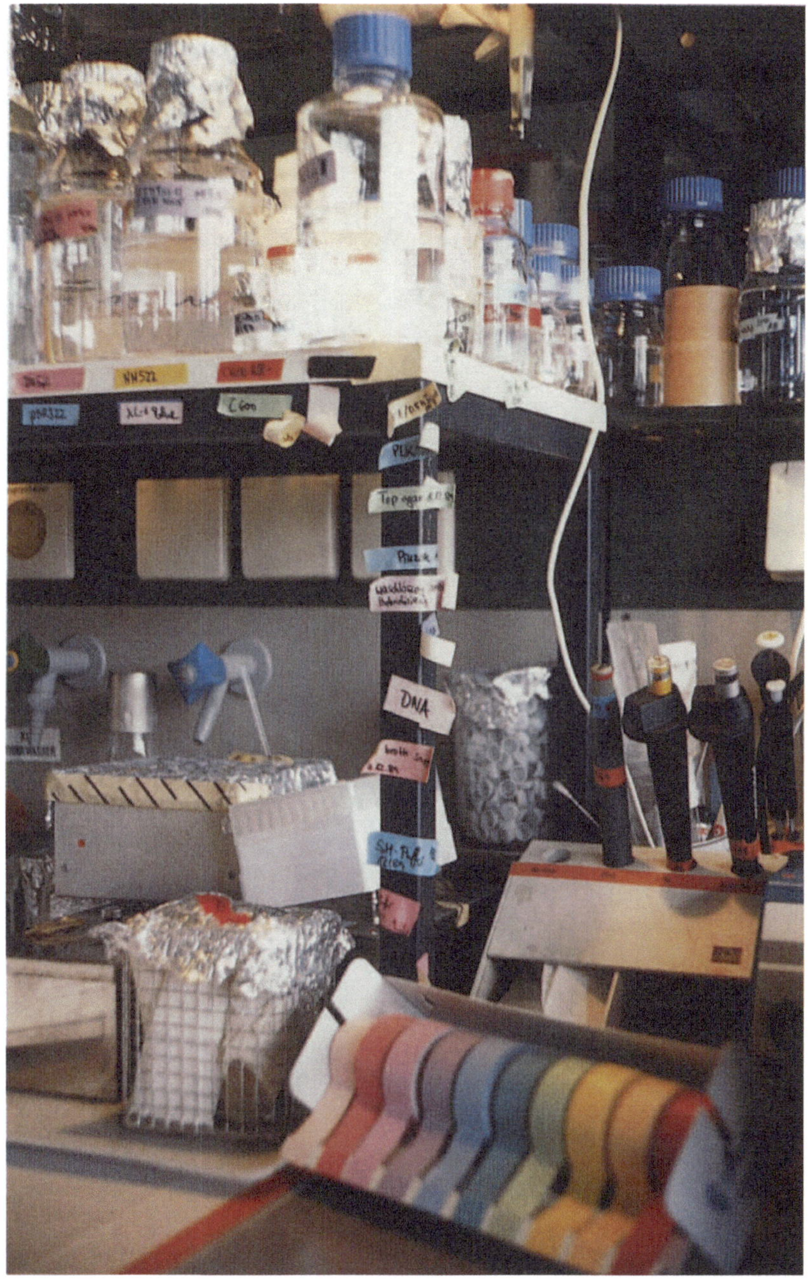

Fig. 47

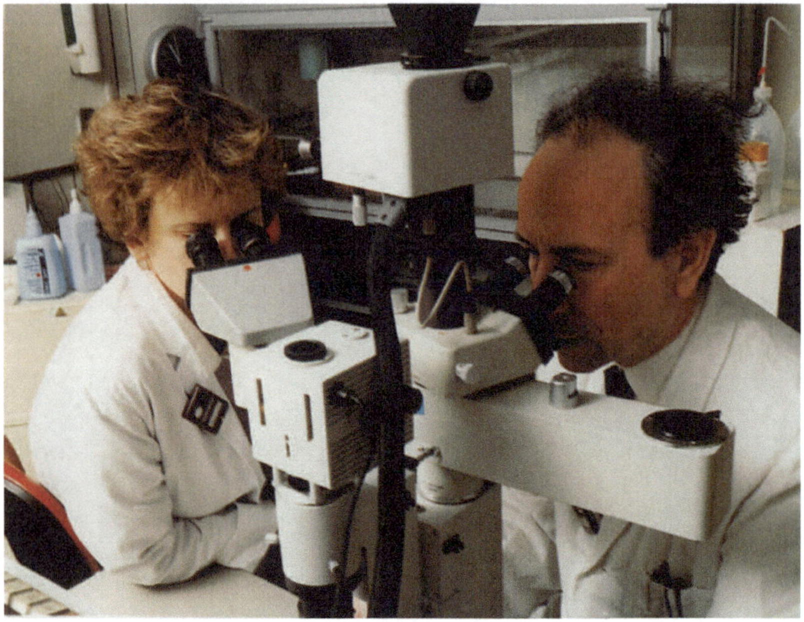

Fig. 48
Odilia Popanda and Heinz Walter Thielmann screen cell cultures of fibroblasts in the microscope.

the binding site for the DNA template and that for the base that is to be integrated. Both functional centers can be characterized experimentally with antibodies or inhibitors.

DNA polymerases can replicate the DNA template only in one direction (from the 5' end to the 3' end). Since, however, the two DNA strands have opposite orientation, the new strands have to be synthesized in opposite order as well. It can therefore be supposed that the catalysis is carried out by enzyme complexes with different polymerization activities. In fact, we know of two DNA polymerases, α and δ. DNA polymerase δ catalyzes the continuous synthesis on the 5' to 3' strand, whereas DNA polymerase α synthesizes small DNA fragments on the 3' to 5' strand (thus producing Okazaki fragments).

During synthesis, the integration of every DNA base is checked by proofreading. If the base is not complementary, it is removed. Only after this verification, which is integrated into the synthesizing process, is polymerization continued. The correcting enzyme, a 3' to 5' exonuclease, is a subunit of DNA polymerase δ.

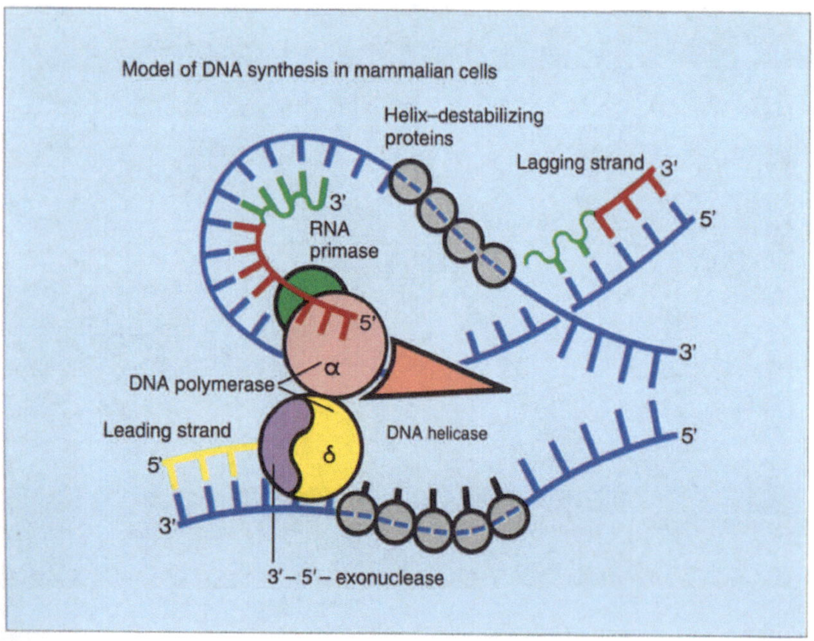

Fig. 49
This is what a DNA replication fork in mammalian cells might look like. First, DNA helicase and helix-destabilizing proteins separate the two parent DNA strands. With the aid of the DNA polymerase δ, the synthesis is continuous on the leading strand. On the lagging strand DNA Synthesis is discontinuous: It requires a primer (produced by RNA primase), which is subsequently elongated by the DNA polymerase-α.

Experimental Characterization of the DNA Replicative Complex

Presently, we are far from understanding the complex structure of the replicative complex; nevertheless, with the help of purified DNA polymerases (which are the main units of the replicative complexes) and their subunits, we can try experimentally to elucidate the mechanism of reaction which determines the fidelity of replication.

So far, the influence of carcinogens on the accuracy of the DNA replicative complex has been studied on ovary cells of the Chinese hamster. The cultivated cells were treated with methylating carcinogens; the replicative complex was isolated after the SOS induction time by careful purification methods (such as immunoaffinity chromatography) and compared to the replicative complex of untreated control cells.

Our DNA replicative complexes consisted of the subunits DNA polymerase α and δ, RNA primase, as well as other elements. Size, shape and molecular mass of the enzyme activities were determined by analysis of the sedimentation rate as well as gel filtration.

The DNA replicative complexes that had been isolated from cells treated with carcinogens had almost the same molecular masses as the complexes of untreated cells. There was no difference with regard to sedimentation and diffusion coefficients. There was also no difference in the reaction of the active centers of the DNA polymerase α with antibodies and specific inhibitors. The only fact indicating that a treatment with carcinogens does have an influence was that the activity of the RNA primase was higher in treated than in untreated cells.

For an exact comparison between the DNA replicative complexes of cancer cells and normal cells, MORRIS liver tumors of rats are particularly well suited, because they occur with different degrees of malignancy in rats fed with carcinogens. Our hypothesis is that malignancy might be correlated with the extent of changes in biochemical properties, particularly in that of the DNA polymerases.

A comparison of the DNA replicative complex from rat liver with that of hepatoma cells revealed differing molecular masses, as well as differing properties of the binding sites for DNA and for bases, which clearly correlated with the degree of malignancy of the hepatomas. The differences in the binding sites (determined by inhibition through antibodies and inhibitors) became apparent by the fact that the replicative complexes from cancer cells bound more closely to the DNA template, and that the chosen bases were selected less specifically. This may mean that, on the one hand, the DNA template may be read and replicated more quickly, but that, on the other hand, the base-pairing is less accurate, which in turn may lead to a reduced fidelity of replication.

Determination of the Fidelity of Replication

The question now arises of whether the mutation of normal cells to cancer cells under the influence of carcinogens is indeed accompanied by a change in the properties (in particular, the accuracy of replication) of the DNA replicative complex. This question can only be answered by determining the fidelity of replication.

There are two test methods: the ΦX174 reversion assay and the M13mp2 forward mutagenesis assay. In both assays a circular phage DNA with a single-stranded section is offered as a template to the DNA polymerases that are to be analyzed; the goal is the in vitro replication of the phage DNA. Erroneous replication alters the genetic information of the phage DNA, as can be seen from the altered enzymatic properties of the phages after multiplication in host bacteria. The ratio of altered to normal phages indicates the frequency of mutation, which is a measure for the fidelity of replication.

The difference between the two test methods is the length of the single-stranded fraction of the DNA to be replicated. The reversion assay monitors whether a section of three bases of the DNA template is incorrectly replicated, which would result in an exchanged base in the product of synthesis. With this assay, we have analyzed DNA replicative complexes from Chinese hamster ovary cells treated with carcinogens and from the corresponding control cells with respect to their fidelity of replication. The error frequency of the enzymes from both preparations was almost identical (about one base mispairing per 500 000 replicated bases).

This result, however, has to be interpreted very cautiously. On the one hand, there might be differences in the fidelity of replication that are beyond the detection limit of the reversion assay: its accuracy is $1{:}10^6$, which means

Fig. 50
The forward mutagenesis assay tests the fidelity of replication of DNA polymerases in a three-step procedure.

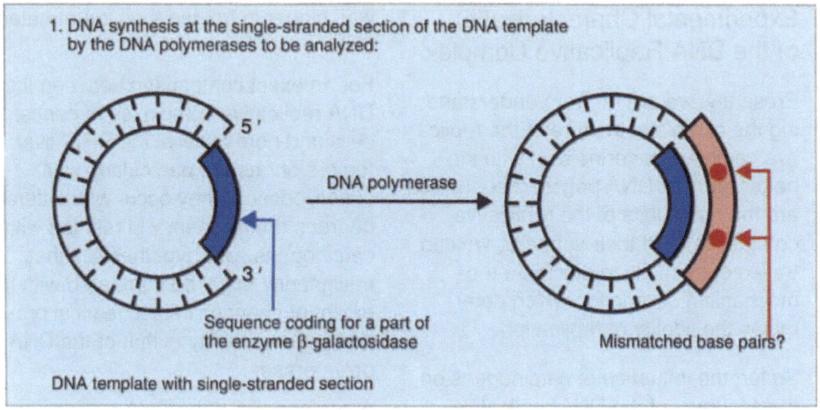

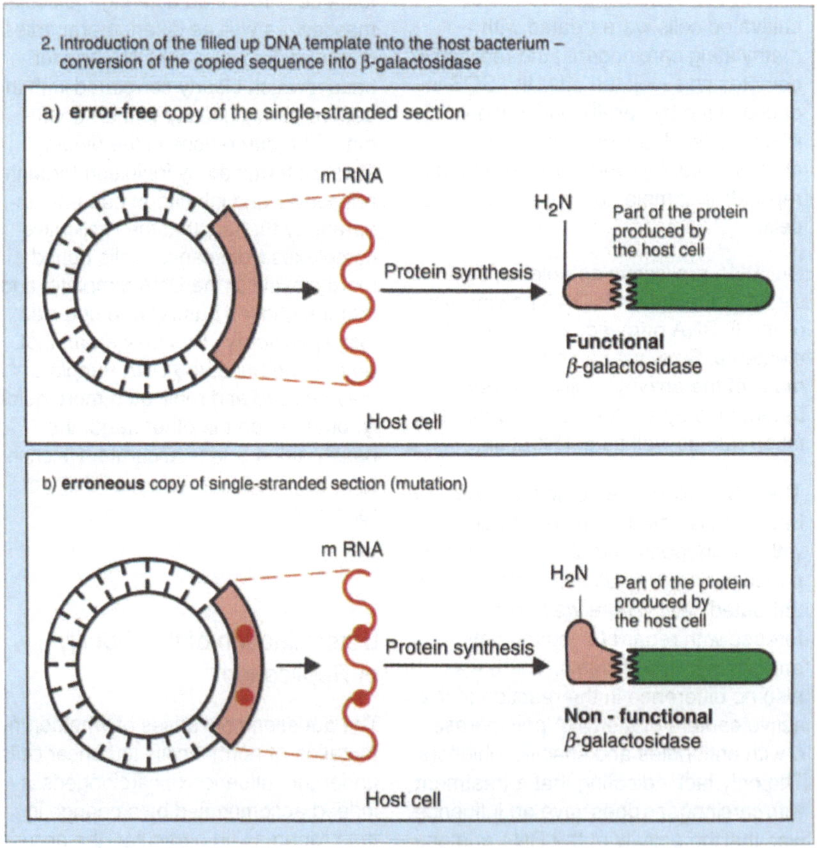

that it detects one mispairing base per million polymerized nucleotides; the physiological fidelity limit, however, is $1:10^9$ to 10^{11}. In a strict sense, our assay would only be meaningful if it showed a difference in the fidelity of replication. Identical values for fidelity of replication, however, indicate rather a lack of sensitivity of the test method. In addition, the reversion assay only monitors specific types of mispairing, mainly the incorporation of wrong bases. Deletions or insertions of extra nucleotides or DNA frame-shift mutations cannot be detected. But it is exactly this type of mutation which might be induced by the SOS mechanism.

The forward mutagenesis assay, which we will now be using to measure the fidelity of the replicative complexes, monitors all possible mutations. The test method: A circular DNA molecule of the E. coli phage M13mp2 containing a larger single-stranded gap is offered to the DNA polymerase as a template for in vitro synthesis. This test DNA is constructed from the viral circular M13mp2 single strand to which a shorter complementary linear fragment is annealed in such a way that we obtain a double-stranded phage with a single-stranded section of 390 bases. The linear fragment is produced in a separate preparation, in which the double-stranded M13mp2 phage is cut by two restriction enzymes (Pvu I and II) thus, losing 390 base pairs from its total length.

The single-stranded section of the hybrid phage is the complementary

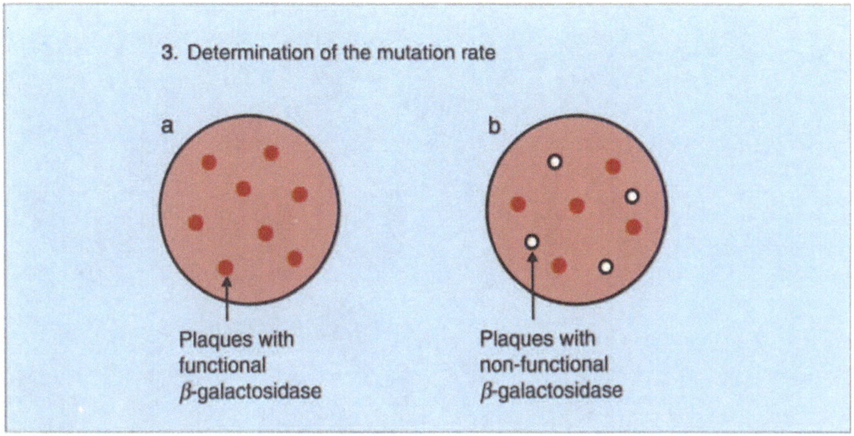

form of a DNA sequence containing the genetic information for a part of the enzyme β-galactosidase (lacZ gene). As soon as the single-stranded region is filled up to a double strand (in vitro) by the DNA polymerase to be analyzed, the product of this synthesis is transfected into an E. coli host bacterium for further analysis. This host strain contains the part of the β-galactosidase gene missing in the phage, but lacks the information carried by the latter.

Functional β-galactosidase can therefore be produced in the host bacterium only if the transfected phage DNA contributes the gene sequence lacking in the host. Each of the two separate gene fractions produces an inactive protein; these combine to form a fully active β-galactosidase. The latter can be detected by a reaction in which a blue dye is released enzymatically from an indicator substance. A blue color thus indicates the presence of an active enzyme, whereas an inactive enzyme remains colorless.

If the DNA polymerase under investigation correctly completes the single-stranded phage section, the host cell produces functional β-galactosidase, blue phages emerge. If, however, the polymerase does not replicate correctly, a biologically spoiled enzyme portion is produced that is unable to complete the host cell's β-galactosidase part, and the phage colonies thus remain colorless.

The ratio of the number of colorless and blue colonies is a measure of the fidelity of replication of a DNA polymerase. In addition, phage DNA can be recovered from the colorless colonies which contain phages with errors in the partial β-galactosidase gene. We use sequence analysis to determine the nucleotide sequence in the multiplied DNA. The type of mutation that has taken place can be determined by a comparison with the genuine sequence, which can be used to produce an intact protein fragment. Unfortunately, this method is expensive: for each polymerase preparation, about 100 such analyses are needed to determine whether replicative complexes taken from cells treated with carcinogens or from tumor cells cause DNA replication errors that do not occur in untreated or normal cells.

The project is supported by the Deutsche Krebshilfe, Dr. Mildred Scheel Foundation for Cancer Research.

Dr. Odilia Popanda
Priv.-Doz. Dr. Dr. Heinz Walter Thielmann
Division of Interaction of Carcinogens with Macromolecules in Biological Systems

Participating scientists

Dr. Angelika Brucker
Dipl.-Biol. Ingrid Ensch-Simon

In collaboration with

Lawrence A. Loeb
The Joseph Gottstein Memorial Cancer Research Laboratory,
University of Washington,
Seattle, Washington, USA

Thomas A. Kunkel
Laboratory of Genetics,
National Institute of Environmental Health Sciences,
Research Triangle Park,
North Carolina, USA

Selected publications

Popanda, O., Thielmann, H. W.: DNA polymerase α from normal rat liver is different than DNA polymerase α from MORRIS hepatoma strains. Eur. J. Biochem. 183, 5–13 (1989)

Brucker, A., Loeb, L. A., Thielmann, H. W.: DNA polymerase α-primase complexes from carcinogen-treated Chinese hamster ovary cells. Cancer. Res. 50, 6894–6901 (1990)

Popanda, O., Thielmann, H. W.: The function of DNA polymerases in DNA repair synthesis of UV-irradiated human fibroblasts. Biochim. Biophys. Acta, 1129, 155–160 (1992)

4.6 Cultivated Liver Cell Lines as a Model for Prestages of Hepatoma

by Doris Mayer

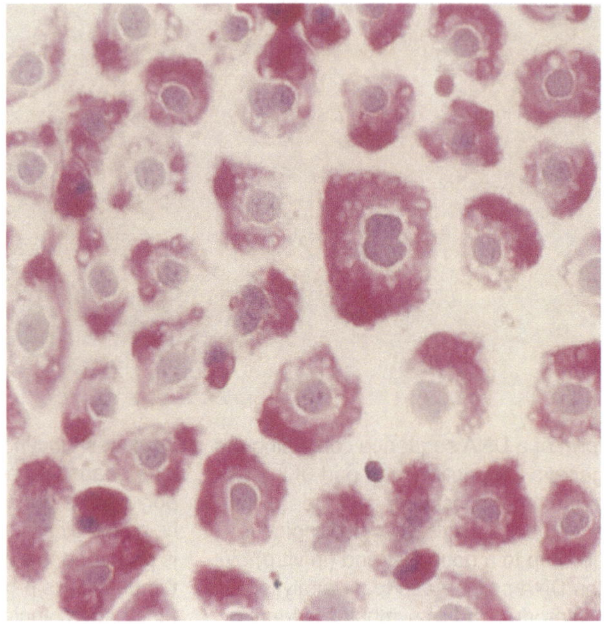

Introduction

The development of tumors in the liver is a multi-stage process. Most hepatomas develop from prestages consisting of focally arranged cells, which differ in their microscopic appearance from normal liver cells (hepatocytes), and which store an excess of glycogen, the liver's reserve carbohydrate. Within a few months, in laboratory animals, such glycogen-storing cells develop into hepatomas; in humans the latency period is probably several decades. These liver tumors are generally low in glycogen.

Cells showing alterations which can be graded as early stages of cancer growth (carcinogenesis) are of particular importance for the clarification of biochemical and molecular-biological mechanisms leading to tumors and their prestages. However, at the beginning of carcinogenesis, the number of such preneoplastic cells is very small. For example, glycogen-storing cells account for, at most, 3% of the total liver tissue in rats treated with chemical carcinogens. Biochemical studies, however, require uniform populations of glycogen-storing cells. For these examinations, it is not possible to use the liver as a whole, since all "contaminations" with normal cells or with cells that have already changed too much would lead to false results.

Several methods are available to obtain glycogen-storing cells for studies in test tubes. One such method is to isolate these cells from carcinogen-treated rat livers. For this, the liver is perfused with collagenase, a proteolytic enzyme, and the liver cells are isolated by dissociating the contacts between the cells. Subsequently, the glycogen-storing cells can be enriched using various centrifugation techniques. However, the yield is extremely low, and despite many efforts undertaken by numerous laboratories, the isolation of a uniform population of preneoplastic cells has not been successful to date.

Establishment and Characterization of Cell Lines

We have chosen a different method and tried to establish glycogen-storing cells as cell lines in culture. It has been known for some time that liver cells in culture can be rendered immortal. Such liver cells are no longer normal hepatocytes, but may have gone through several phases of transformation in the culture dish (in vitro). Several groups have reported that, in some rare cases, such liver cells in culture spontaneously become malignant and may grow as tumors after transplantation into newborn animals of the same strain or into nude mice, whose immunological rejection, due to their innate immunodeficiency, is poor. We therefore concluded that liver cell cultures in which tumor cells can

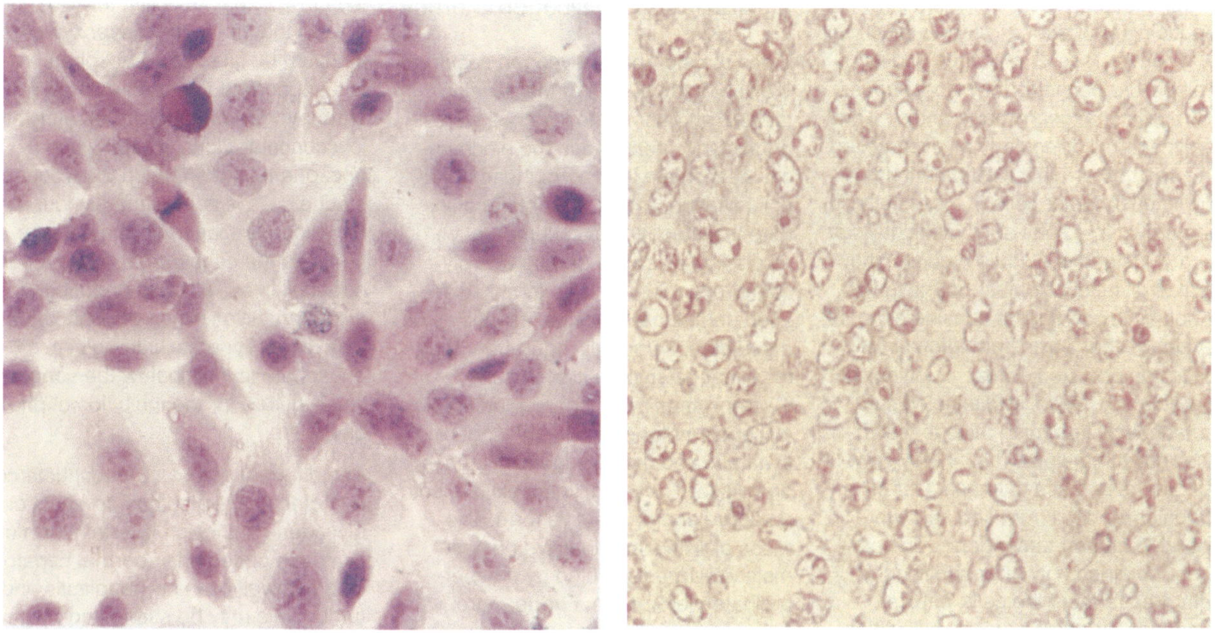

Fig. 51
Various liver cell lines established in cultures (left to right): (1) glycogen-storing cells (enlarged 100 times), (2) glycogen-poor cells (enlarged 100 times), (3) tumor (enlarged 160 times) growing after transplantation of the cells into an animal.

develop spontaneously, should also contain cells corresponding to tumor prestages, i.e. preneoplastic cells. The criterion for the selection of these cells was the storage of glycogen as observed in carcinogen-treated animals ("in vivo").

Liver cells of healthy animals not treated with carcinogens were isolated with collagenase and subsequently cultured. Most hepatocytes of adult animals do not grow in culture and die after 10 to 14 days. Some cells, however, begin to divide; several weeks later, the cultures have a very heterogeneous cell picture. The hepatocytes then have to be selected, since the liver is a very complex organ containing not only hepatocytes, but also other cell types, such as bile duct cells, connective tissue cells (fibroblasts) and endothelial cells, some of which tend to grow well in culture. By single cell cloning, a technique which guarantees that cell lines derived from one single cell are obtained, several cell lines were established. From these cell lines were selected those that were considered to be derivatives of hepatocytes. One major criterion was that they were epithelial cells (in the liver, the only cells of epithelial origin are hepatocytes and bile duct cells; all other cell types are of mesenchymal origin). This could be established by the immunocytochemic identification of cytokeratins, a group of filamentous proteins not present in mesenchymal cells. In addition, the cultivated cell lines had to show hepatocyte-specific properties. One example is the enzyme glucose-6-phosphatase, whose activity can be shown electron-microscopically in the endoplasmic reticulum of hepatocytes and in some of our cell lines. We obtained both glycogen-storing and glycogen-poor cell lines derived from hepatocytes that can be kept in vitro permanently. The advantages of such cell lines are that they supply very uniform material once they are established and that they can be grown in any quantity.

One of our glycogen-storing cell lines degenerates after longer cultivation (approximately 150 passages, corresponding to about 1.5 years) in such a way that it loses its glycogen and its cell picture becomes inhomogeneous. The cells change in shape and size and begin to grow irregularly all over, covering each other. This phenomenon is common in tumor cells. If these cells are grown in a semi-solid medium ("soft agar") instead of a liquid medium, they form individual colonies. Formation of colonies in soft agar is considered to be evidence that a transformation of the cells has occurred. These colonies can be isolated, grown, and injected subcutaneously into nude mice to test if they are tumorigenic (i.e., if they grow as tumors in these animals). Our cell colonies isolated from soft agar were found to be non-tumorigenic. Tumors were obtained only after additional in vitro treatment of the cells with carcinogens, or after very long cultivation (approximately 400 to 500 passages, corresponding to several years of permanent cultivation). The tumor yield was extremely low. Presently, we are developing a technique for enriching and selecting the tumor cells that develop spontaneously in vitro in order to increase the yield and to reduce the latency period.

Most tumors obtained up to now show a very undifferentiated appearance. However, we have also observed tumors that morphologically can be compared to hepatocellular carcinomas as seen in the laboratory animal after treatment with chemical carcinogens. The conclusion can therefore be drawn that the transformation of hepatocytes in vitro follows similar patterns as in vivo, which is from a glycogen-storing cell via a glycogen-poor cell to the tumor.

Mechanisms of Glycogen Storage

Since the storage of glycogen occurs at the very early stages of the development of a tumor in the liver, we were particularly interested in the biochemical mechanism leading to these metabolic changes. We were able to elucidate this mechanism in comparative studies on glycogen-storing and glycogen-poor cell lines, on freshly isolated normal hepatocytes, as well as on a dedifferentiated, glycogen-free hepatocellular carcinoma kept in culture. Two enzymes mainly participate in the glycogen metabolism: the glycogenic synthase and the glycogenolytic phosphorylase. These enzymes exist in both an active and an inactive form. The ratios of active and inactive enzyme molecules are regulated by a superordinate mechanism. Furthermore, various isoenzymes of phosphorylase have been detected. Isoenzymes are enzymes that all catalyze the same reaction, though they are different protein molecules which, as is the case for phosphorylase, are read from different genes and which differ in their composition of amino acids. These isoenzymes, however, are regulated differently by products of the cell metabolism or by hormonal influences. Three isoenzymes of phosphorylase are known: the muscle type, the liver type, and the brain type. Hepatocellular carcinomas do not express the liver isoenzyme, but instead express an isoenzyme that at least is very similar, if not identical, to the brain type. Using isoenzyme-specific antibodies, it could be shown that, not only tumors, but also non-tumorigenic, glycogen-storing and glycogen-poor cultivated cell lines produce the brain type of phosphorylase. It is a special property of this isoenzyme that its active form (in contrast to that of the liver isoenzyme) is inhibited by glucose 6-phosphate, which is an important intermediate within the carbohydrate metabolism at relatively low concentrations. The glucose 6-phosphate concentration in glycogen-storing cells is approximately four times the concentration in normal rat liver and 10 times the concentration in glycogen-poor cell lines, which is enough to inhibit the active form of phosphorylase. In glycogen-poor cells the glucose 6-phosphate level is below the concentration required for the inhibition of phosphorylase.

The different glucose 6-phosphate content of the cells also has an effect on glycogen synthesis. A certain form of synthase observed in normal hepatocytes as well as in preneoplastic and tumor cells may be stimulated by glucose 6-phosphate. The glucose 6-phosphate concentration required for stimulation, however, is only measured in normal hepatocytes and glycogen-storing cells. Glycogen synthesis does not occur in glycogen-poor cells, probably due to the shortage of glucose 6-phosphate.

The mechanism of glycogen storage is thus probably based on both an increased synthesis of glycogen and on an inhibition of the glycogen degradation. Both phenomena are due to an extraordinarily high intracellular glucose 6-phosphate concentration. The reason for this accumulation of glucose 6-phosphate is still not totally clear. It also still remains to be clarified why and how, in preneoplastic liver cells and in carcinoma cells, the gene for the liver-specific isoenzyme of phosphorylase is inactivated and why and how the gene for the tumor or brain type is activated.

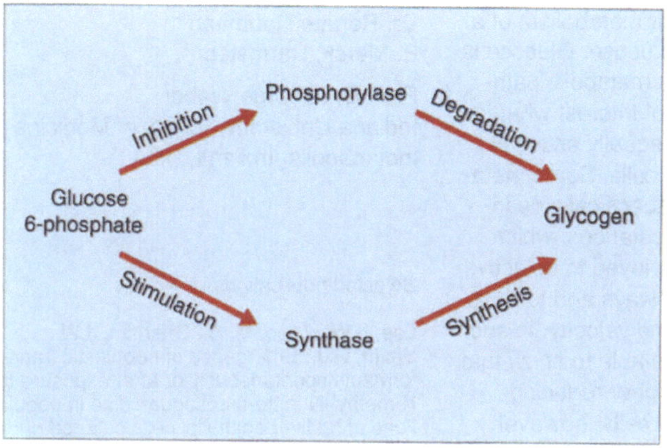

Fig. 52
Mainly, two enzymes participate in the glycogen metabolism: the glycogen-anabolizing synthase and the glycogen-degrading phosphorylase.

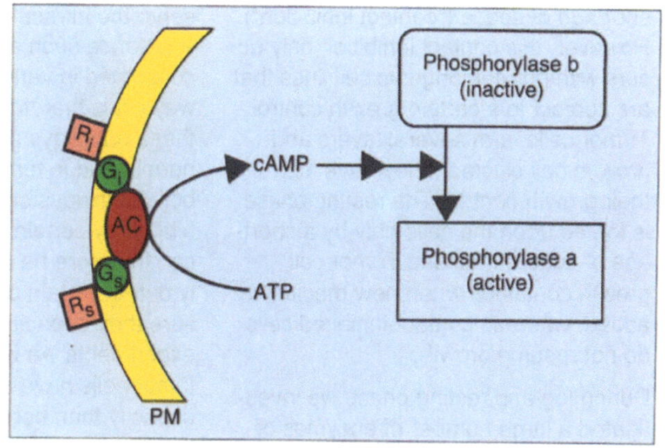

Fig. 53
Both the synthase and the phosphorylase exist in an active form and in an inactive form. Phosphorylase is activated by a superordinate enzyme system.

In our opinion, our cell culture model will be well suited to investigate the regulation of gene expression in tumor cells and their prestages.

Regulation of Adenylate Cyclase

Now we shall describe another principle of the regulation of enzyme activity by means of the example of adenylate cyclase. Adenylate cyclase plays a central role in signal transmission within the cell. Recent findings show that defects or changes in signal transmission are of general importance for tumor development. Adenylate cyclase is an enzyme system located within the cell's plasma membrane, which, via its product cyclic adenosine monophosphate (cAMP), regulates a large number of metabolic pathways, such as the activation of glycogen phosphorylase. Compared to its activity in normal tissue, the activity of adenylate cyclase in most tumors, including tumors of the liver, is reduced. However, not only tumors, but also the non-tumorigenic cell lines described above, as well as preneoplastic lesions induced in vivo also show significantly reduced adenylate cyclase activity, as compared to normal liver cells.

Adenylate cyclase consists of several components. The catalytic subunit is responsible for the actual reaction, i.e., for the conversion of adenosine triphosphate (ATP) into cAMP. The activity of the catalytic subunit is controlled by so-called G-proteins that may have either an inhibiting (Gi) or a stimulating (Gs) effect on the catalytic subunit. The state of activation of the G-proteins depends on whether they receive a signal from a neighboring receptor. The reduction of the activity of adenylate cyclase in our cell lines may be explained by the finding that the amount of catalytic subunit is not reduced, but instead that of inhibitory protein is increased significantly. However, the regulation of adenylate cyclase is much more complex, since alterations are also observed in the stimulating proteins.

Growth-Dependent and Transformation-Dependent Processes

Tumors induced in laboratory animals and their prestages always have a certain number of cells in the growing (proliferating) and resting phases. Thus, it is sometimes extremely difficult to decide whether certain changes in the activity of enzymes observed in such lesions are connected with cell proliferation, or whether they are directly correlated with the transformation, i.e., with the conversion of normal cells into tumor cells. Cell cultures are very useful tools for the differentiation of these effects. After seeding into culture dishes, cells first pass through a lag or adaption phase; then they enter a phase of exponential growth (log phase), until they merge into a plateau or resting phase. This latter phase is entered when the cells that have been growing as a monolayer stop dividing due to a shortage of space ("contact inhibition"). However, this contact inhibition only occurs with non-tumorigenic cell lines that are subject to a certain growth control. Tumor cells form several layers and grow in cell clusters; they have lost their growth control. The resting phase is forced upon the cells only by a shortage of culture medium. Tumor cell growth continues when new medium is added, whereas contact-inhibited cells do not resume growth.

During log and resting phase we investigated a large number of enzymes of the nucleic acid and carbohydrate metabolisms in our cell lines. We chose so-called key enzymes of both metabolic pathways that in normal tissue have only low activities and which limit the rate of metabolic turnover. We observed that, compared to normal liver cells, the activity of the anabolic enzymes of both metabolisms is significantly increased during the cell's resting phase, whereas the activity of the catabolic enzymes is reduced. These alterations of activity observed in resting, transformed cells are considered to be correlated to the transformation. They apparently are part of the genetic program characteristic of tumor cells. In addition, during the proliferation phase the activity of the enzymes of the nucleic acid biosynthesis is strongly increased, whereas that of the enzymes of the carbohydrate metabolism is not. The biochemical regulatory mechanism responsible for these different behaviors still remains to be clarified.

Intracellular metabolic turnover

As compared to whole organs, cultured cells can be used more easily to observe the intracellular metabolism of a substance such as glucose. Glucose is consumed in various metabolic pathways; it is therefore of interest whether these pathways are equally active in normal and in tumor cells. Some metabolic pathways can specifically be inhibited by certain substances, which can therefore be employed to selectively detect certain pathways and to measure their capacity and velocity. In such experiments we were able to show that tumor cells have a higher reducing capacity than normal cells; however, the metabolism in normal cells is faster than in tumor cells.

The examples given above show the importance of cultivated preneoplastic liver cell lines for the investigation of changes in the metabolism of liver cells during the neoplastic cell transformation. Cell lines always constitute an artificial system, which, however, render possible the investigation of problems that cannot be studied in the organism as a whole.

Dr. Doris Mayer
Division of Cell Pathology

Participating staff
Prof. Dr. Peter Bannasch
Bettina Burk
Dr. Hans Jörg Hacker
Dr. Fritz Klimek
Iris Letsch
Dr. Gabriele Seelmann-Eggebert

In collaboration with

Dr. Lutz Edler
Research Program Bioinformatics,
Deutsches Krebsforschungszentrum

Dr. Renate Naumann
E. Merck, Darmstadt

Prof. Dr. George Weber,
Indiana University School of Medicine,
Indianapolis, Indiana, USA

Selected publications

Lee, L.W., Tsao, M.-S., Grisham, J.W., Smith, G.J.: Emergence of neoplastic transformants spontaneously or after exposure to N-methyl-N'-nitro-nitrosoguanidine in populations of rat liver epithalial cells cultured under selective and non-selective conditions. Am. J. Pathol. 135, 63–71 (1989)

Mayer, D., Klimek, F., Hacker, H.J., Seelmann-Eggebert, G., Bannasch, P.: Carbohydrate metabolism in hepatic preneoplasia. In: Bannasch, P., Keppler, D., Weber, W. (eds.) Liver Cell Carcinoma. Kluwer Academic Publishers, Dordrecht, Boston, London, pp. 329–345 (1989)

Mayer, D., Letsch, I.: Glucose-6-phosphate plays a central role in glycogen accumulation in a glycogen-storing rat liver cell line. Cell Biochem. Funct. 7, 243–256 (1989)

Mayer, D., Natsumeda, Y., Ikegami, T., Faderan, M., Lui, M., Emrani, J., Reardon, M., Oláh, E., Weber, G.: Expression of key enzymes of purine and pyrimidine metabolism in a hepatocyte-derived cell line at different phases of growth cycle. J. Cancer Res. Clin. Oncol. 116, 251–258 (1990)

Mayer, D., Naumann, R., Edler, L., Bannasch, P.: Investigation by amperometric methods of intracellular reduction of 2,6-dichlorophenolindophenol in normal and transformed hepatocytes in the presence of different inhibitors of cellular metabolism. Biochem. Biophys. Acta 1015, 258–263 (1990)

Naumann, R., Mayer, D., Edler, L., Bannasch, P.: Evaluation of the kinetics of the intracellular reduction of 2,6-dichlorophenol-indophenol in normal and transformed hepatocytes measured by amperometric methods. Biochem. Biophys. Acta 1015, 253–267 (1990)

Mayer, D., Letsch, I.: Resolution of glycogen phosphorylase isoenzymes in precast PhastSystem polyacrylamide gels. Electrophoresis 12, 297–302 (1991)

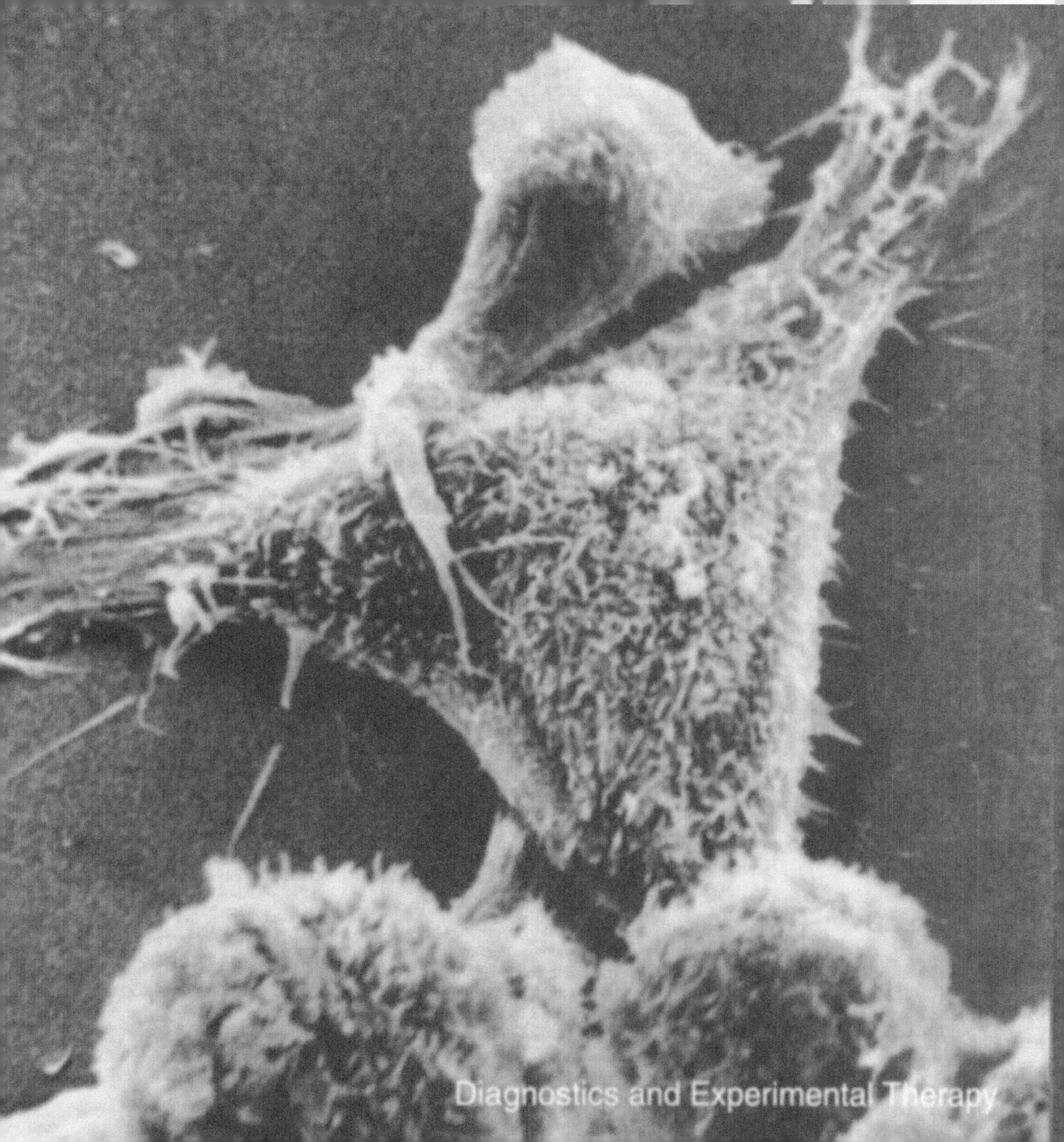
Diagnostics and Experimental Therapy

5

Diagnostics and Experimental Therapy

It is the goal of the Research Program to make new molecular-biological developments in the areas of cell biology, virology, and immunology accessible for cancer diagnosis and therapy.

The Division of Histodiagnostics and Pathomorphological Documentation is responsible for all the centralized histopathological examinations within the Deutsches Krebsforschungszentrum. Its research activities include the expansion of computerized image analysis aiming at quantitatively describing the nucleus's morphology, on the basis of which the structural and cellular heterogeneity of tumors may be characterized. For this purpose, the division utilizes a most advanced image processing system.

Closely related to these morphological evaluations are investigations with transgenic mice serving as model systms for diseases in humans, the elaboration of a catalog of experimental tumors, and the tumor bank of the Deutsches Krebsforschungszentrum. The latter keeps numerous established animal tumor models at the disposal of the Center's researchers.

The research done by the Division of Cell Growth and Division mainly focuses on the examination of molecular processes during cell division using biochemical, histochemical and cytochemical techniques, as well as on in-situ hybridization.

The malignant transformation of cells is usually accompanied by alterations in the structure and number of chromosomes. Defects in the distribution of chromosomes become visible during or after cell division, when the mitotic spindle separates the chromosomes into chromatides. In this process the centromere, visible as a constriction in the chromosome, plays an important role. The process is controlled by specific proteins.

The Division of Perinatal Toxicology deals with cancer chemotherapy. One focus is the development of strategies to overcome therapy resistance in ovarian tumors. The researchers are particularly interested in the role which intracellular enzymes play in the development of resistance and the importance of selective inhibitors of these enzymes. These studies are based on animal experiments and on the examination of human ovarian carcinomas. A further objective is the investigation of the mechanism of action of new metal complex compounds. In cooperation with the Neurosurgical Clinic of the University of Heidelberg, this division is also involved in the development of new carrier systems which, after surgical implantation, slowly release medications.

Antitumor and antivirus mechanisms are the focus of work of the Division of Molecular Biology of DNA Tumor Viruses. It concentrates on intracellular signal transmission systems which regulate the growth of tumor cells, and which may also be used by viruses for proliferation. Presently, a new class of intracellular signal transmission inhibitors is being studied. Further research includes the investigation of the effects of biomodulators in combination with chemical substances that both enhance the desired effect of body effector substances and simultaneously reduce their adverse side effects.

The Division of Applied Immunology analyzes the activation processes of human T-lymphocytes, which are responsible for tumor control and defense. One focus of research is the analysis of receptor-mediated intracellular signal transmission processes which control genes that are relevant for differentiation and growth.

Cytoplasmic enzyme systems are characterized molecularly in order to develop new growth-inhibiting and immunomodulatory substances. Another focus of work is the clarification of the cell-to-cell-interaction. The processes taking place there are of major importance in the defense against tumor cells. Tumor cells alter their interaction structures and thus behave abnormally, which allows them to escape detection by defense cells. Endogenous biomodulators (cytokines) are tested with regard to their effect on the expression of interaction structures and adhesion molecules. Monoclonal antibodies against functional determinants of these molecules are produced; they serve to establish new diagnostic reagents which may be used for investigating the tumor cell's phenotype. Current clinical activities at the division focus on improving the control of transplant rejection (a reciprocal model of tumor defense), as well as on the improvement of vaccination strategies against viral infections favoring tumor growth.

The new Division of Molecular Pharmacology will deal with the molecular and functional characterization of an endogenous class of signal transmission components, the so-called G-proteins. These proteins are a central component in the regulation of cell growth and differentiation.

The overall concept of the Research Program also includes future Clinical Cooperation Units, which will be divisions of the Deutsches Krebsforschungszentrum that closely cooperate with the Clinics of the University of Heidelberg. This is to ensure that new clinical strategies in cancer diagnosis and therapy can be introduced quickly and efficiently into the treatment of patients. Presently, the first clinical cooperation units are being established in the Medical Clinic V (Medical Polyclinics; head: Prof. Dr. Werner Hunstein) and in the University Pediatric Clinic (head: Prof. Dr. Hans Joachim Bremer). In view of the new dynamic developments in the field of hemato-oncology, it is planned that the new units will first focus their work on research in this area.

Coordinator of the Research Program:
Prof. Dr. Stefan Meurer

Divisions and their heads:

Histodiagnostics and Pathomorphological Documentation:
Prof. Dr. Dymitr Komitowski

Perinatal Toxicology:
Prof. Dr. W. Jens Zeller

Molecular Pharmacology:
Priv.-Doz. Dr. Peter Gierschik

Cell Growth and Division:
Prof. Dr. Neidhard Paweletz

Molecular Biology and DNA Tumor Viruses:
Prof. Dr. Gerhard Sauer

Applied Immunology:
Prof. Dr. Stefan C. Meurer

5

5.1 Adhesion Molecules: Key Structures for Tumor Directed Immune Defenses

by Stefan Meuer and Reinhard Wallich

The fact that the immune system can contain the development of cancer is underscored by the fact that malignant diseases arise more often and spread faster if immunodeficiencies exist.

However, it is not only impairments of the immune system itself that allow tumor cells to survive immunologic attacks. Very often malignant tumors, for example, are surrounded by a wall of defense cells, which, however, do not prevent the cancer tissue from growing and forming metastases. It is assumed that, in these cases, cancer cells develop strategies to block and/or circumvent the immune system and thus to prevent their detection and elimination.

Only recently has it been possible to gain insight into the molecular interactions between defense cells (lymphocytes) and tumor cells. The development of monoclonal antibodies and new methods of genetic engineering have considerably furthered this development. Since the success of fighting cancer immunologically depends on

Fig. 54
The information for the formation of adhesion molecules is coded in the sequence of genetic elements, which is analyzed here.

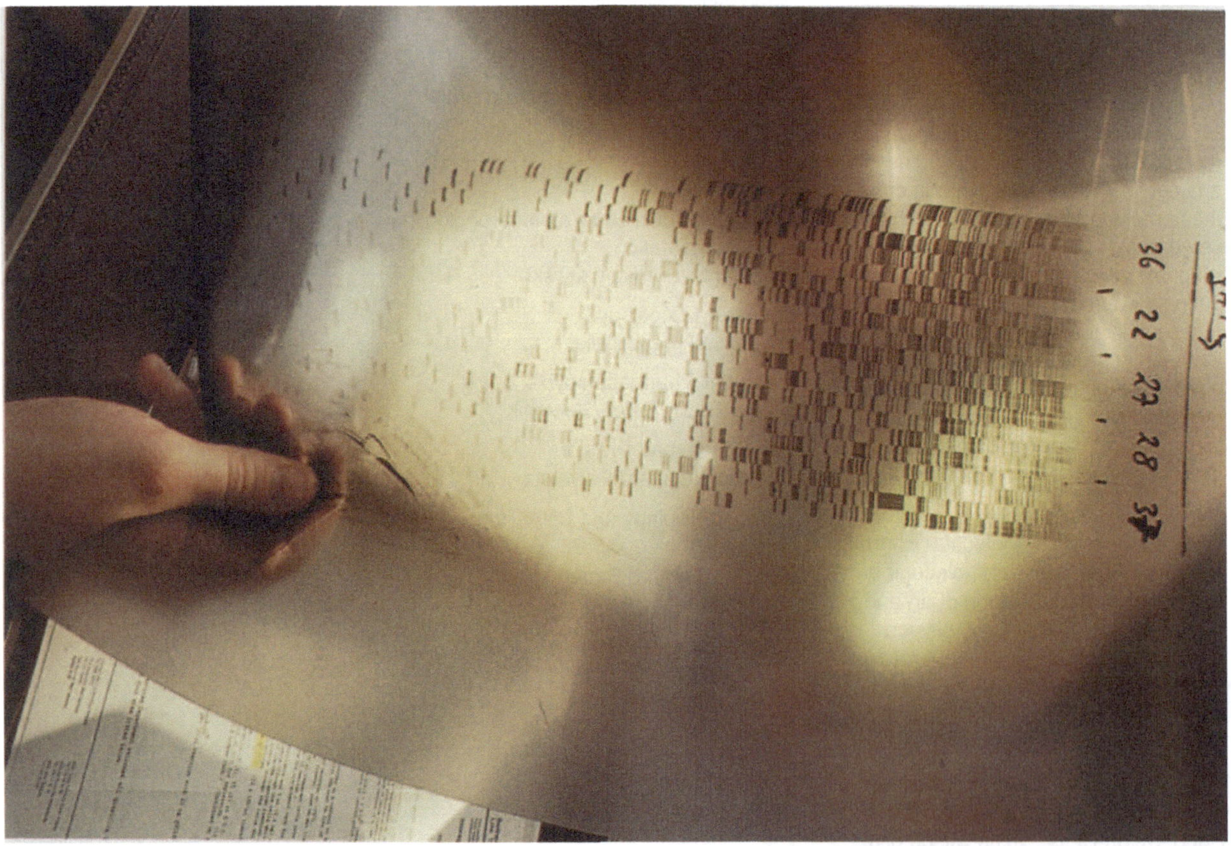

complex cellular interactions, two aspects of "immunodeficiency" must be considered. One is the weakened immune function itself, the other is the tumor's capability to prevent the action of defense cells in spite of the normal functioning of the immune system.

Apart from the specific recognition structures (protein molecules which are present in the membrane of T-lymphocytes, which are, in turn, important for fighting tumors) that have been known for some years, researchers have only recently discovered additional glycoprotein molecules that can be found on the surface of many of the body's cells. The cells of the immune system carry special receptors (which are surface protein molecules, too), with the aid of which they bind to receptor structures. This adhesion is of crucial importance, both for the circulation of leucocytes through the organism (which makes it possible for the lymphocytes to reach the tumor), as well as for the activation of the lymphocytes with the object of destroying a malignant cell.

The proteins LFA-3 (lymphocyte function associated molecule 3) and ICAM-1 (intercellular adhesion molecule 1) are examples of such adhesion molecules. Today, it is known that they are of special importance in the interaction between defense cells and tumor cells. For instance, their concentration on the surface of tumor cells is correlated with the degree of a tumor's malignancy and with its likelihood to metastasize. If such adhesive structures are missing or altered, it is impossible for the T-lymphocytes to attack the tumor cells.

There are two ways that would allow tumors to escape the immune system's surveillance on the level of adhesive structures:

1) Tumor cells might make adhesion molecules disappear from their surface by "retracting" them.

2) Tumor cells might release soluble fragments of adhesion molecules that are normally firmly bound in the cell membrane. It might be possible that soluble forms of adhesion molecules bind to the corresponding receptors of the defense cells and thereby prevent interaction with the adhesion molecules bound to the membrane.

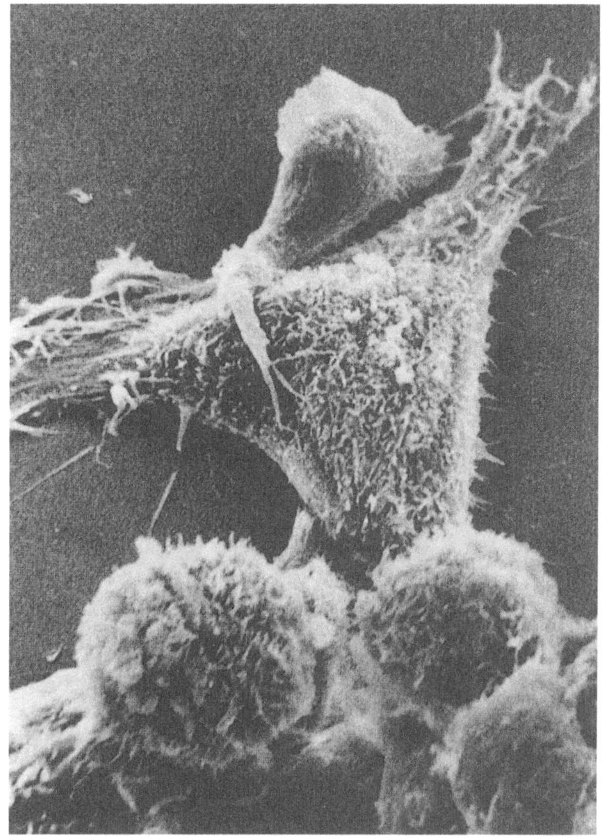

Fig. 55
A stimulated lymphocyte (above) probes an intact cancer cell with an offshoot, called uropode, and thus initiates the destruction of the cancer cell.

Studies on several malignant forms of T-cell leukemia have indeed proven that tumor cells use the first escape from surveillance. If one compares the degree of the leukemia in a patient's blood to the concentration of the adhesion molecules LFA-3 and ICAM-1 on

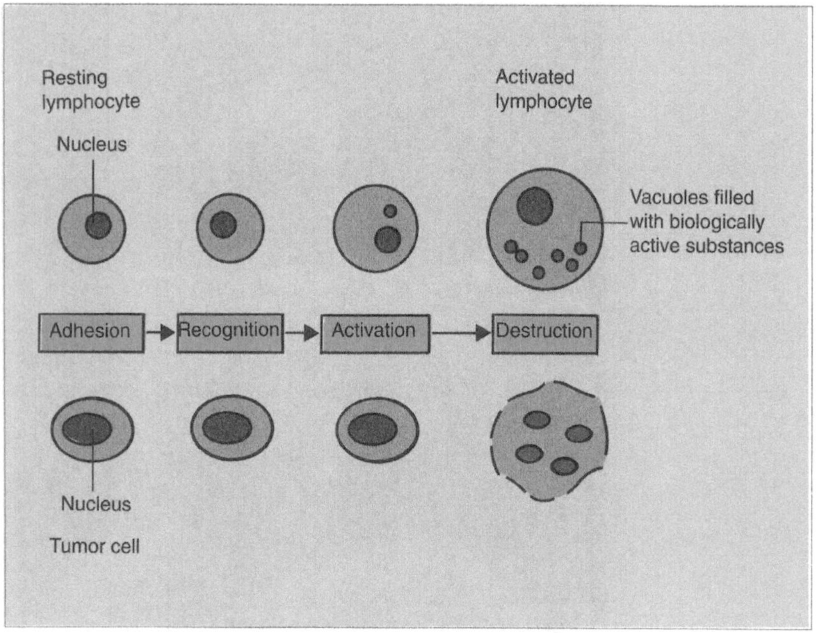

Fig. 56
The first step towards destroying a tumor cell is adhesion. The immunocompetent cell is activated after having identified the tumor cell.

the surface of such tumor cells, one finds a statistically highly significant correlation: the lower the surface concentration of these adhesion molecules on the tumor cell, the more severe is the leukemia (i.e. the number of malignant white blood cells in the patient's blood). Endogenous tumor-specific lymphocytes (killer cells) cannot recognize and destroy cancer cells that carry only few adhesion molecules on their surface. Artificially produced immunological messenger substances (e.g. tumor necrosis factor), however, can increase the surface concentration of LFA-3 and ICAM-1 on tumor cells. If tumor cells are exposed to such messenger substances (mediators), the immune function is re-activated by the expression of adhesion molecules.

Up to now, these correlations have only been shown in vitro. In the future, they might become the basis of new clinical strategies for the immune therapy of malignant diseases. This example shows that, in order to be efficient, endogenous biological agents must be used, both with respect to the tumor and with respect to the immune system. Controlling only one parameter will not be effective.

Whether tumor cells also use the second way is presently under investigation. Very recently and for the first time, a human adhesion molecule, LFA-3, was identified in soluble form in the blood plasma. A method for the determination of its concentration in body fluids was also developed. It is still not known, however, if, in the case of certain malignant diseases, higher amounts of these soluble adhesion molecules are indeed present in the cancer tissue, and if they prevent immune cells from adhering successfully.

Even though it has not yet been proven fully in vivo that tumors can escape recognition by producing soluble adhesion molecules, it is worthwhile speculating about how it might be possible to eliminate or by-pass these potential inhibitory factors. One way is the use of special monoclonal antibodies. Genetic engineering and specific biochemical methods make it possible to produce so-called bifunctional antibodies, which simultaneously bind to both the tumor and the defense (killer) cell. Such antibodies establish a close cell-cell interaction and thus provide an essential prerequisite for the destruction of tumor cells. Presently, research is under way to investigate this clinical perspective.

The strategies which are used by malignant tumors to evade destruction by the immune system might very well be beneficial in other clinical situations, e.g., when it is necessary to specifically suppress the functioning of defense cells. This is the case in organ graft rejection. The observation of an "escape mechanism" successfully used by tumors paved the way to an important new development in transplantation medicine: genetic engineering has recently made it possible to produce a soluble form of the extracellular domain of the human adhesion molecule LFA-3. This protein can hardly be distinguished from the natural LFA-3 molecule. In very low concentrations it has all the predicted functional properties: geneti-

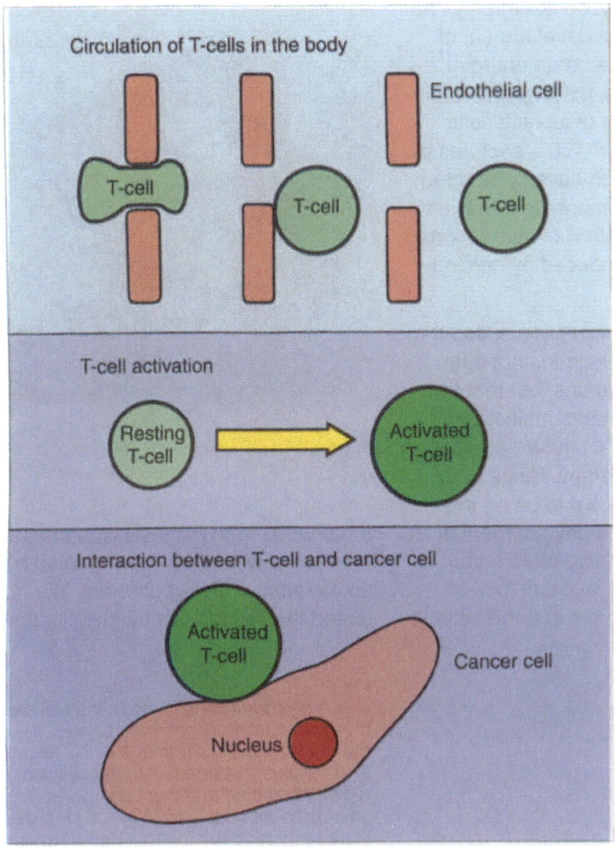

Fig. 57
Adhesion molecules participate in a host of processes within the organism.

cally engineered soluble LFA-3 prevents lymphocytes from binding to LFA-3-carrying cells and thus prevents killer cells from attacking and destroying their target cells. The same molecule also blocks a process that is essential for the rejection of organ transplants, i.e., the binding of lymphocytes to endothelial cells and their mutual activation. These properties make the artificial adhesion protein LFA-3 a promising new weapon in fighting the undesirable rejection reaction following transplantation.

In addition to the significance for the development of basic strategies for the therapy of malignant diseases with endogenous biologic agents, the research projects described above have provided us with new concepts for the treatment of undesirable rejection reactions. The observation of nature's strategies, which in some cases even promote diseases, may open up new pathways to the development of new and effective biological therapies.

Prof. Dr. Stefan Meuer
Dr. Reinhard Wallich
Division of Applied Immunology

Participating scientists

Dipl.-Biol. Marion Albert-Wolf
Dr. Matthias Roux
Dr. Albrecht Schirren
Dipl.-Biol. Heiko Völpel

In collaboration with

Dr. Barbara Endler-Jobst
Division of Biotechnology,
BASF AG,
Ludwigshafen

Dr. Klaus Schollmeyer
Bioresearch Corporation,
Boston, Massachusetts, USA

Selected publications

Albert-Wolf, M., Meuer, S.C., Wallich, R.: Dual function of recombinant human CD58: inhibition of T cell adhesion and activation via the CD2 pathway. International Immunology 3, 1335–1347 (1991)

Schirren, C.A., Völpel, H., Meuer, S.C.: Adhesion molecules on freshley recovered T leukemias promote tumor directed lympholysis. Blood 79, 1–6 (1992)

5.2 Increased Incidence of Drug Resistant Lung Tumors in Smokers

by Manfred Volm

It is a common phenomenon that malignant tumors develop chemoresistance, not only with regard to a single substance, but also to quite different drugs. In the past, various molecular aspects of this multidrug resistance have been investigated. The studies have shown that the over-expression of a cell membrane protein (P-glycoprotein) plays an important part in the development of multidrug resistance. In an energy-dependent process, the P-glycoprotein – which is, because of its molecular weight, also called P-170 – secretes cytostatic agents which have penetrated into the cell. An increased expression of this P-glycoprotein was also reported in rat liver tumors induced by carcinogenic substances.

From these findings, we concluded that environmental carcinogens not only cause tumors in humans, but that they also make these tumors multidrug resistant, a fact which frustrates all attempts at chemotherapy. Since cigarette smoking is known to be an important factor for the development of lung cancer, pulmonary tumors should be more frequently resistant to cytostatics than tumors in non-smokers.

If our working hypothesis was true, this resistance would be accompanied by an increase of P-glycoprotein. We tested this hypothesis by investigating

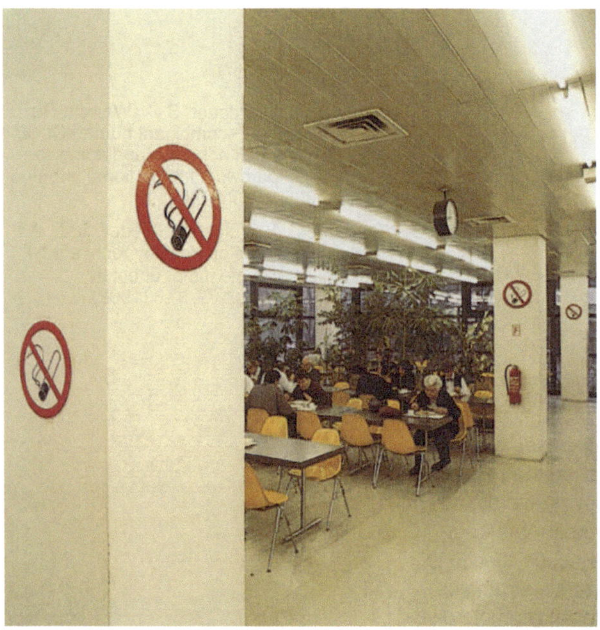

Fig. 58
Ninety percent of all persons that die of lung cancer are smokers. In the Deutsches Krebsforschungszentrum, smoking is prohibited.

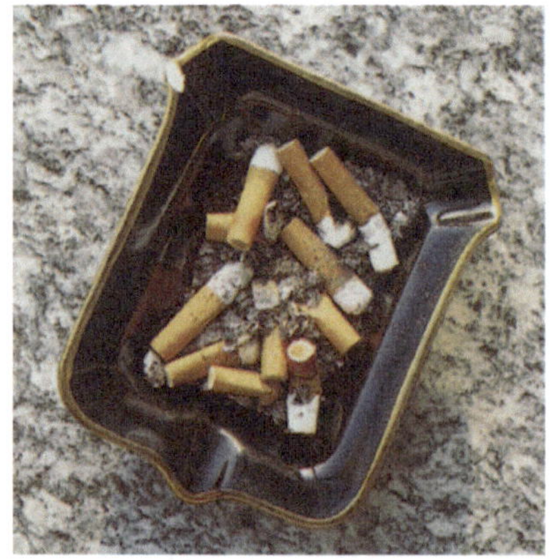

Fig. 59

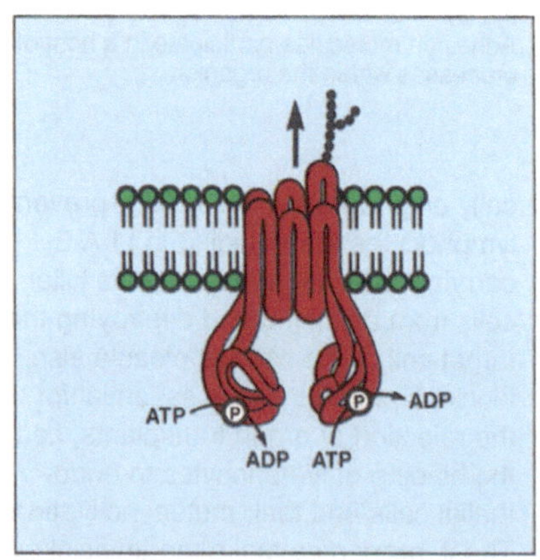

Fig. 60
The P-glycoprotein is found in the cell membrane. In multidrug- resistant tumors, it removes cytostatics from the cell. The part of the protein that extends into the cell contains regions that bind to the energy carrier adenosine triphosphate (ATP). ATP provides the energy required for transport (arrow).

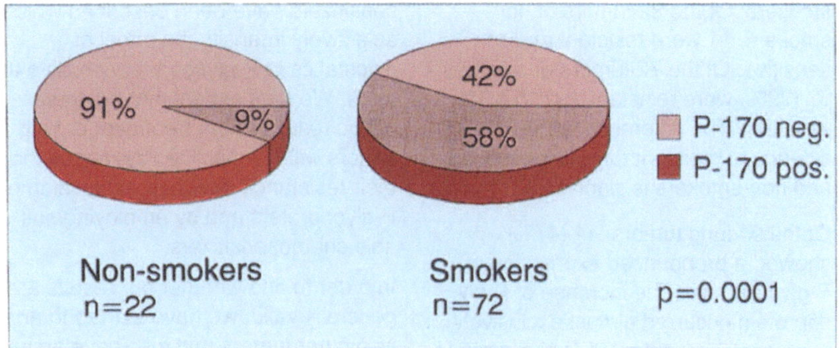

Fig. 61
Lung tumors found in non-smokers rarely show an increased P-glycoprotein (P-170) level, which, in contrast, is observed in more than half of the lung tumors of smokers.

the resistance of lung tumors and the expression of P-glycoprotein in smokers and non-smokers.

All of our patients were operated on in the Clinic for Thoracal Diseases of the Landesversicherungsanstalt Baden in Heidelberg-Rohrbach. Since most of the patients did not receive additional drug therapy, the resistance could be investigated only in vitro. We thus used an in vitro test to measure the resistance of all of the tumors. The test allows us to measure the drug-resistance of tumors with an accuracy of 95%. P-glycoprotein was immunohistochemically measured in tumor specimen with the help of a monoclonal antibody against that protein.

The tumors responded very differently to the drugs. 68 (72%) out of 94 lung tumors were classified resistant, 26 tumors (28%) as sensitive. Of the 94 patients, 72 were smokers and 22 non-

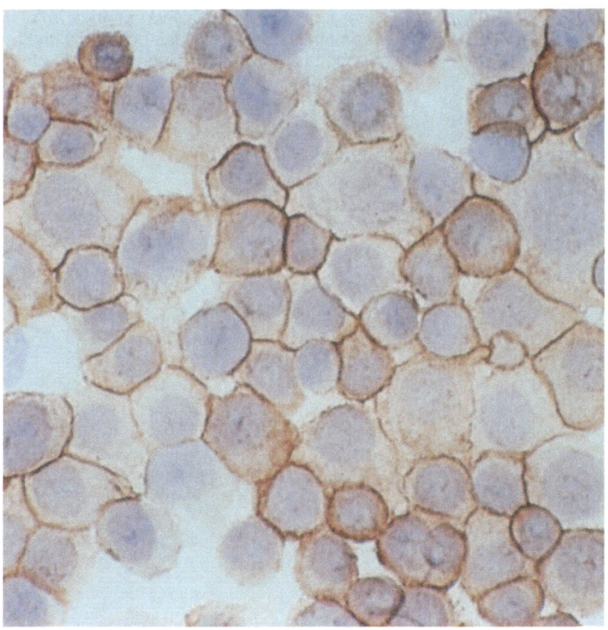

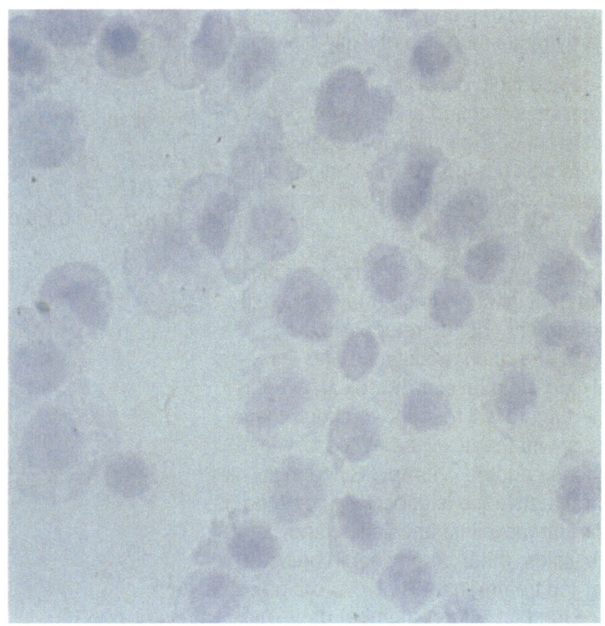

Fig. 62
These lung tumor cells (SA 180 cells) were stained with a monoclonal antibody against P-glycoprotein. The cell membrane of the multidrug-resistant cells (left) is stained brown. It contains a significant amount of P-glycoprotein. In drug-sensitive cells (right), no P-glycoprotein is found.

smokers. Of the 22 tumors of non-smokers, 11 were resistant and 11 sensitive. Of the 72 tumors of smokers, 57 (79%) were resistant and 15 (21%) sensitive. The difference in the incidence of resistant tumors in smokers and non-smokers is significant.

Of the 94 lung tumors, 44 (47%) showed a pronounced expression of P-glycoprotein. The increase of P-glycoprotein occurred almost exclusively in smokers (42 out of 44 P-glycoprotein positive tumors). This difference in the expression of P-glycoproteins in smokers and non-smokers is also significant.

We found a significant correlation between the resistance and the P-glycoprotein ($p < 0.0001$). 60% of the resistant tumors were found to have an increased expression of P-glycoprotein, whereas only 12% of the sensitive tumors showed such an expression. The increase of resistant bronchial carcinoma in smokers can thus be explained partly by an increase of P-glycoprotein.

A relationship between the number of cigarettes smoked and the number of resistant or P-glycoprotein positive tumors was not found. The findings were independent of age and sex, as well as of tumor stage.

Knowledge of these mechanisms of resistance in lung tumors may lead to the development of more specific therapies. The tumor resistance and the P-glycoprotein level may indicate whether the tumors will respond to chemotherapy or whether it will be necessary to choose another therapy. Since multidrug resistance is especially common for anthracyclins, antibiotics, and alkaloids, other drugs should be used for the treatment of P-glycoprotein positive tumors. A large number of chemosensitizers have been described which selectively intensify the effect of cytostatics in P-glycoprotein positive tumors. We thus expect that the therapeutic results of the treatment of lung tumors will be improved by measuring their resistance and their expression of P-glycoprotein and by employing suitable chemosensitizers.

In order to find whether our results are generally valid, we have started to analyze other tumors that also have an increased incidence in smokers (such as tumors of the bladder and of the kidneys). Additionally, we have also begun to analyze other resistance mechanisms to find out whether our results are restricted to P-glycoprotein.

Prof. Dr. Manfred Volm
Division of Oncological Diagnostics and Therapy

Participating scientists

Dr. Jürgen Mattern
Dr. Barbara Samsel

In collaboration with

Prof. Dr. Ingolf Vogt-Moykopf
Prof. Dr. Peter Drings
Thorax Clinic Heidelberg-Rohrbach

Selected Publications:

Volm, M., Wayss, K., Kaufmann, M., Mattern, J.: Pretherapeutic detection of tumour resistance and the results of tumour chemotherapy. Eur. J. Cancer 15, 983-993 (1979)

Thorgeirsson, S.S., Huber, B.E., Sorrell, S., Fojo, A., Pastan, I., Gottesman, M.M.: Expression of the multidrug-resistance gene in hepatocarcinogenesis and regenerating rat liver. Science 236, 1120-1122 (1987)

Volm, M., Bak, M., Efferth, T., Lathan, B., Mattern, J.: Immunocytochemical detection of a resistance-associated glycoprotein in tissue culture cells, ascites tumors and human tumor xenografts by Mab 265/F4. Anticancer Res. 8, 531-536 (1988)

Volm, M., Efferth, T., Bak, M., Ho, A.D., Mattern, J.: Detection of the multidrug resistant phenotype in human tumours by monoclonal antibodies and the streptavidin-biotinylated phycoerythrin complex method. Eur. J. Cancer Clin. Oncol. 25, 743-749 (1989).

Volm, M., Mattern, J., Efferth, T.: P-Glykoprotein als Marker für Multidrug-Resistenz in Tumoren und Normalgewebe. Tumordiagn. u. Ther. 5, 189-197 (1990)

Volm, M., Zerban, H., Mattern, J., Efferth, T.: Overexpression of P-glycoprotein in rat hepatocellular carcinomas induced with N-nitrosomorpholine. Carcinogenesis 11, 169-172 (1990)

5.3 Rational Development of Inorganic Antitumor Metal Complexes

by Walter Jens Zeller, Stefan Fruehauf and Bernhard K. Keppler

Many cytostatics (anticancer drugs) are analogues, i. e., compounds which are derived from a basic substance without significant changes in the mechanism of action. Examples are the nitrogen mustard compounds (such as mechlorethamine, “nitrogen mustard”), the group of the 2-chloroethylnitrosoureas (such as BCNU), the anthracyclines (such as doxorubicin), or the vinca alcaloids (such as vincristine).

For another group of compounds, the platinum complex compounds (derived from cisplatin), we use a rational preclinical strategy of investigation that avoids animal experiments. As a consequence of the introduction of cisplatin (DDP) into the therapy of certain cancers, such as testicular or ovarian carcinomas, clinical oncology has made a big leap towards healing these two types of tumors. Presently, there are two main drawbacks to cisplatin therapy: the frequently developing resistance and the significant toxicity (especially nephrotoxicity). These two shortcomings stimulate the search for other metal complexes with different mechanisms of action and toxicity profiles.

Although the mechanism of action of cisplatin is not completely known, there are indications that the cytostatic action is mediated mainly via a DNA interstrand cross-linkage and DNA intrastrand cross-linkage. DNA-protein cross-linkage apparently plays only a minor role in the chemotherapeutic action of this substance. On the other hand, DNA-protein cross-linkage is thought to be a main cause for undesired side effects. For example, it is known that the nephrotoxic compound cisplatin induces a high rate of DNA-protein cross-linkage and binds strongly to plasma-proteins. Less nephrotoxic platinum analogues, such as carboplatin, display a weaker plasma-protein binding. Thus, it is possible to attribute positive and negative components of the activity profile to underlying molecular mechanisms. Further work may then concentrate on eliminating the structural causes of the negative aspects of the activity profile.

Such a procedure seems to be useful also for other classes of cytostatics. For example, 2-chloroethylnitrosoureas (type BCNU) have both a desired DNA interstrand cross-linking as well as an undesired hydroxyethylating component of action. Since the latter appears to be mainly responsible for mutagenicity and cancerogenicity and hardly contributes to the therapeutic effect of this class of substances, it seems desirable to reduce or eliminate it as much as possible. Since cross-linkage and hydroxyethylation can be determined in vitro, it is possible to develop new and better substances without in vivo experiments. The dose-limiting toxicity of the anthracyclines (cardiotoxicity) is attributed to the formation of oxygen radicals and lipid peroxidation in myocardial cells. In vitro methods that measure both the formation of oxygen radicals and the therapeutic activity of a compound relative to the mother substance doxorubicin, may be successful in the development of less toxic analogues.

Our investigation of new platinum complex compounds using an experimental ovarian tumor was aimed to establish an in vitro system which may serve to detect promising new compounds of this class.

We investigated therapeutic and toxic profiles by means of genotoxicity experiments (DNA interstrand cross-linkage, DNA- protein cross-linkage, and DNA single-strand breaks) and cell proliferation studies. Conclusions on metabolism and certain pharmacologic properties of the substances, such as the rate of activation or sensitivity towards hydrolysis, may be derived from comparing short-term and long-term exposure assays. Three new platinum analogues are presented here. Results

Fig. 63
Comparison of the effect of four platinum-complex compounds on ovarian cancer cells. The abbreviation, ID70, stands for the dose which is necessary to inhibit the growth of the colony by 70%.

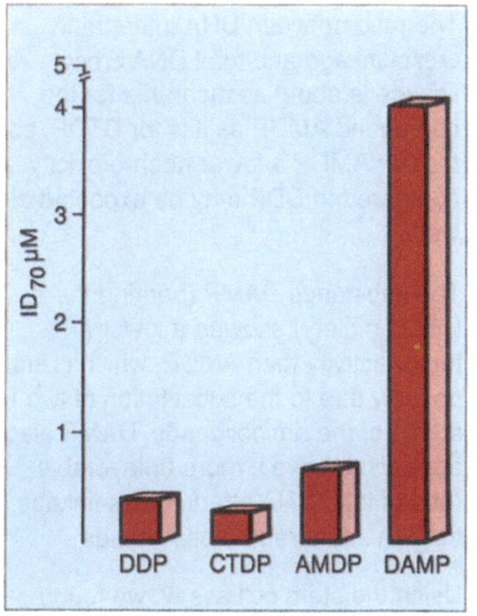

on other metal complex compounds (titanium and ruthenium compounds) have been published elsewhere.
As can be seen from Figure 63, the bis-dicarboxylate-platinum compound CTDP was the most effective of all analogues. During long-term incubation at equimolar concentration in the ovarian tumor line O-342, its activity was comparable to that of cisplatin. The genotoxic profile of CTDP is equally promising. The ratio of total DNA cross-linkage to DNA interstrand cross-linkage was about five for DDP and about one for CTDP. This shows that CTDP does not induce DNA-protein cross-linking. As a consequence, a reduced nephrotoxicity can be expected. The compounds AMDP and DAMP contain an osteotropic phosphonate and a cytostatically active platinum moiety and have been developed primarily for the treatment of bone tumors or bone metastases. Our results indicate a significant effect of both phosphonate-linked analogues on the ovarian tumor line O-342.

The ratio between DNA interstrand cross-linkage and total DNA cross-linkage is about as favorable for the compound AMDP as it is for CTDP, so that for AMDP a lower nephrotoxicity compared to DDP may be expected as well.

The substance DAMP (bearing the DACH moiety) showed a lower antitumor activity than AMDP, which is supposedly due to the substitution of two H atoms of the aminoligands. DAMP also appears to have a more unfavorable ratio of total DNA strand cross-linkage to DNA interstrand cross-linkage .

Using the stem cell assay, we found that differences in the sensitivity between resistant and sensitive tumor cell lines can be uncovered much more convincingly by long-term (>7 days) exposure of the tumor cells to the cytostatic compound than by short-term exposure (1 hour). For example, the ratio of the ID_{70} values (inhibitory $dose_{70}$: colony formation reduced to 30% of the control value) of cisplatin in the resistant line (ID_{70}: 33.5 μM) to cisplatin in the sensitive line (ID_{70}: 11.8 μM) was only 2.8 after short-term exposure. After long-term exposure, however, this ratio was tenfold higher (28), the ID_{70} values being 8.7 μM and 0.31 μM for the resistant and the sensitive cell lines, respectively. During long term exposure, the resistant line is apparently much more efficient in blocking the cisplatin effect than the sensitive line.

In summary, it can be concluded that new platinum complex compounds may be effectively characterized by in vitro experiments. It also seems possible to develop less toxic analogues (without loss of therapeutic activity) by determining various parameters of their genotoxicity and by comparing them with those of clinical reference compounds with a known profile of activity.

Prof. Dr. Walter Jens Zeller
Division of Perinatal Toxicology

Dr. Stefan Fruehauf
Medical University Clinic and Outpatient Clinic,
University of Heidelberg

Priv.-Doz. Dr. Dr. Bernhard K. Keppler
Inorganic-Chemical Institute,
University of Heidelberg

Selected publications

Zeller, W.J., Frühauf, S., Chen, G., Keppler, B.K., Frei, E., Kaufmann, M.: Chemoresistance in rat ovarian tumors. Eur. J. Cancer 27, 62–67 (1991)

Frühauf, S., Zeller, W.J.: In vitro evaluation of platinum, titanium and ruthenium metal complexes in cisplatin-sensitive and -resistant rat ovarian tumors. Cancer Chemother. Pharmacol. 27, 301–307 (1991)

Frühauf, S., Zeller, W.J.: New Platinum, Titanium and Ruthenium Complexes with different Patterns of DNA Damage in Rat Ovarian Tumor Cells. Cancer Res. 51, 2943–2948 (1991)

Keppler, B.K., Berger, M.R., Heim, M.E.: Neue tumorhemmende Metallkomplexe. In: Erhöhung des therapeutischen Index durch Reduktion der Toxizität, Hrsg. W.J. Zeller, K. Hellmann, B.T. Hill, M.R. Berger, D. Schmähl. Aktuelle Onkologie 61, 237–258 (1991)

5.4 Towards a Receptor-Mediated Chemotherapy

by Wilfried Hefter and Martin Berger

Up to now, no chemical substances are known that damage tumor cells exclusively. All antineoplastic agents in use today are also toxic to normal tissue. The therapeutic possibilities of a given substance therefore mainly rely on the difference in sensitivity of the tumor cells relative to the other body cells. There are about 200 different tumor types, all of which respond quite differently under chemotherapy; even within one tumor type significant differences in sensitivity may exist. For this reason, much work has been put into a more precise characterization of tumors in order to be able to select the most effective substances for chemotherapy. However, by optimizing chemotherapy this way, the unspecific mode of action and the resulting toxic side-effects are not expected to be altered dramatically. Current chemotherapy research therefore aims at developing substances that take advantage of the specific properties of certain tumor types for selective therapy.

The most common malignant tumor in women is cancer of the breast. Although breast cancer responds to chemotherapy at an advanced stage in 60–70% of the patients with a remission (i.e., a significant reduction or temporary disappearance of the tumor and its metastases, the effect of the therapy does not translate into an increased mean survival time of the affected women. 60–70% of the tumors have hormone receptors. These are receptors for a certain class of hormones (the steroid hormones), which, in their function as messenger substances, bind very specifically to cell molecules (the receptors) and thus initiate cell processes. This is the way, for example, in which the growth and differentiation of the glandular cells in normal breast tissue are controlled. It is a characteristic feature of steroid hormones that its receptors do not develop on the surface of the cell, as is the case for other hormone receptors; instead, the hormone enters the cell and acts, in conjunction with its receptor, directly on the DNA in the nucleus. In recent years, chemotherapeutic agents that are to act through these hormone receptors have been synthesized and tested.

Nitrosoureas are cytotoxic agents which, by virtue of their damaging action on the cell DNA, act in a highly antineoplastic way, but also have severe toxic side-effects. In order to increase the selectivity of a therapy with nitrosoureas, some of these cytotoxic drugs were chemically linked to steroid hormones. By means of the hormones, the cell-damaging agent should be preferentially introduced into those tumor cells containing corresponding receptors in order to specifically damage the DNA, whereas the normal tissue containing no or few receptors should be largely spared.

In the following, one of these hormone-linked agents was chosen as an example to demonstrate how far we have progressed in realizing this concept.

The substance is HECNU-succinyl-dihydrotestosterone (HS-DHT) (Fig. 1). The nitrosourea HECNU is linked by a "spacer", the succinic acid, to the male sex hormone dihydrotestosterone (DHT). DHT binds to its corresponding receptors and, in very high concentrations, also to the receptors for the female sexual hormone estradiol. If the conjugate of DHT and nitrosourea at least partly maintains an affinity towards the receptors, the result could be a more extensive damage of cells containing the corresponding receptors than of receptor-negative cells. The effect of the substance was therefore studied with the aid of two cell lines: the DHT and estrogen receptor-positive MCF-7 cells, a human breast cancer cell line, and the receptor-negative KB cells that stem from a human oral cavity carcinoma. Both cell lines can be bred continuously and thus are suited for comparative studies.

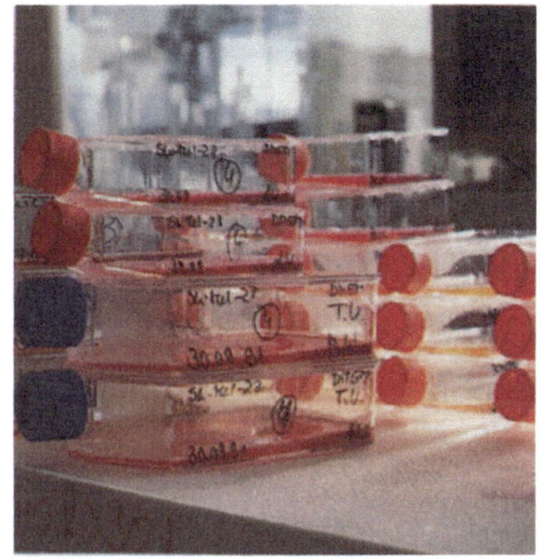

Fig. 64
Cultures of receptor-positive breast cancer cells and receptor- negative cells of a carcinoma in the oral cavity. In the Division of Carcinogenesis and Chemotherapy, conjugates from a chemotherapeutic agent and a steroid hormone are tested; they will selectively develop their cytotoxic effect via hormone receptors.

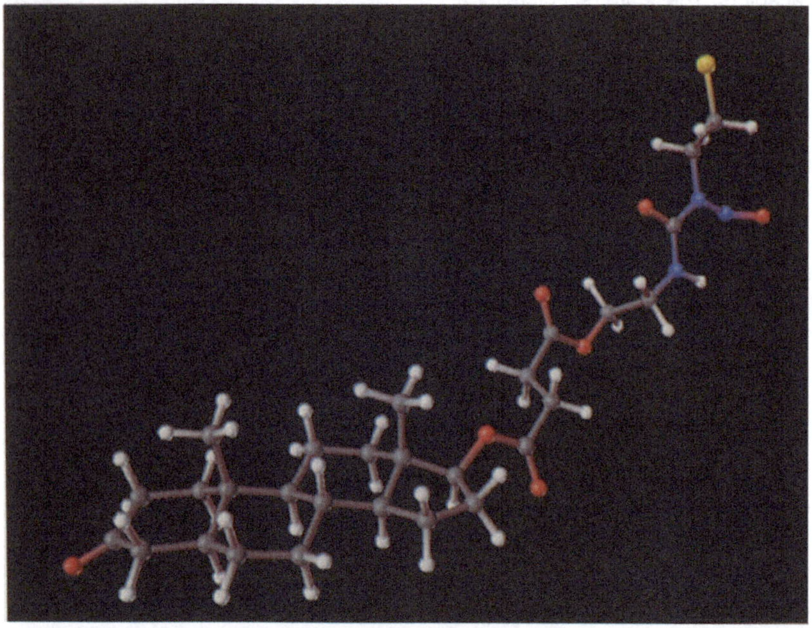

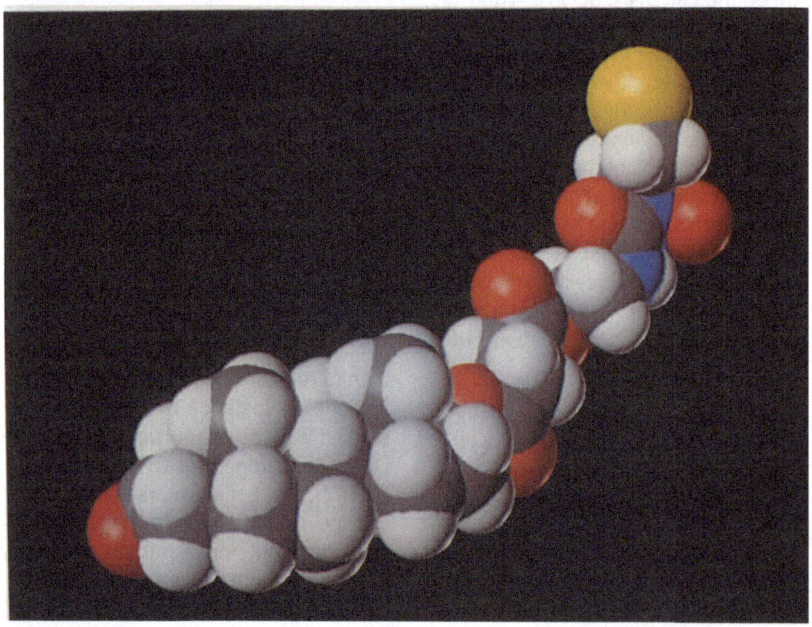

Fig. 65
Two different molecular models of a conjugate made from a chemotherapeutic agent and a steroid hormone, coupled together by a "spacer". In this way, the cytotoxic substance is introduced selectively into receptor-containing tumor cells.

Both, the conjugate HS-DHT and the mixture of the nitrosourea linked to the "spacer" (HS) and the hormone (DHT), as well as the effects of HS and DHT separately were investigated in the cell lines at comparable dosages, and after different incubation times. The growth of the cells was determined 4 days after the beginning of the treatment.

The conjugate HS-DHT exerts a similarly strong inhibition of the cell growth on both the MCF-7 and the KB cells. After an incubation time of only 6 hours, the growth of the cells is completely inhibited. In contrast to this, the growth inhibition by the mixture HS plus DHT is significantly weaker for both cell lines. Only after an incubation time of 4 days is the growth inhibiting effect of the mixture on the MCF-7 cells as pronounced as that of the conjugate.

DHT is distinctly less active than the mixture for both cell lines. Here, too, a strong growth inhibition can only be observed after long-term incubation (4 days).

The nitrosourea derivative HS is less active in the MCF-7 cells than in the KB cells. In the mixture, its effect adds up to that of DHT, yielding a cumulative inhibition of cell growth. This becomes especially obvious for the KB cells, since these cells are more sensitive to HS.

As a consequence, the difference in growth inhibition between the conjugate

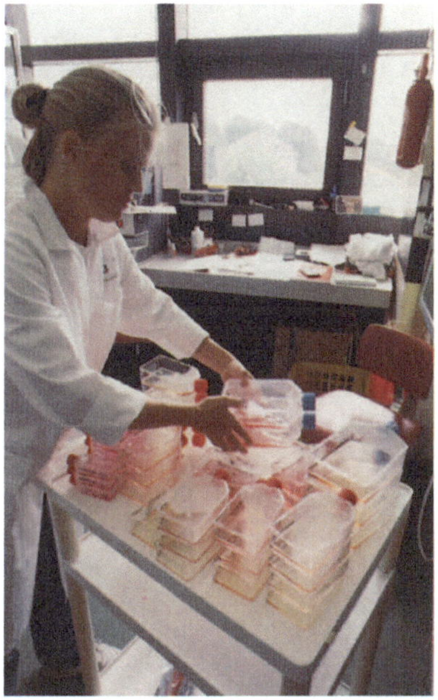

Fig. 66
Preparation of samples for high-pressure liquid chromatography, which gives clues about the efficacy of the tested medications.

HS-DHT and the combined mixture HS plus DHT is larger in the MCF-7 cells after up to 6 hours of incubation. Thus, the increase in response to HS-DHT is greater in the receptor-positive cells, which is an indication for a receptor-mediated mode of action.

In order to find out if the better effect of HS-DHT compared to that of the mixture in the MCF-7 cells is due to an additional receptor-mediated mechanism of action, we simultaneously incubated both cell lines with the conjugate and the hormones estradiol (E2) and dihydrotestosterone (DHT). The hormones occupy the receptors or replace the conjugate on the receptors under this condition. Thus, if the hormonal receptors were of importance for the action, the effect of the conjugate on the receptor-positive MCF-7 cells should diminish, whereas for the receptor-negative cells it should remain unchanged.

E2 can reduce the growth inhibition of small HS-DHT concentrations in a dose-dependent manner. Up to three-quarters of the action of the conjugate can thus be neutralized. The growth inhibition of the higher concentration is antagonized to a smaller extent. This is due to the fact that the effect of the conjugate is dominated at a higher dose by an unspecific action rather than by the receptor-mediated action.

The effect of HS-DHT can also partly be neutralized by DHT; however, less efficiently than with E2.

In contrast to these results, in the receptor-negative KB cells the effects of HS-DHT in both concentrations were not able to reduce either E2 or DHT.

The MCF-7 and KB cells were examined in order to verify if the action of the conjugate does indeed, as expected, result in higher receptor-mediated DNA damage caused by the nitrosourea.

The nitrosourea introduces strand breaks in the DNA, the extent of which can be measured. Under the given conditions, neither a dose of 100 μM HS nor of HS plus DHT causes detectable strand breaks; thus, we compared the effect of 500 μM HS with that of 100 μM HS-DHT.

Since KB cells are more sensitive to HS than MCF-7 cells, the rate of DNA strand breaks in the former is significantly higher than in the latter. For the conjugate, however, the situation is exactly the reverse. In the KB cells, 100 μM HS-DHT produced only about the same number of strand breaks as 500 μM HS, whereas in the receptor-positive MCF-7 cells the rate of strand breaks caused by the conjugate is five times greater than for 500 μM HS, which is significantly more than in the KB cells. The hormonal linkage of HS thus excessively increases the DNA damage in the MCF-7 cells. This means that, in accordance with the assumed mechanism of action, a comparatively higher effect of the conjugate on the receptor-positive cells can be shown, not only through differences in growth inhibition, but also on the level of the DNA.

The sum of all these results indicates an at least partially hormonal receptor-mediated action of HS-DHT in the receptor-positive MCF-7 cells.

In principle, it thus seems possible to utilize the receptors of steroid hormone receptor-positive tumors for therapy. It has to be taken into account, though, that all experiments were performed under laboratory conditions. But in animal experiments as well, HS-DHT proved to be more effective in the therapy of mammary tumors in rats than the mixture of HS and DHT, or than each of these substances separately.

Nevertheless, the substance examined is still far from developing its action in an ideal way. Very low concentrations suffice for the hormones to bind to their receptors. In order to achieve a receptor-mediated effect, however, the dose of the hormone-linked cytostatic has to be 1000 times higher; this, of course, reduces the action's selectivity and might induce unwanted side-effects, either by the substance itself or by its decay products. Several research groups, therefore, are synthesizing and examining compounds with presumably still higher receptor affinity in order to develop a therapy with lowest-possible dosage and best possible effect.

In summary, it is unlikely that this research will yield a chemotherapeutic agent for the treatment and healing of all types of breast cancer, since this disease is extremely varied in its manifestations. But it seems that it will be possible to develop a more effective therapy with less severe side-effects, compared to chemotherapy with today's agents.

Dr. Wilfried Hefter
Priv.-Doz. Dr. Martin Berger
Division of Carcinogenesis and Chemotherapy

Participating staff

Michaela König
Birgit Kaiser

In collaboration with

Prof. Dr. Gerhard Eisenbrand
Department of Food Chemistry and Environmental Toxicology, University of Kaiserslautern

Selected publications

Berger, M. R., Floride, J., Schmähl, D., Schreiber, J., Eisenbrand, G.: Estrogen-linked 2-chloroethylnitrosoureas: Anticancer efficacy in MNU-induced rat mammary carcinoma, uterine activity in mice and receptor interactions. Eur. J. Cancer Clin. Oncol. 22, 1179–1191 (1986).

Brix, H.P., Berger, M.R., Schneider, M.R., Tang, W.C., Eisenbrand, G.: Androgen-linked alkylating agents: biological activity in methylnitrosourea-induced rat mammary carcinoma. J. Cancer Res. Clin. Oncol. 116, 538–549 (1990).

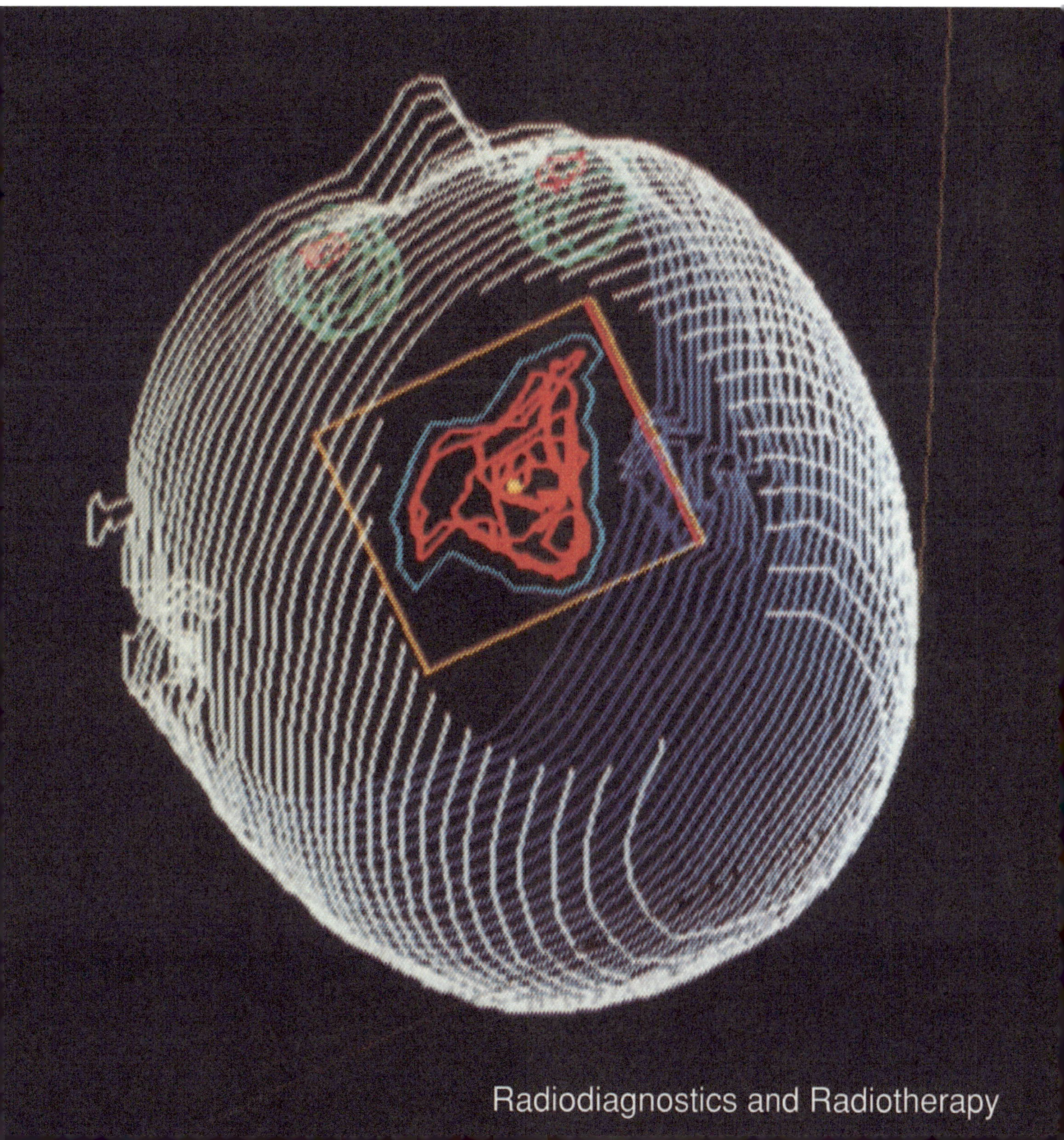
Radiodiagnostics and Radiotherapy

6

Radiodiagnostics and Radiotherapy

Radiology is one of the most important specializations in medicine for the detection, treatment, and follow-up of cancer diseases. Today, radiology not only encompasses conventional radiological methods of diagnosis and therapy, but also advanced techniques that make use of non-ionizing forms of radiation.

Research in Radiological Diagnostics

In the fight against cancer, diagnostics is of strategic importance. Failures in diagnosis can hardly be compensated by therapy.

Tumor diagnostics basically has the following tasks:

1. Detection of the tumor in the earliest possible stage;
2. Determination of its size, localization, relationship to organs, and spread ("staging");
3. Characterization of the tumor tissue through morphological, physiological, and biochemical parameters;
4. Control of the course of therapy, and
5. Diagnostic postoperative care.

The decisive first step in treating the individual cancer disease is the earliest possible detection of the tumor. Diagnostic procedures should put little strain on the patient so that they can be used as soon as suspicion arises. In general, the tumor develops without symptoms for several years before it is detected. At the time it is detected or when symptoms become evident, it has usually grown to a size of more than 1 centimeter. This means that, even in the case of an early detection, several million tumor cells have already grown.

After tumor detection, the next important diagnostical step is the determination of the tumor stage (staging). Staging is the basis for both the planning of the therapy and the evaluation of its success. Each tumor type requires the use of specific examination methods to determine its size, its spatial relationship to other structures, and its spread within the organism. Here, computed tomography has proven to be of great value. Computed tomography also is the basis for calculating advanced radiotherapy plans. Another goal of diagnostics is to find out the tumor's individual characteristics and its "internals". This is done by evaluating the tumor's histological properties in the microscope and, if necessary, in the electron microscope (grading). Recent approaches aim at detecting and quantifying physiological and biochemical parameters such as blood circulation and metabolism within the tumor, in the healthy surrounding tissue, and in metastases. This data provides important information for therapy planning and for the evaluation of the success of the therapy.

Modern diagnostic methods that make it possible to exactly monitor the effect of a therapy considerably help to optimize the treatment. The tumor's response to therapy can now be detected more precisely and earlier than it could have been 20 years ago. In the case of poor response, the treatment plan can thus be altered at an earlier stage of the therapy. After successful removal or apocatastasis of the tumor, the patient has to be continuously monitored in order to detect local relapses or metastases as early as possible. In follow-up examinations, of course, non-invasive methods that do not strain the patient are preferred over invasive techniques.

Various diagnostic methods are available for the detection and evaluation of the cancer disease:

1. Biochemical and immunologic examinations of body fluids (blood, urine, discharges, etc.);
2. Detection of tumor tissue with imaging techniques:
   a) radiodiagnostics
   b) endoscopy
   c) ultrasound diagnostics
   d) computed tomography
   e) magnetic resonance tomography
   f) scintigraphy, including immunoscintigraphy
   g) positron emission tomography;
3. Detection of individual tumor cells (cytodiagnostics) in the sputum, in smear, or in puncture fluid;
4. Pathological detection of tumor cell clusters through sampling of suspicious tissue.

Imaging techniques make it possible to detect tumors and metastases that are larger than 1 to 2 centimeters. Due to physical and biophysical limitations, however, it cannot be expected to enhance the resolution in the near future. Instead, the development in diagnostics is aimed at better specifying the characteristics of the detected foci.

In the recent past, diagnostic research focused on improving the evaluation of the tumor's size, its structure, and its functional performance on the basis of newly developed, advanced radiological methods. Such examinations have now become possible with magnetic resonance tomography and positron emission tomography.

Magnetic resonance tomography (MRT) images a specified portion of the body slice-by-slice; the slice images can then be evaluated by the physician. For the examination, the patient is placed in a strong magnetic field. Certain atomic nuclei, which have an intrinsic angular momentum (spin), behave like small magnets and align with the external magnetic field. They may be excited by radio waves whose frequency corresponds to the nuclei's precession frequency. The excited nuclei emit high-frequency signals that give information on the state of the tissue they are located in. However, these signals have to be decoded with the help of modern data processing methods. The use of even stronger magnetic fields makes it possible to also investigate specific metabolic processes occurring in the tissue (magnetic resonance spectroscopy).

Parallel to and supplementing MRT, the tumor tissue is also examined with positron emission tomography (PET). PET renders slice images of the distribution of radiolabeled organic substances within the body. A radiolabeled molecule, in which one of its atoms is replaced with a radioactive atom of the same kind, has the same biological properties as the corresponding unlabeled molecule. A fact of great importance for the analysis of metabolic processes is that radiolabelling makes it possible to measure quantitatively.

Positron emission tomography and magnetic resonance tomography make it possible to non-invasively measure important metabolic parameters (perfusion, metabolisms of glucose, phosphorus, and proteins, catabolism) of cancer drugs in the tumor. By comparing the treatment data with the data collected prior to and at the beginning of the treatment, the physician can draw conclusions about the success of the therapy or optimize the treatment protocol.

Therefore, both techniques are used in the search for tumors, in tumor staging, for monitoring the course of therapy and, most importantly, for the characterization of tumor tissue in the living organism.

Radiological Therapy Research

The term "cancer" does not mean one specific disease but is a comprehensive term for a multitude of different tumor types. Thus, it cannot be expected that all malignant tumors can be influenced or cured with one and the same therapy. One basic difficulty for some therapeutic techniques comes from the fact that the tumor cell has developed from a normal cell. Consequently, much lesser differences to normal cells can be exploited for therapy than, for example, in the case of bacteria.

There are various approaches to cancer therapy: surgical removal of the tumor tissue, radiotherapy, hyperthermia, hormone therapy, chemotherapy, and immunotherapy. Surgery and radiotherapy are local tumor treatments. They cannot be used, however, if the tumor has infiltrated vital organs, as a consequence of which radical removal or destruction of the tumor is no longer possible without damaging the healthy tissue. Preliminary results show that radiotherapy of various tumors can be effectively supplemented by local hyperthermia.

Chemotherapy is used for several types of solid tumors after they have metastasized. Chemotherapy has shown important results in the treatment of malignant diseases of the hematopoietic tissue (leukemia). Positive effects on primarily malignant tumors of the lymph nodes can be achieved through radiotherapy and/or chemotherapy, depending on the tumor's stage. In general, hormone therapy is limited to tumors whose cells carry hormone receptors.

In the field of radiotherapy, the activities of the Deutsches Krebsforschungszentrum aim at the complete elimination of the tumor while optimally sparing the neighboring healthy tissue. This objective can be realized by improving radiotherapy planning, in particular, by using computerized tomography and electronic data processing.

A particularly powerful radiotherapeutic technique being developed at the Deutsches Krebsforschungszentrum is photon conformation therapy. In conformation therapy, the tumor is irradiated from various directions, and an adjustable multi-leaf collimator adjusts the shape of the irradiating beam to that of the tumor for each direction of irradiation. Thus, the dose is concentrated and homogeneously distributed within the tumor, while the neighboring tissues are protected.

Another technique used for precision radiotherapy, stereotactic convergent beam irradiation, has been developed for the treatment of small tumors in the brain or in the region of the head and neck. The patient's head is immobilized, and the tumor is irradiated from various directions with highly collimated photon beams. Again, the dose is concentrated within the tumor and the neighboring healthy tissue is spared. This technique is used for single-high-dose irradiations of tumors, metastases and vessel deformations in the brain.

Another research project focuses on interstitial stereotactic brain tumor therapy. A special puncturing device allows the surgeon to precisely introduce a needle into the brain and advance it to a specified target point. The needle then serves to inject liquid or solid radioactive substances into the tumor. This makes it possible to irradiate the tumor from within while sparing the surrounding tissue. This technique also allows the surgeon to inject chemotherapeutic agents or to introduce special antennas, with the aid of which the tumor volume can be locally heated. The combined application of radiation, heat, and cytostatics may improve the success of the therapy.

Radiobiological factors limit the effect of photons and electrons in the treatment of highly differentiated and slowly growing tumors, as well as in the treatment of large tumors with central necroses. The use of high-energy neutrons may improve these results. Researchers of the Deutsches Krebsforschungszentrum have developed an angle-weighted isocentric radiation technique with fast neutrons. This method, too, produces a high dose concentration within the target volume and helps to protect the surrounding tissue. It is being used in the treatment of sialomas, soft-tissue sarcomas, and recurrences of rectal tumors.

Presently, a combined therapy of irradiation and hyperthermia is being tested for the treatment of tumors of the esophagus, the bile duct, the cervix, and the rectum. Controlled local hyperthermia can be produced with special antenna systems.

For many years, pulsed high-energy ultrasound has been used to destroy nephroliths. Experimental studies have shown that a modified form of this technique, in combination with radiation, heat, and chemical substances, is suitable for the local treatment of tumors. Clinical trials are planned to follow these preliminary experiments.

Another promising concept which is being further developed and applied at the Deutsches Krebsforschungszentrum is photodynamic therapy. A photosensitizer is introduced into the tumor via the circulating blood, and the tumor is irradiated with suitable laser light. The resulting chemical processes destroy the tumor from within. Researchers of the Deutsches Krebsforschungszentrum have succeeded in developing photo-sensitive substances with considerably higher accumulation rates in the tumor than has been achieved with previous substances. This method may improve the treatment of superficial tumors.

Clinical studies on all of the mentioned techniques are being carried out in close cooperation with the clinics of the Tumor Center Heidelberg/Mannheim and the Department of Stereotactic Neurosurgery of the University of Cologne.

Coordinator of the Research Program:
Prof. Dr. Walter Lorenz

Divisions and their heads:

Oncological Diagnostics and Therapy:
Prof. Dr. Gerhard van Kaick

Biophysics and Medical Radiation Physics:
Prof. Dr. Walter Lorenz

Radiochemistry and Radiopharmacology:
Dr. Wolfgang Maier-Borst

6.1 Positron Emission Tomography of Malignant Tumors in the Region of ENT and in the Lung

by Uwe Haberkorn and Michael Knopp

Developments in measurement techniques and medical diagnostics have made it possible to introduce positron emission tomography into clinical practice as a complementary imaging technique.

Radiodiagnostics use x-rays of various energies, whereas conventional nuclear medicine mainly relies on so-called gamma emitters as sources of radiation. Positron emission tomography (PET) uses positron-emitting isotopes.

Positron emitters have unstable nuclei that decay into stable forms. In the course of this process, a proton converts into a neutron by emitting a positron and a neutrino. A positron is a positively charged electron. In general, it interacts with the surrounding matter by "hitting" an electron. If this occurs, the particles convert into electromagnetic radiation in the form of two photons, which are emitted at an angle of 180°, and which each carry an energy of 511 keV. This annihilation radiation can be detected with an array of detec-

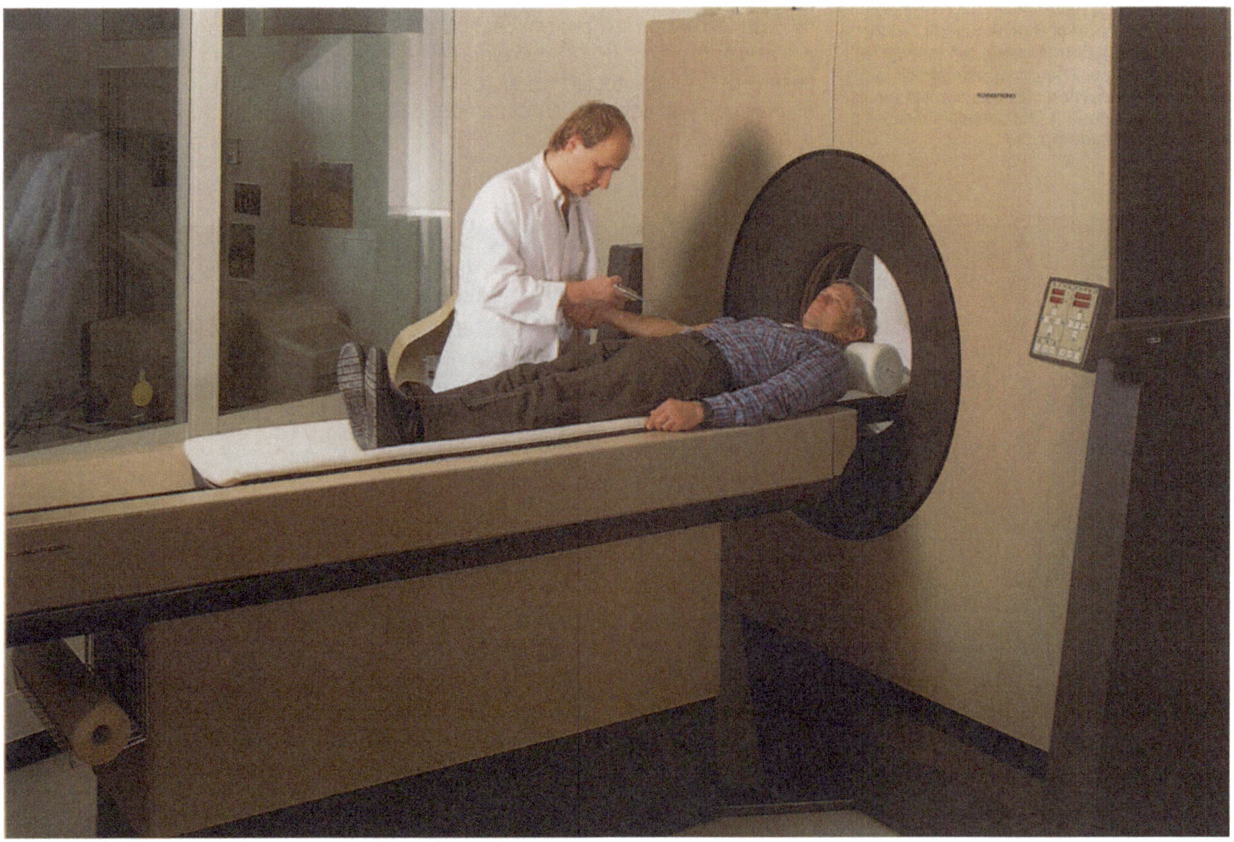

Fig. 67
Preparation of the examination of a patient with the positron emission tomograph, which measures metabolic processes in tumors.

tors arranged on a ring. Only those photons that are registered simultaneously (within a defined time interval) at opposite detectors are accepted as valid counts. This technique makes it possible to measure absolute activity distributions within the examined region and to calculate sectional images by locating the source of radiation.
The isotopes most frequently used are carbon-11 (C-11), nitrogen-13 (N-13), oxygen-15 (O-15) and fluorine-18 (F-18). These have short half-lives of between 2 and 108 min. Since these isotopes are present in organic compounds and can be used as substitutes for hydrogen and hydroxyl compounds, it is possible to study physiological processes in living organisms. After standardization on the basis of the applied activity and of the volume of distribution, absolute measurements permit one to make comparative measurements in the same patient or in various patients at different points in time.

The goal of our working group is the investigation of the tumor's metabolism and perfusion, as well as the observation and therapy planning for patients receiving radiotherapy or chemotherapy. The following radiopharmaceuticals are presently used: (F-18)-deoxyglucose (FDG), O-15-labeled water, (C-11)-aminoisobutyric acid, (N-13)-glutamate and (F-18)-5-fluorouracil.

Clinical Results for Tumors of the Ear, Nose and Throat (ENT)

Ideally, a diagnostic method should help the examiner to 1) make a decision about the basic disease, and 2) predict the further course of the disease. The diagnostic value of PET has already been proven by making it possible to differentiate between the scar and re-appearing tumors in patients suffering from colon tumors. There have also been indications for a possible prognostic significance of, for example, the accumulation of radioactively labeled deoxyglucose (FDG) in brain tumors in clinical as well as in animal studies. For human brain tumors, a relationship between the uptake of radioactively labeled glucose and the cellularly determined degree of malignancy has been established. Tumors in

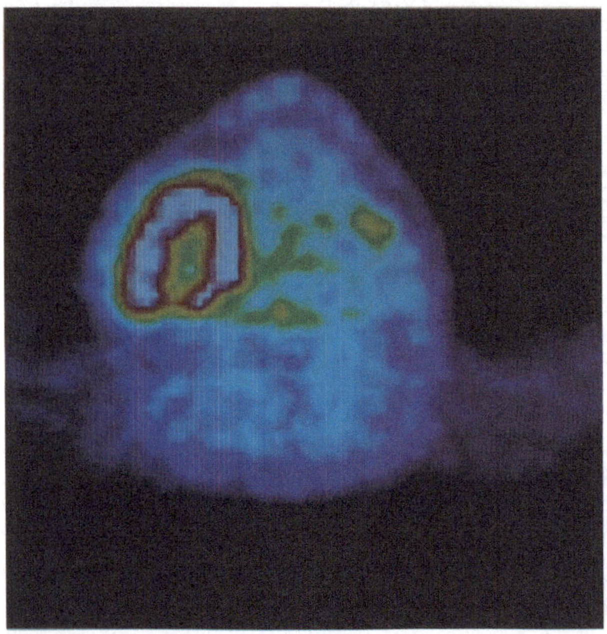

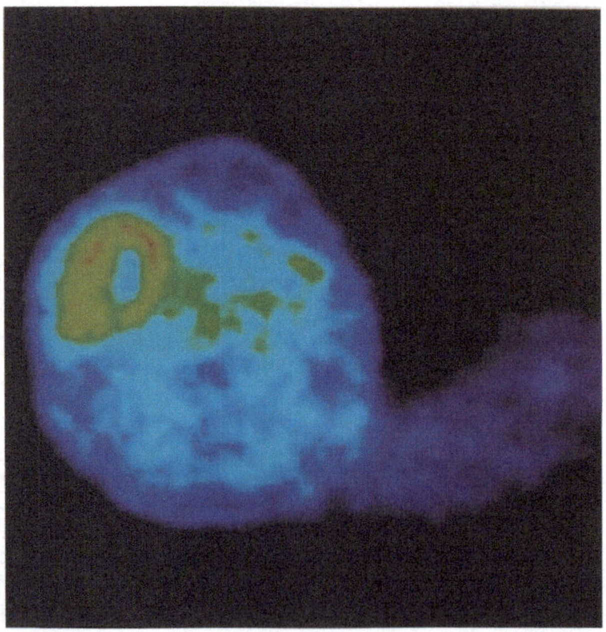

Figs. 68, 69
PET images of a patient with a lymph node metastasis of head and neck cancer – prior to (Fig. 68) and after (Fig. 69) the first cycle of chemotherapy. The evaluation shows a pronounced reduction of the accumulation of fluorodeoxyglucose (FDG), which indicates a response to the therapy.

Fig. 70
The green columns show a sufficient decrease in the FDG uptake in the patients responding to therapy; the red columns show an insufficient decrease or even an increase if the response to therapy is insufficient.

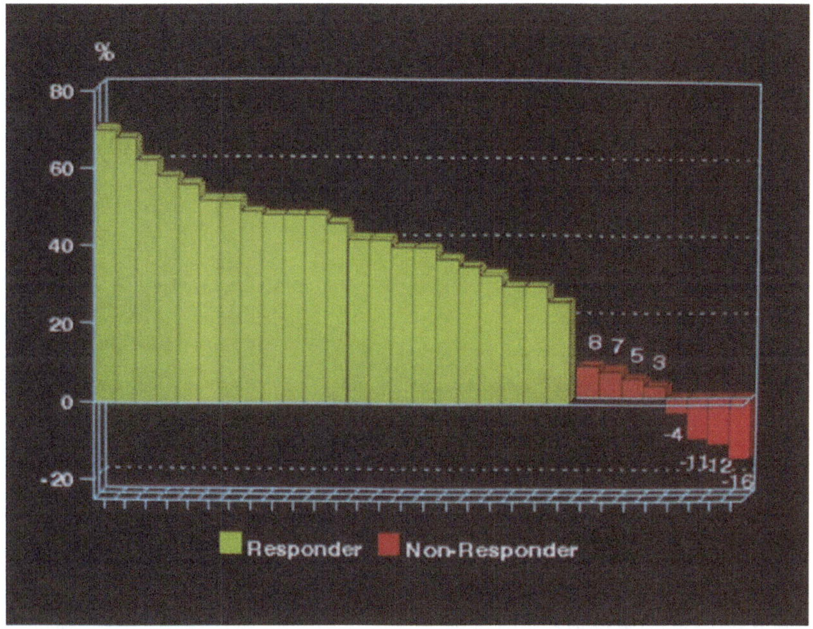

the rat brain showed that the regional glucose consumption depends on the synthesis of deoxyribonucleic acid (DNA). It was thus assumed that, in these tumors, the increased uptake and metabolization of glucose are mainly needed for the synthesis of DNA. Our own study on ENT tumors revealed the existence of two groups with differing FDG accumulation behavior. In addition to using PET, the proliferation rate, a measure of tumor growth, was determined by flow cytometry. This method permits one to rapidly determine the cell cycle phase distribution of the tumor cells. On the basis of these results, the proliferation rate can be calculated. In both groups, considerable changes in the proliferation rate were associated with only slight alterations in the accumulation of FDG. This finding shows that the synthesis of DNA alone does not sufficiently explain the increased accumulation of glucose. Recent studies in the field of molecular biology indicate that activated oncogenes may be another causal factor.

The observation of the therapy of ENT tumors is another important field of application for PET. In our institute, we carried out PET and computer tomographic (CT) examinations on patients subjected to combined chemotherapy. From the CT images, we determined the tumor volume prior to and after the first therapy cycle in order to calculate the tumor growth rate under therapy. The parameter used for PET was the accumulation of FDG, which was assumed to be lower in the case of effective therapy and constant or even increased in the case of ineffective therapy. The validity of these assumptions is supported by reports of animal experiments and preliminary clinical studies on tumors treated with radiotherapy and chemotherapy. As a result, our data indicated a decrease in the FDG accumulation after the first cycle of chemotherapy in only 43% of the cases. This finding corresponds to clinical response rates. However, a comparable change in the FDG accumulation was related to different growth rates for tumors and lymph nodes, which is also known in clinical practice. We conclude that the accumulation behavior of FDG as measured with PET can be used for the observation of chemotherapy patients. The possibility to evaluate the efficiency of the therapy at a very early point in time can help the assisting oncologist to match the therapy to the individual patient's needs.

Clinical Results for Lung Tumors

In non-invasive diagnostics of bronchogenic tumors, the introduction of modern sectional imaging techniques such as computer tomography and magnetic resonance tomography have led to significant advances in the clarification of bronchial masses. However, these sectional imaging techniques only make it possible to evaluate the form, location, and density of a given mass.

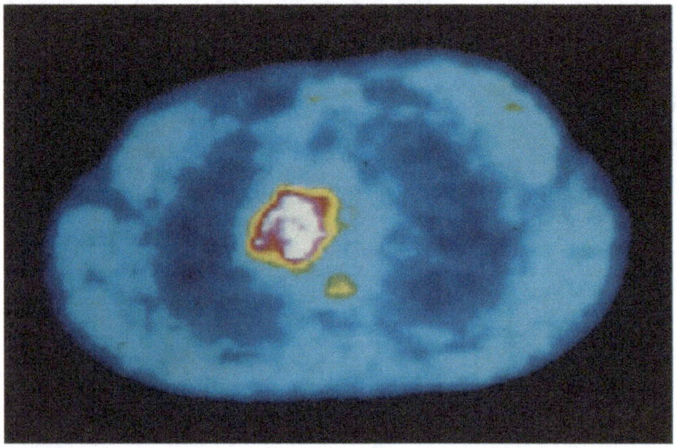

Fig. 71
PET image of a section through the thorax, showing an intensively accumulating bronchial tumor (red).

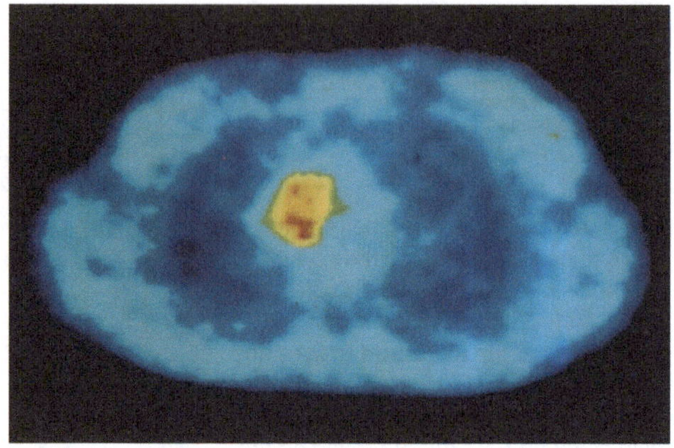

Fig. 72
Image of the metabolic activity. Its decrease after therapy is an indication for the response to therapy.

The injection of contrast media into blood vessels allows the examiner to draw conclusions about the perfusion. In contrast to this, PET provides information on metabolic processes if used with metabolically active substances such as fluorine-18-labeled deoxyglucose; furthermore, this information can be presented in sectional images. This metabolic data can be used for the differentiation of malignant tumors, inflammatory or scar alterations. By standardizing the examination and calibrating, it is possible to determine whether the metabolism of part of the examined tissue section is increased. Thus, precise measurement data on the metabolic activity can be obtained. Possible changes in these measurement values may then be used as observational parameters in follow-up examinations as a basis for the evaluation of the therapeutical success.

An important criterion in medical imaging is provided by the contrast behavior of a specific focus as compared to the surrounding tissue. The normal metabolic activity of lung parenchyma is, due to the large volume of air, relatively low. The metabolic activity of inflammatory alterations is higher than normal, but still lower than in malignant masses and with a more irregular pattern of distribution. For diagnostic clarification, it frequently does not suffice to detect the tumor; it may also be necessary to evaluate the lymph outflow tracts. PET makes it possible to differentiate between inflammatory hypertrophied lymph nodes and metastatic lymph nodes within the thorax. Presently, however, the device-dependent detection limit for the lymph nodes is a minimum diameter of 1 centimeter. Our results have shown that, in doubtful cases of tumor-affected lymph nodes, PET can considerably improve the classification of the tumor stage. PET can provide important information for the evaluation of the tumor stages, in particular, through the direct imaging of active tumor masses and their anatomical relations. This is of particular importance if the morphological findings do not permit one to differentiate unambiguously between the tumor and its inflammatory neighboring regions.

Another important field of application for PET is the observation of a tumor's biological behavior under therapy. It is possible to measure the response of a tumor even before a change in its volume is observed, by comparing the tumor's PET data under therapy to those acquired before therapy. We carried out follow-up examinations of thoracic masses in patients receiving chemotherapy and/or radiotherapy. Early detection of the tumor's response to therapy is of even greater importance as more treatment methods become available. If, at an early stage in therapy it becomes evident that it does not produce the desired result, it is possible to decide on another treatment protocol.

In a preliminary investigation as part of a case control study, we examined 21 patients with PET prior to and during therapy. All those patients for whom the applied therapy protocol was successful (14/21) showed a clearly decreased FDG accumulation. The remaining patients (7/21), who did not respond to the therapy protocol, did not show a considerable change in the FDG accumulation. Thus, if a PET examination reveals at an early point in time that the tumor does not respond to the chosen protocol, the unsuccessful therapy can be discontinued in order to avoid possible side-effects.

PET can also help to determine whether the tumor has been entirely destroyed or if an active residual tumor remains present. If PET reveals the presence of an active residual tumor, the treating physician can decide whether an additional treatment protocol should be applied.

Conclusion

The results achieved during recent years in cooperation with various study groups have established the significance of PET for the diagnostic clarification of masses and possible lymphatic metastatic spread. Its diagnostic application in the clarification of uncertain masses is particularly important if other non-invasive techniques produce ambiguous findings. Another important feature is that PET, for the first time, makes it possible to non-invasively observe the metabolism of tumors under therapy and to do so at a time that is too early to permit precise conclusions based on volume change of a tumor alone. This additional information significantly advances therapy follow-up and makes it possible to individually optimize the therapy protocol, the goal being to objectively determine the best possible therapy protocol and to make it possible to realize the most promising therapy.

Dr. Uwe Haberkorn
Dr. Michael Knopp
Division of Oncological Diagnostics and Therapy

Participating scientists

Priv. Doz. Dr. Ludwig G. Strauss
Prof. Dr. Gerhard van Kaick
Division of Oncological Diagnostics and Therapy

Dr. Josef Doll
Prof. Dr. Walter J. Lorenz,
Dr. Hermann Ostertag
Division of Biophysics and Radiation Physics

Dr. Wolfgang Maier-Borst
Dr. Franz Oberdorfer
Division of Radiochemistry and Radiopharmacology

In cooperation with

Dr. Helge Bischoff
Thorax Clinic Heidelberg

Dr. Christof Reisser
Clinics for Diseases of Ear, Nose, and Throat of the University of Heidelberg

Selected publications

Strauss, L.G., Clorius, J.H., Schlag, P., Lena, P., Kimmig, B., Engenhard, R., Marin-Grez, M., Helus, F., Oberdorfer, F., Schmidlin, P., van Kaick, G.: Recurrence of Colorectal Tumors: PET Evaluation. Radiology, 170, 329–332 (1989)

Knopp, M.V., Strauss, L.G., Dimitrakopoulou, A., Haberkorn, U., Blatter, J., van Kaick, G.: Positron Emission Tomography for the diagnostic work up in thoracic oncology. Nuklearmedizin Hrsg. H. Schmidt et al., 58–60 (1990)

Haberkorn, U., Strauss, L.G., Reisser, Ch., Haag, D., Dimitrakopoulou, A., Ziegler, S., Oberdorfer, F., Rudat, V., Kaick, G.: Glucose uptake, perfusion and cell proliferation in head and neck tumors: relation of positron emission tomography to flow cytometry. J. f. Nucl. Med. 32, 1548–1555 (1991)

6.2 Precision Radiotherapy of Tumors in the Region of the Head and Neck: A New Approach to Tumor Therapy

by Wolfgang Schlegel
and Günther Gademann

The Significance of Local Tumor Treatment

In Germany, every year about 250 000 persons fall ill with cancer. One of the most important treatment methods is radiotherapy, which is used in about half of all cases. In spite of significant successes in local cancer treatment, which is able to heal about 35% of all cancer patients, about 30% of all patients still die of a locally growing tumor.

These tumors are mostly locally growing tumors in the regions of the brain, skull, and neck. Since, in general, they cannot be totally resected by surgical intervention, the operation must be followed by an irradiation of the tumor or its remnants. The close vicinity of radiosensitive organs, such as the optic nerves, the spinal cord and the brain stem, often means that with conventional irradiation techniques it is not possible to apply a sufficiently high dose to the tumor without inducing serious damage to the healthy tissue.

One focus of the Research Program Radiological Diagnostics and Therapy of the Deutsches Krebsforschungszentrum is the improvement of the radiotherapeutic possibilities of newly developed methods and powerful computer techniques. These are based on advanced imaging techniques such as computed tomography (CT) and magnetic resonance tomography (MRT). The technique of precision radiotherapy of tumors in the region of the head and neck, which is presented here, was developed at the former Institute of Radiology and Pathophysiology of the Deutsches Krebsforschungszentrum. In collaboration with the Radiological Clinic of the University of Heidelberg it is already used in the treatment of patients. Precision radiotherapy concentrates the highest possible dose in the region of the tumor, while sparing as much as possible the neighboring, sometimes extremely radiosensitive, normal tissue.

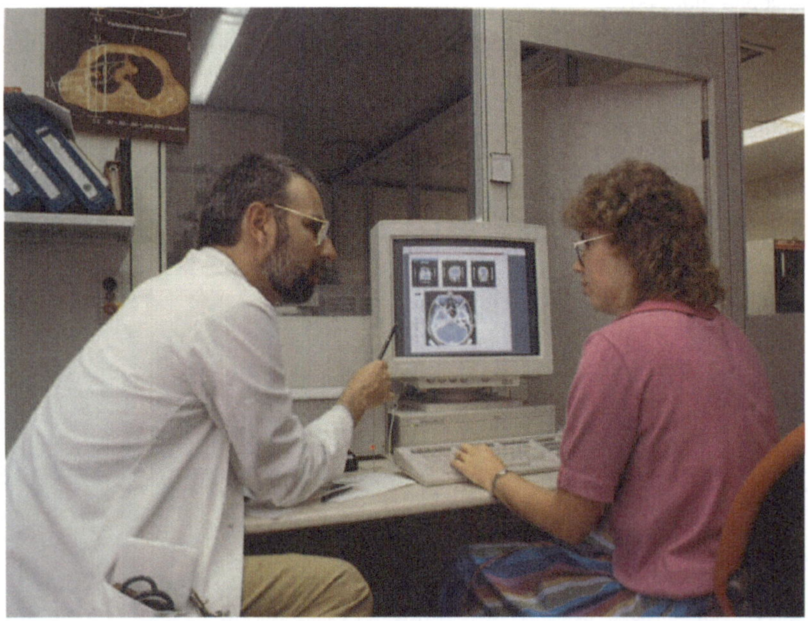

Fig. 73
A radiotherapist and a medical informatician planning treatment.

New Ways for Improving the Exactness of Radiotherapy

One way to protect the normal tissue is to spread the applied dose over a period of several weeks. This, however, requires that for each treatment the patient is positioned in exactly the same way. This can be achieved with a head mask, which is individually fabricated for each patient. Prior to the beginning of the treatment, the mask is used for the CT examination which is used to display the tumor on the computer screen. In many cases, however, the tumor can be more safely delineated in MRT images. This examination, too, requires the use of the head positioning mask.

Computer Methods for Radiotherapy Planning

The computer superimposes MRT and CT images. In the MRT images, the physician delineates the tumor target area, which is then transferred into the CT images. Only on the basis of CT data can the physical dose distribution in the patient be calculated. Organs at risk, which are to be spared during treatment, are also delineated electronically in the computer images. The computer now has complete spatial information on the position and the shape of the target area and the organs at risk. The target area, the organs at risk and the perimeter of the patient's head can be viewed under any angle on the computer screen, in order to check the data.

After these preparations, the treatment can be planned. In precision radiotherapy, a concentration of the dose to the target area is achieved by using two tricks. First, the patient is irradiated from not less than three directions, which are selected in such a way that organs at risk are spared. This makes it possible to concentrate the dose in the area of intersection of all the irradiating beams. Second, a variable collimator is used to exactly match the shape of the irradiating beam to the tumor's contour. The surrounding normal tissue is thus optimally shielded.

After the directions of the irradiation and the shape of the collimator have been set, the computer calculates the resulting dose distribution. On the monitor, the dose distribution, which is represented either as a set of colored isodose lines or as colored areas, is superimposed over the CT images. The radiotherapy plan is optimized and recalculated until the dose distribution best matches the target area and until the surrounding tissues, in particular the organs at risk, are optimally spared.

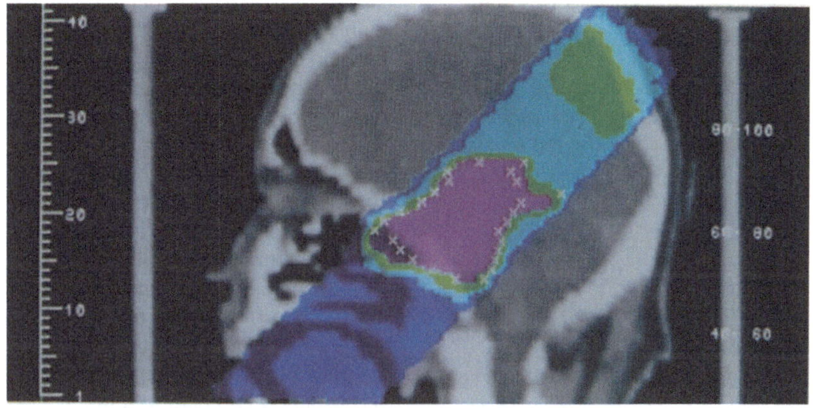

Fig. 74
The computer calculates a side view of the head. This makes it possible to plan unusual irradiation schemes.

Development and Use of High-precision Mechanical Devices

Another prerequisite for the introduction of precision radiotherapy at the Deutsches Krebsforschungszentrum, aside from advanced computer software, was the development of suitable mechanical parts. A stereotactic fixing device, to which the patient's head mask is attached, guarantees that for all individual irradiations the patient positioning can be reproduced with an accuracy in the range of millimeters. Another important development of the Deutsches Krebsforschungszentrum is the above-mentioned beam collimator consisting of many individually adjustable tungsten leaves. Prior to the irradiation the multi-leaf collimator, which is attached to the linear accelerator, is set to outline the contour of the tumor. The irradiating beam thus always matches the shape of the tumor as seen from the direction of irradiation. High-precision radiotherapy is applied daily over a period of 5 to 7 weeks.

Fig. 75
Spatial images (here of a brain tumor) allow the radiotherapist to exactly match the irradiating beam to the shape of the tumor (blue line around red tumor).

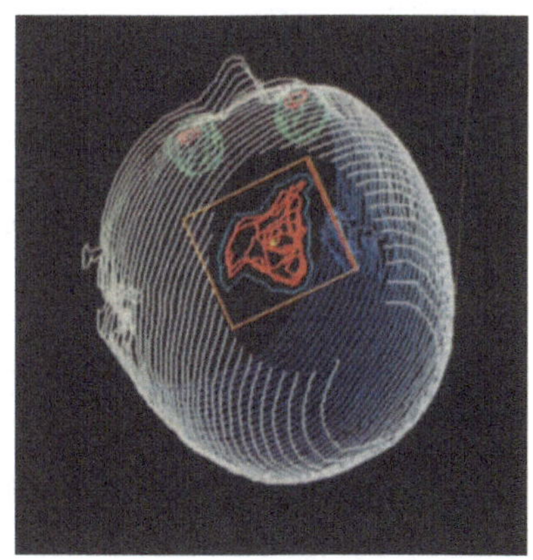

First Clinical Experiences with Precision Radiotherapy

During the past 3 years, 160 patients were treated with precision radiotherapy. Many of the treated tumors, such as the more benign tumors of the meninges and perinuria, but also slowly growing brain tumors, are known to be rather radioresistant. However, first results indicate that during the observation period of an average of 12 months, in 90% of the patients the tumor did not continue to grow. In most cases, tolerance towards precision radiotherapy was extremely good. Due to the concentration of the irradiation inside the patients, even local loss of hair was rarely observed. In about one-third of the patients, the symptoms improved visibly during and after treatment.

The clinical experiences with this new method are only preliminary and may not be overestimated. However, the results obtained so far indicate that, in spite of applying radiodoses which by far exceed those acceptable with conventional techniques, treatment is in most cases well tolerated and the growth of the tumors can be inhibited.

Fig. 76
An individually shaped plastic mask is attached to the metal bars of the stereotactic aiming device. The linear accelerator's laser positioning device allows the radiotherapist to exactly adjust the spatial coordinates.

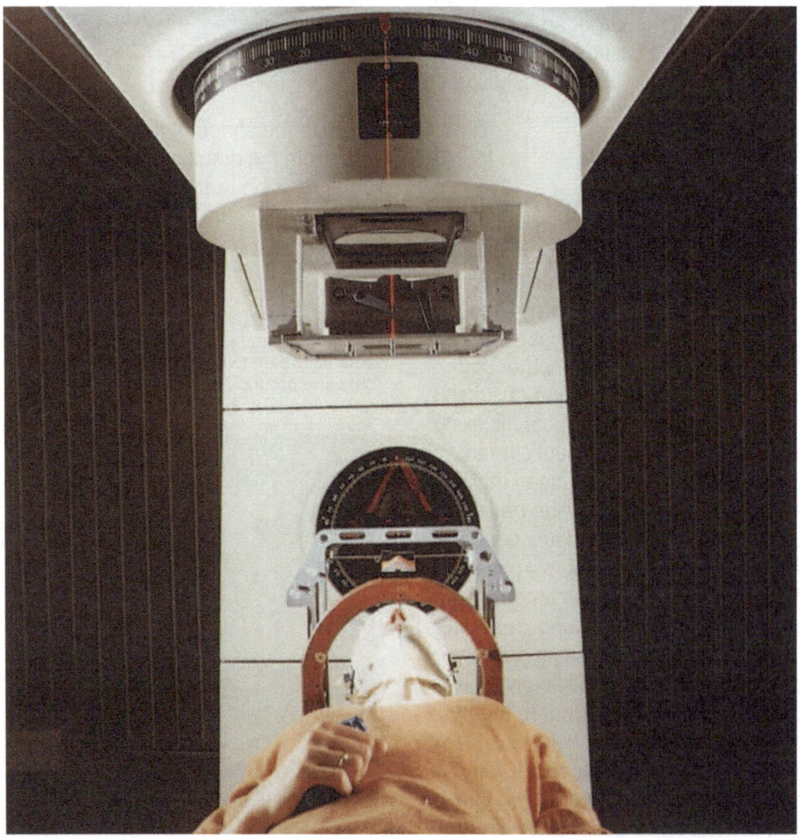

Future Goals: Extension and Propagation of the Treatment Technique

Precision radiotherapy was developed and clinically applied by a closely cooperating research group of physicians, scientists, and technicians of the Deutsches Krebsforschungszentrum and the University of Heidelberg's Radiological Clinic. The work is sponsored by the Tumor Center Heidelberg/Mannheim. It is planned to generalize the methods developed for the head and neck region for radiotherapy of tumors in the body.

Another important aspect is to clinically test the developed methods in other hospitals. After the clinical significance has been demonstrated, the precision radiotherapy should be made available for general use. Presently, the funds supplied by the German Cancer Aid (Deutsche Krebshilfe) allow us to distribute our advanced three-dimensional computer planning programs to other radiotherapeutic institutions and hospitals and to adapt it to local conditions and requirements. Presently, our software is installed at the university hospitals of Würzburg, Berlin, and Hamburg, at the Royal Marsden Hospital in London and at the Heavy Ion Accelerator Laboratory (LBL) in Berkeley, California, USA. Presently, joint projects with the university hospitals of Tübingen, Freiburg, Erlangen, and the Paul Scherrer Institute in Villingen, Switzerland, are being planned. After professional retouching of the software and of the mechanical components by a medical company, the technique will soon be available to all interested radiotherapeutic hospitals.

Improving local radiotherapy also means considering the use of other types of radiation, such as charged particles. The Deutsches Krebsforschungszentrum is actively participating in several such projects in Europe. It is foreseen that the range of tumor types and localizations that can be effectively treated with advanced methods will grow significantly in the future.

Priv.-Doz. Dr. Wolfgang Schlegel
Biophysics and Medical Radiation Physics

Priv.-Doz. Dr. Günther Gademann
Clinical Radiology Department, Radiotherapy, Radiological University Clinic Heidelberg

Participating scientists

Dr. Sabine Behrens
Dipl.-Inform. Med. Rolf Bendl
Dr. Thomas Bortfeld
Dr. Josef Doll
Dr. Karl-Heinz Höver
Dr. Sylvia Otto-Oelschläger
Ing. Otto Pastyr
Division of Biophysics and Medical Radiation Physics

Dr. Josef Bürkelbach
Dr. Rita Engenhart
Dr. Jürgen Romahn
Clinical Radiology Department, Radiotherapy, Radiological University Clinic Heidelberg

Selected publications

Bauer-Kirpes, B., Schlegel, W., Boesecke, R., Lorenz, W. J.: Display of organs and isodoses as shaded 3-D objects for 3-D therapy planning. Int. J. Radiat. Oncol. Biol. Phys. 13, 135–140 (1987)

Boesecke, R., Doll, J., Bauer, R., Schlegel, W., Pastyr, O., Lorenz, W. J.: Treatment Planning for conformation therapy using a multi-leaf collimator. Strahlentherapie und Onkologie 164, 151–154 (1988)

Gademann, G., Schlegel, W., Becker, G., Rohmahn, J., Höver, K. H., Pastyr, O., van Kaick, G., Wannenmacher, M.: High precision radiotherapy of head and neck tumours by means of an integrated stereotactic and 3D planning system. Int. J. Radiat. Oncol. Biol. Phys. 19, suppl. 1, 135 (1990)

Schlegel, W.: Computer Assisted Radiation Therapy Planning. In: 3D Imaging in Medicine, Ed. K. H. Höhne, NATO ASI Series Vol. F60. Springer, Berlin pp. 399–410 (1990)

6.3 A New Method for the Visualization of Blood Vessels: Magnetic Resonance Angiography

by Wolfhard Semmler and Andreas H. Gamroth

In recent years, a magnetic resonance (MR) technique has been developed that makes it possible to image blood vessels without a contrast medium.

The new method exploits the fact that MR signals of tissue at rest differ from those of blood in motion. Several techniques create high-contrast sectional images of blood vessels (Fig. 78), while the stationary tissue remains dark.

With the aid of modern computer technology these high-contrast sectional images can be combined to form a three-dimensional model of the vascular tree. If a projection ray is made to penetrate these sections, high signal intensities from flowing blood can be registered. As a result, a selective three-dimensional image of all vessels with blood flow is obtained (maximum intensity projection, MIP). This volume can then be viewed three-dimensionally from various orientations and the physician can view the rotating vascular tree of the examined body region. Thus, additional images taken from different angles are no longer needed.

Fig. 77
Magnetic resonance tomographer with control unit for the supervision of the examination by the physician.

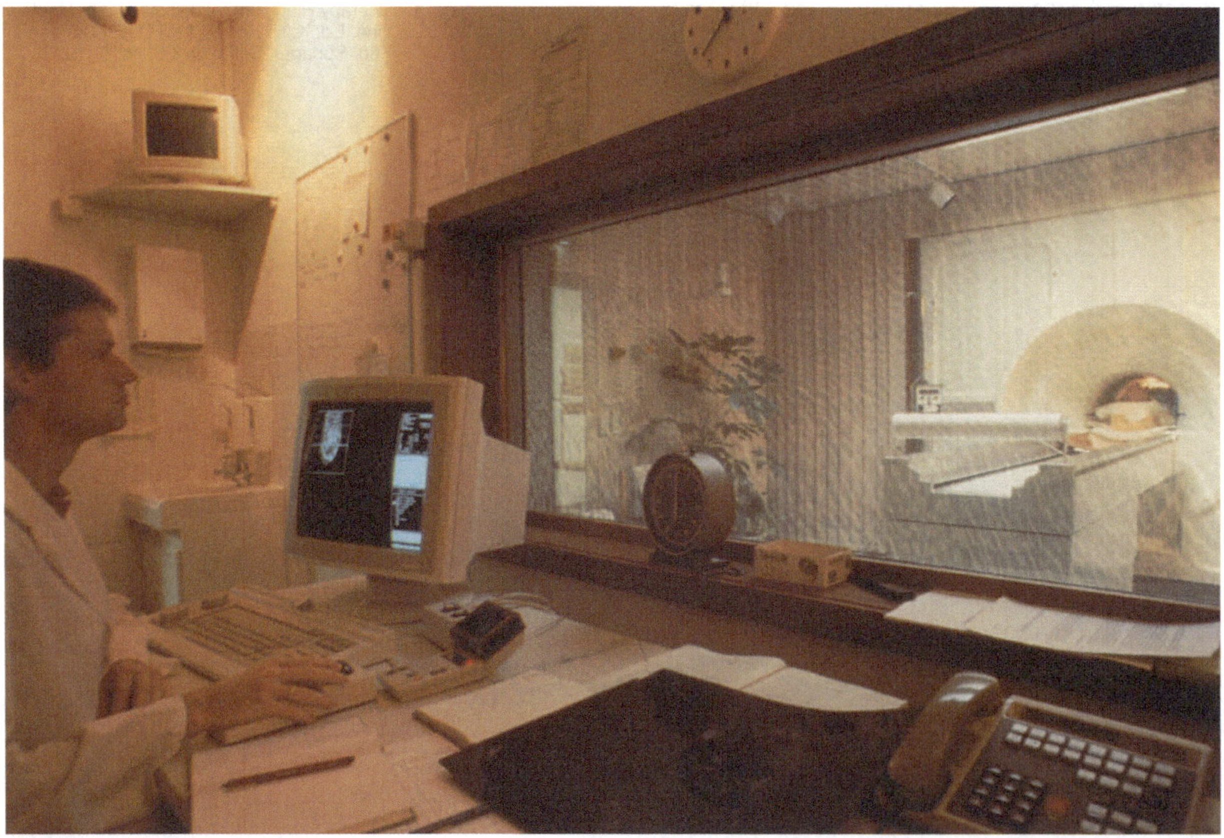

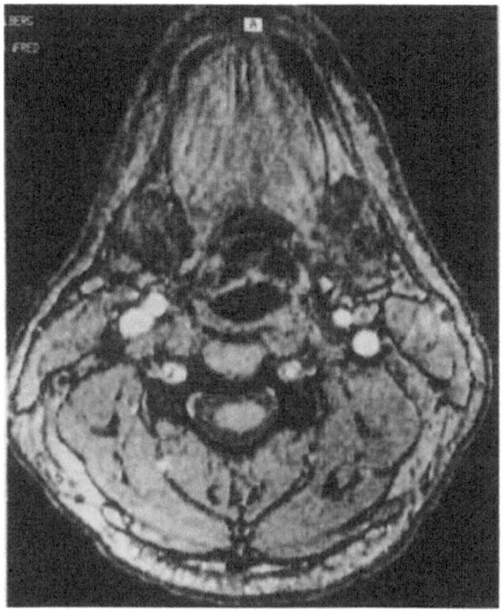

Fig. 78
High-contrast magnetic resonance angiographic image of the blood vessels in the region of the neck.

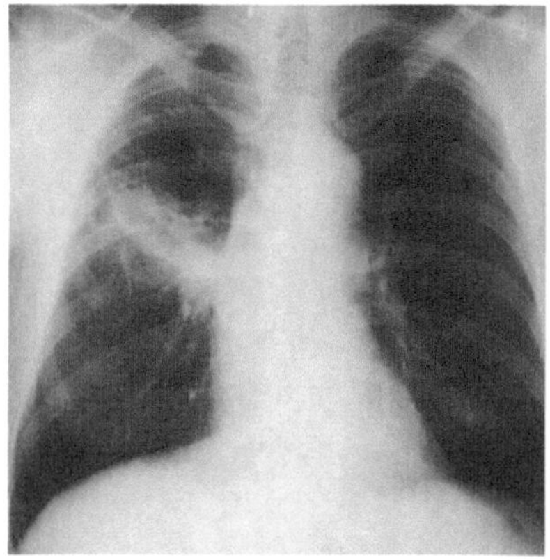

Fig. 79

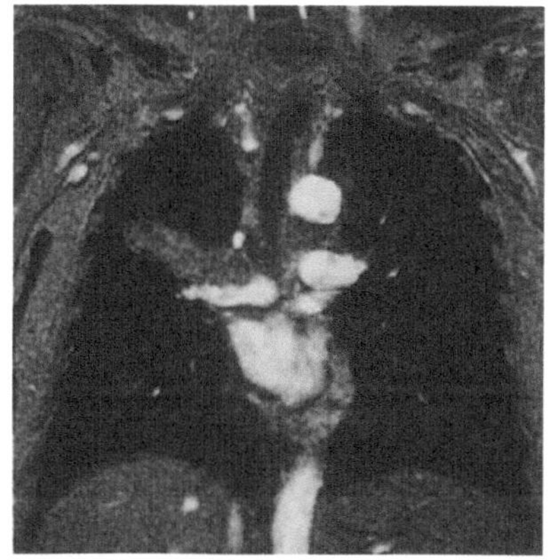

Fig. 80

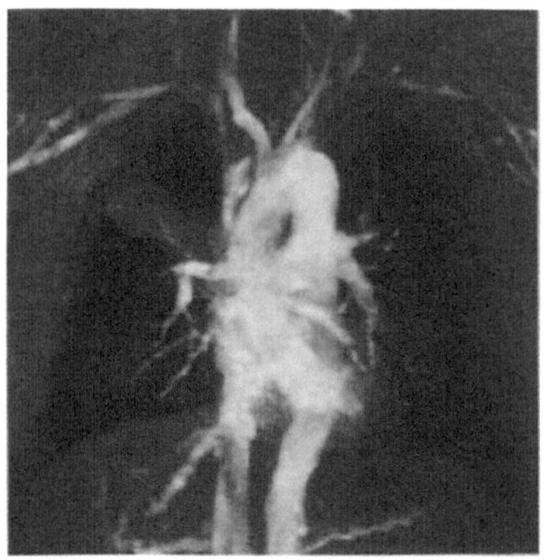

Fig. 81

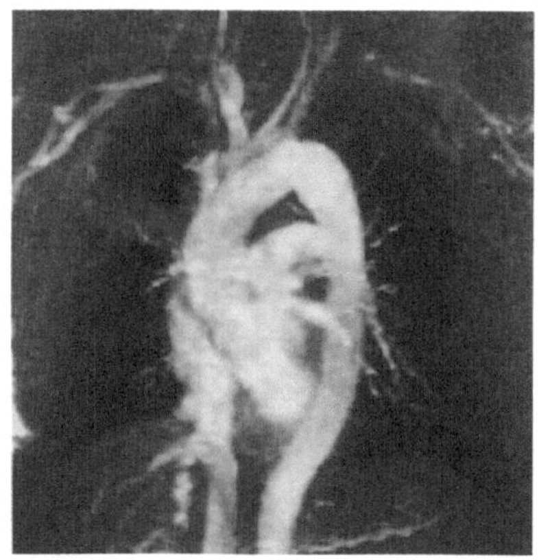

Fig. 82

What purpose does this new technique serve? Will it be of importance for cancer diagnostics?

In cooperation with our clinical partners from the Tumor Center Heidelberg/Mannheim, we employed this new technique on patients suffering from various types of tumors. The strain on the patients was low, since they only had to undergo an MR examination lasting between 15 and 30 minutes. A contrast medium was not administered.

In cooperation with the Thorax Clinic Heidelberg-Rohrbach we examined patients suffering from lung cancer. Therapists, surgeons in particular, are interested in knowing to what extent the tumor has displaced or occluded blood vessels. Figure 79 shows a conventional x-ray image of the lung of a patient with right central bronchial carcinoma. The tumor, neighboring inflammatory alterations, and large vessels cannot be discerned. In contrast, MR angiography (MRA) provides high-contrast images of the large vessels and of the heart cavities (Fig. 80). It is apparent that the right pulmonary artery is being compressed by the tumor (arrow). Figures 81 and 82 demonstrate the advantage of three-dimensional projection. Figure 81 shows a sagittal projection of the vascular tree, which in Figure 82 is rotated by about 35° to the right, thus allowing the viewer to look into the "aorto-pulmonary window," the space between the large thoracic aorta and the main pulmonary artery.

One further application of MRA resulted from our cooperation with the Radio-

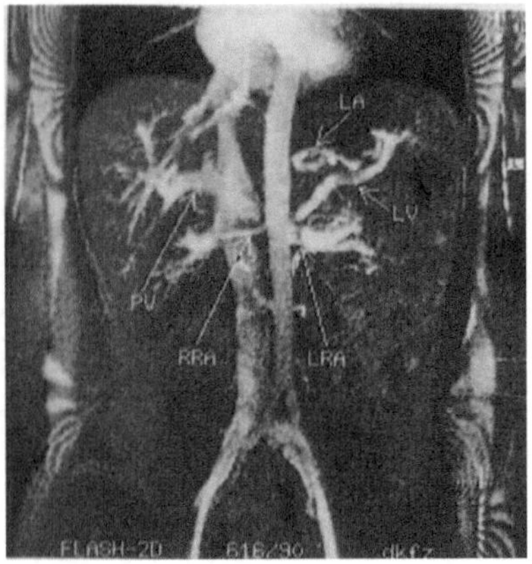

Fig. 83

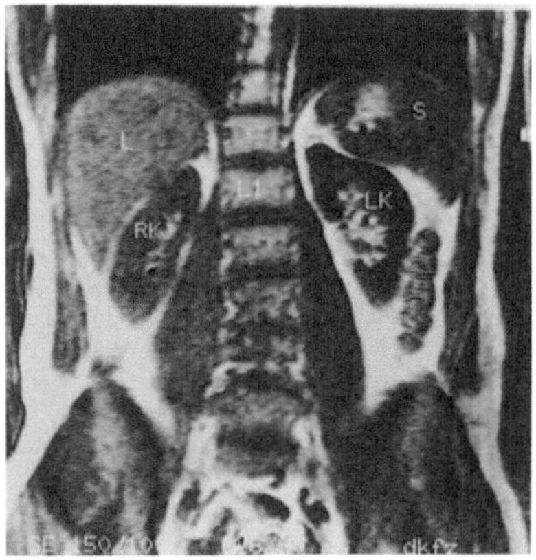

Fig. 84

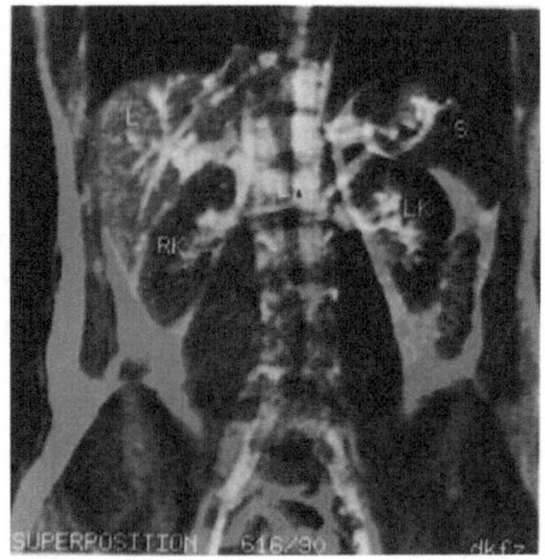

Fig. 85

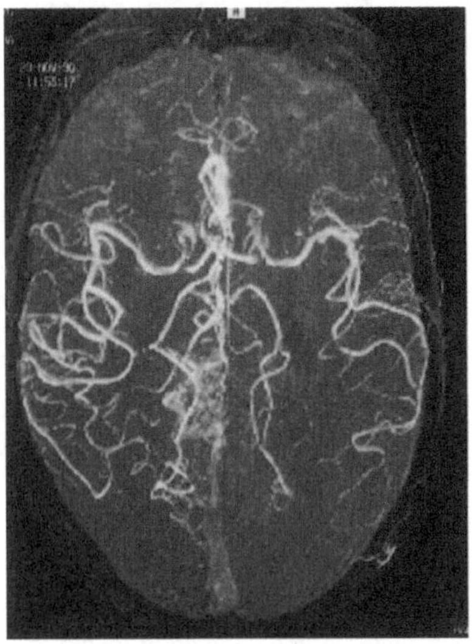

Fig. 86a

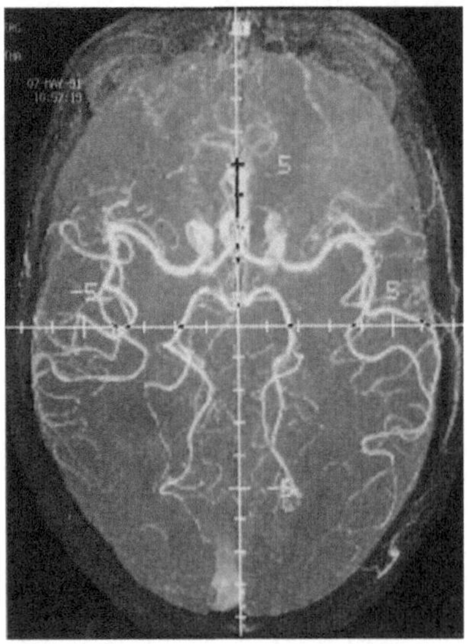

Fig. 86b

logical Clinic of the University of Heidelberg. It was shown that MRA can also be used in radiotherapy planning, particularly in the case of malignant diseases of the lymphatic system. These diseases are commonly treated by irradiating the lymph tracts of the abdominal cavity. Since the lymph tracts are located in the immediate vicinity of the blood vessels, MRA can be of practical help in treatment planning (Fig. 83). An additional MR tomogram, i. e., a series of sectional images, allows the therapist to determine the extension of the spleen (which is to be included in the radiotherapy) and of the kidneys (which are to be shielded against radiation) (Fig. 84). If one superimposes an MR sectional image of the entire abdominal cavity, showing spleen and kidneys, with an MR angiogram of the same region, displaying the vessels, one obtains a global image that reveals the position of all structures of interest for radiotherapy treatment planning (Fig. 85). Invasive administration of contrast media, which in the past was used for vessel visualization, is no longer necessary.

Yet another application of MRA resulted from our group's cooperation with the Radiological Clinics of the University of Heidelberg. Patients suffering from certain malformations of the cerebral vessels (arteriovenous malformations) have to be treated with radiotherapy if surgery or embolization are not possible. These patients run a high risk of brain hemorrhage; the radiation primarily irritates the intima, which can later lead to an occlusion of the affected vessels.

The success of such a radiotherapeutic treatment must be verified until the desired vascular occlusion is shown, which means that patients have to be submitted to continuous follow-up examinations. Until now, this was done using invasive methods of contrast angiography. Our first findings indicate that our new technique allows us to abolish invasive methods in follow-up examinations. Figures 86a and 86b illustrate the course of the disease in a 30 year old female patient. In this case, the pathologically altered vessels occluded 18 months after radiotherapy, as a consequence of which the neurological symptoms receded almost entirely.

Priv.-Doz. Dr. Wolfhard Semmler
Dr. Andreas H. Gamroth
Division of Oncological Diagnostics and Therapy

Participating scientists

Prof. Dr. Gerhard van Kaick
Division of Oncological Diagnostics and Therapy

Prof. Dr. Walter J. Lorenz
Priv.-Doz. Dr. Lothar Schad
Division of Biophysics and Medical Radiation Physics

In collaboration with

Prof. Dr. Dr. Michael Wannenmacher
Dr. Angelika Köster
Clinical Radiology and Radiotherapy, Radiological Clinic of the University of Heidelberg

Priv.-Doz. Dr. Siegfried Tuengerthal
Dr. Hans-Peter Herb
Radiological Department,
Thorax Clinic Heidelberg-Rohrbach

Selected publications

Kauczor, H.-U., Layer, G., Müller-Schimpfe, M., Tuengerthal, S., van Kaick, G.: Clinical applications of MR Angiography in Intrathoracic surgery. J. Comput. Assist. Tomogr. 15, 409–417 (1991)

Müller-Schimpfe, M., Brix, G., Köster, A., Kimmig, B., Schad, L., Semmler, W., van Kaick, G.: MR-Tomography and MR-Angiography for individual treatment planning of subdiaphragmal radiation therapy. J. Comput. Assist. Tomogr. 16, 110–119 (1992)

6.4 Bone Marrow Involvement in Malignant Systemic Diseases – Recognition by Magnetic Resonance Tomography

by Andreas H. Gamroth
and Gunnar Brix

An infiltration of malignant tumor cells into the medullary space leads to either a local involvement or to a diffuse affection of variable-sized bone marrow regions.

Conventional x-ray diagnostics and computer tomography generally produce satisfying images of the cortical bone (i.e., the corticalis) and the trabeculae (the spongiosa), but not of the medullary space.

Bone marrow scintigraphy is time-consuming (average time needed for an examination: 45 to 60 min) and only images the red marrow; the yellow fat marrow remains invisible.

MR tomography (MRT) has opened new perspectives for the imaging of bone marrow alterations. In the slice images, healthy red and yellow marrow, as well as tumorous infiltrates, are rendered with high contrast. MRT is thus of diagnostic value, even in cases of localized involvement of the medullary spaces. Sampling by iliac crest or sternal biopsies only renders information about a small, and not always representative part of the bone marrow. In addition, these are much more unpleasant for the patient than an MRT examination.

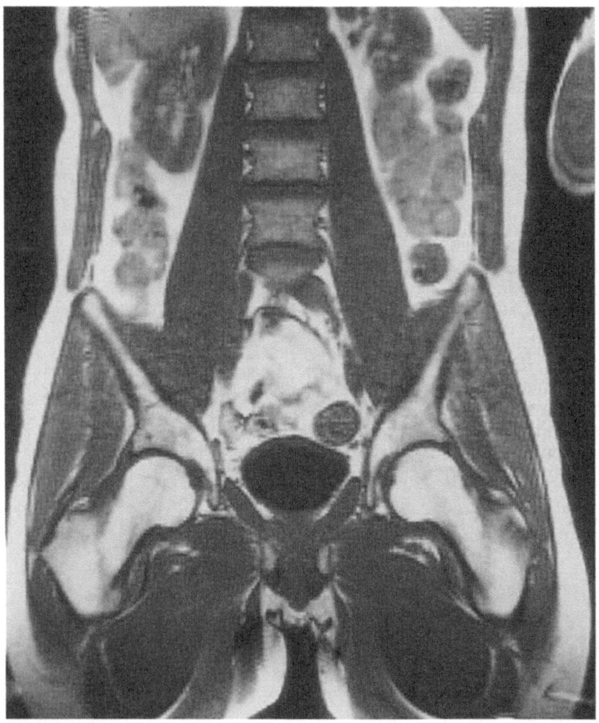

Fig. 87

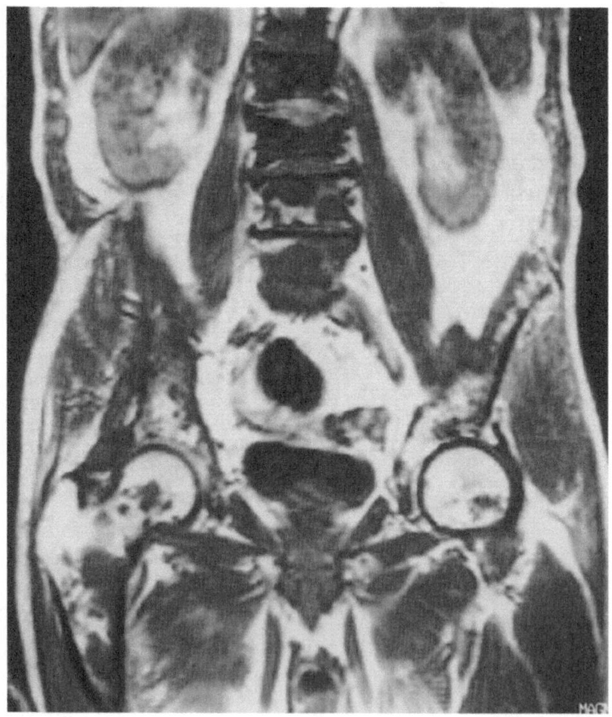

Fig. 88

Previous Developments and Results in Bone Marrow Diagnostics by Magnetic Resonance Methods

From 1988 to 1991 we conducted, in collaboration with our clinical partners of the Tumor Center Heidelberg/Mannheim, prospective studies on the bone marrow involvement of several types of tumors. For these studies, which were run parallel to therapy, the bone marrow of patients with malignant lymphomas (Hodgkin and non-Hodgkin tumors) and leukemias (acute myeloic leukemia and hair cell leukemia) was examined with MRT. The results were then compared to clinical data and bone marrow biopsies. To evaluate the success of the therapy, we are presently observing the development of bone metastases of bronchial carcinomas before, during, and after therapy.

A new approach in MR bone marrow diagnostics is the calculation of separate fat and water images. The latter better allow the therapist to delineate tumor infiltrations that are low in fat than in conventional MRT images. The MRT working group of the Deutsches Krebsforschungszentrum has developed a method that makes it possible to quantitatively assess the fat and water portions. Figure 87 shows a normal medullary space in a representative section in the region of the lumbar vertebral column, the pelvis and the femur, which was acquired with the conventional technique. As a comparison, Figure 88 shows a diffuse bone marrow involvement of a hair-cell leukemia, and Figure 89 shows an image of a focal finding in the left femur in the case of a bronchial carcinoma. The involved medullary spaces are clearly lower in signal (darker).

The morphological appearance can be divided into two groups. The first group includes the localized, circular low-signal (dark) foci as they are observed in the case of metastases of a bronchial carcinoma. The second group is characterized by a diffuse infiltration, as is the case in some forms of leukemia. In the conventional MR sectional image, fatty tissue is bright, whereas tumor tissue, which contains much water, is generally dark (T_1 weighted imaging). In the course of a successful therapy the proportion of healthy, fatty bone marrow cells that previously had been displaced by the tumor cells increases. The combination of conventional MR imaging with subsequent fat-water-separation in a representative slice is thus a novel method that allows the therapist to evaluate morphologically the effectiveness of the therapy. Figures 90 and 91 show the remission of a bone marrow involvement in the case of an acute myeloic leukemia under therapy over 3 weeks.

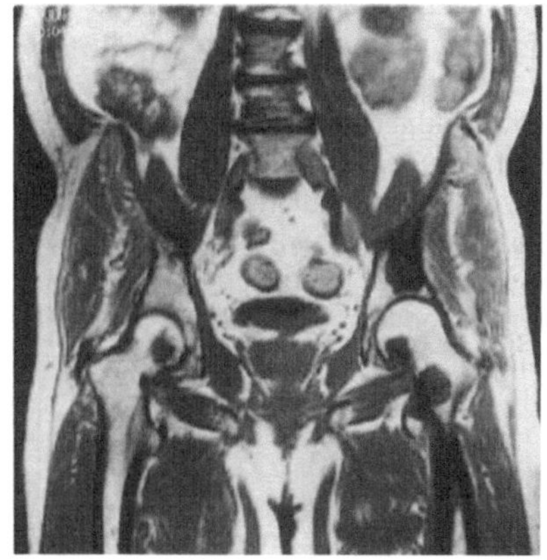

Fig. 89

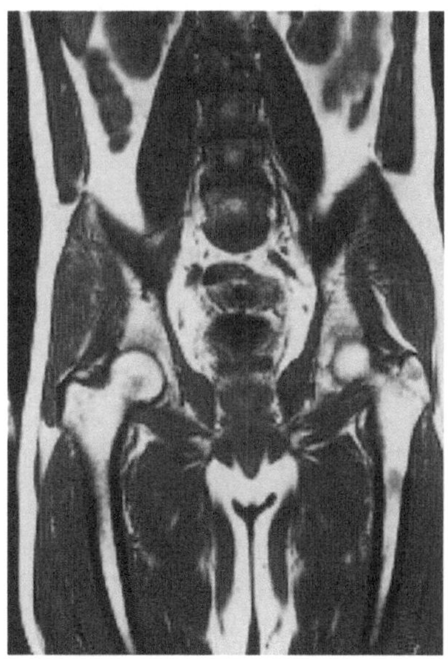

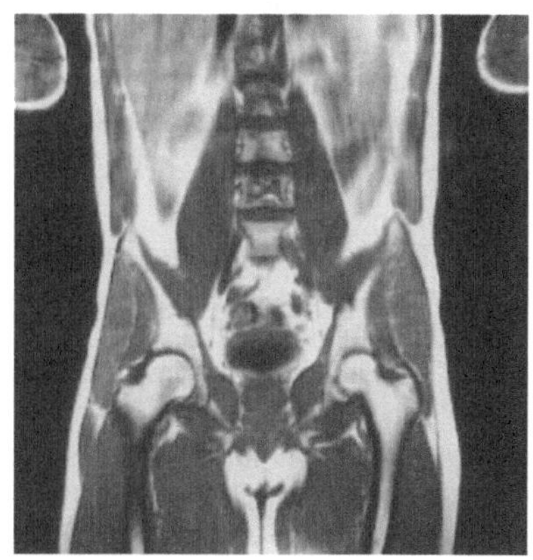

Figs. 90, 91
Acute myeloic leukemia. A pronounced decrease in the involvement of the bone marrow is seen during a three-week course of therapy.

However, it must be noted that neither imaging nor quantitative assessment can serve as a basis to safely differentiate a residual infiltration from a complete remission. Also, connective tissue transformations in the medullary space (fibroses), which may be caused by disease or therapy, cannot be distinguished from tumor tissue in the MR image.

Clinical Significance of MRT for the Assessment of Bone Marrow Infiltrations and Outlook

Initial results of our studies indicate that the majority of the bone marrow infiltrates in the region examined with MRT can be made visible in T_1 weighted measurements. There is a good correlation between the MR findings and the cellular results of the samples taken in the same region. Aside from the fact that MRT also images the structures neighboring the bone marrow (such as muscles and vessels), the following reasons may make it the preferred technique for imaging tumorous medullary foci:

- MRT is a non-invasive and painless method. There is no exposure to x-rays or gamma rays.
- MRT also images well-circumscribed localized foci in regions that often may escape the routine sampling from the iliac crest or the sternum.
- In the case of unclear focal findings, the sampling site can be precisely determined.
- MRT is well-suited for assessing the course of the disease, in particular for evaluating the impact of therapy on the bone marrow involvement.
- Fat-water separation, taken as an additional parameter in the observation of the course of the disease, often makes it possible to additionally quantify the involved areas within a region of interest.

A routine application of MRT might cause a significant reduction in invasive bone marrow sampling. In addition, it might help to make visible the success of a therapy at an early point in time.

Dr. Andreas H. Gamroth
Division of Oncological Diagnostics and Therapy

Dr. Gunnar Brix
Division of Biophysics and Medical Radiophysics

Participating scientists

Priv.-Doz. Dr. Wolfhard Semmler
Prof. Dr. Gerhard van Kaick
Division of Oncological Diagnostics and Therapy

Prof. Dr. Walter J. Lorenz
Division of Biophysics and Medical Radiophysics

In collaboration with

Prof. Dr. Werner Hunstein
Dr. Martin Benz
University Clinic and Outpatient Clinic, University of Heidelberg

Selected publications

Döhner, H., Gückel, F., Semmler, W., van Kaick, G., Ho, A.D., Hunstein, W.: Magnetic resonance imaging of bone marrow in lymphoproliferative disorders: correlation with bone marrow biopsy. Br. J. Haematol. 73, 12–17 (1989)

Gückel, F., Brix, G., Semmler, W., Zuna, I., Knauf, W., Ho, A.H., van Kaick, G.: Systemic bone marrow disorders: characterization with proton shift imaging. J. Comput. Assist. Tomogr. 14 (4), 633–642 (1990)

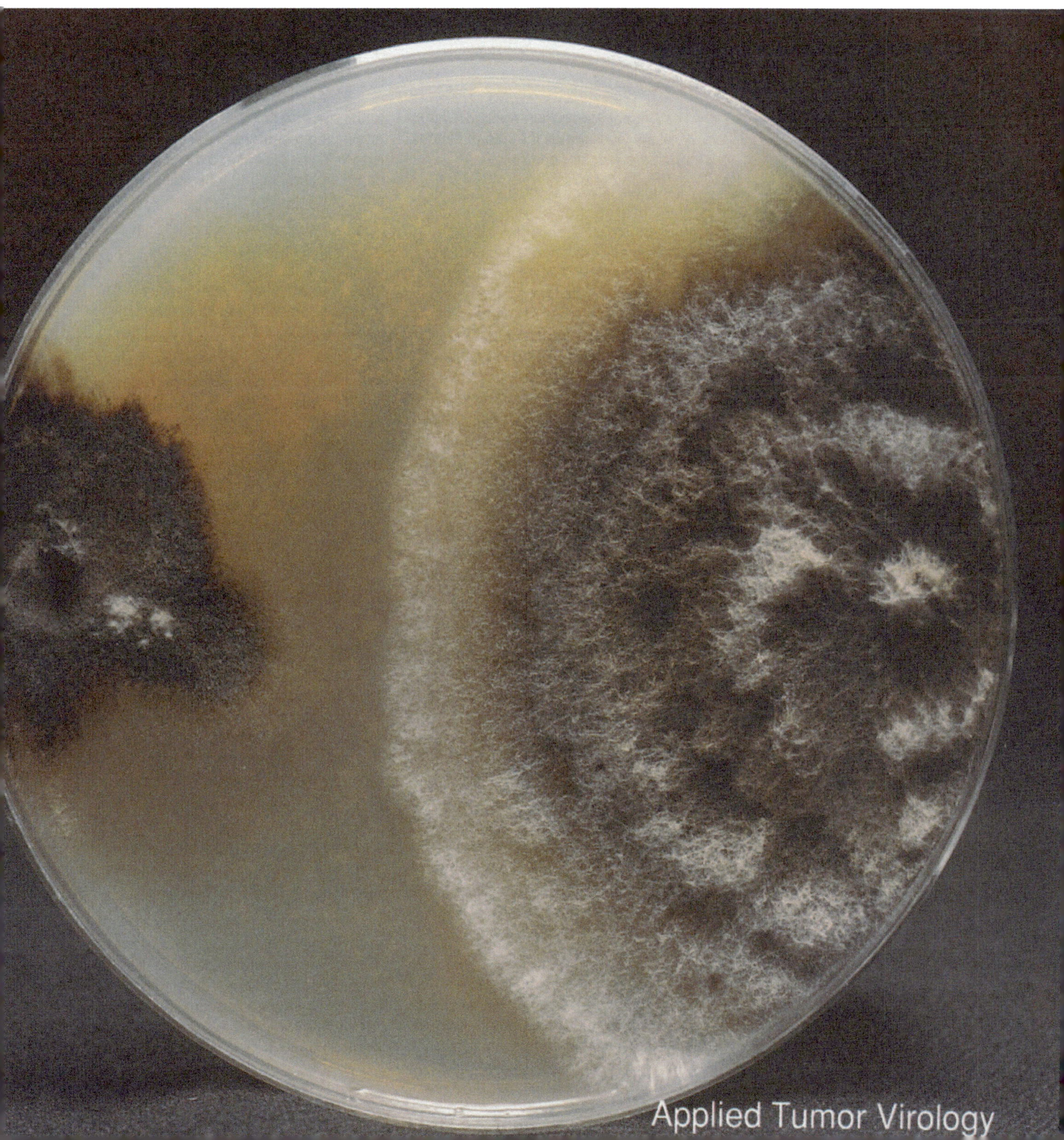

Applied Tumor Virology

7

Applied Tumor Virology

The Research Program Applied Tumor Virology investigates the role of various viruses in carcinogenesis.

One focus of work is the investigation of the relationship between development of genital cancer and infection with human papilloma viruses (HPV). How do the whole organism or individual cells react to an infection with certain papilloma virus types? When does the infection change the cell into a malignant one? Aside from these questions, much emphasis is put on epidemiologic studies on the frequency of HPV infections and investigations on the immune response. They will be the basis on which strategies for the prevention of or the fight against HPV infections will be developed.

The lymphotropic papova virus belongs, together with the papilloma viruses, to the group of small tumor viruses, which contain a double-stranded DNA genome. Experimentally, they can mainly infect cells of Burkitt's lymphoma, a malignant disease of immune cells, which is particularly common among children and adolescents in Africa. The researchers are trying to find out which structures on the surface of the degenerated cells cause these cells to be preferentially infected by the virus.

The vital role played by the hepatitis-B virus (HBV) in the development of liver carcinoma was proven by epidemiologic studies. Researchers investigate certain viral genes to reveal how these viruses contribute to the malignant changes in liver cells.

Epidemiologic studies have also indicated that still unidentified viruses may be related to the development of other tumors. These hints are subject to further research. Presently, for example, the researchers are investigating Hodgkin's disease, a malignant degeneration of certain hematopoietic cells.

Apart from studies on "classic" antiviral substances (such as for example interferons, i. e., messenger molecules of the immune system), scientists work on the development of new therapeutic concepts.

It has been known for some time that the smallest viruses, the parvoviruses, can inhibit cell growth. In epidemiologic studies and with molecular-biological methods the researchers are now attempting to unveil the basic mechanisms of this interaction. They are also trying to produce artificial virus particles which will serve as vehicles to introduce genetic information into cells.

The Research Program also investigates the Human Immunodeficiency Virus (HIV), which is known to cause AIDS. The stages of infection may be the clue to developing a successful vaccine or therapy. Researchers are therefore investigating the role of the envelope protein in viral infection and cell damage. Using antisense RNA, they are elucidating the function of the various viral genes and attempt to selectively inhibit these genes.

A new research group concentrates on the characterization of genes that play a role in inherited human diseases that are frequently related to cancer.

Since cancer is mainly a disease of older people, the Research Program Applied Tumor Virology also investigates the molecular processes of aging from which it hopes to deduce information on the processes that lead to the development of cancer.

Coordinator of the Research Program:
Prof. Dr. Lutz Gissmann

Divisions and their heads:

Tumor Virology:
Prof. Dr. Jean Rommelaere

Genome Modifications and Carcinogenesis:
Prof. Dr. Lutz Gissmann

Tumor Virus Immunology:
N. N.

Virus-Host-Interactions:
Prof. Dr. Claus H. Schröder

Characterization of Tumor Viruses:
Priv.-Doz. D. sc. Ethel-Michele de Villiers

Molecular Biology of Aging:
Dr. Heinz D. Osiewacz

Organization of Complex Genomes:
Dr. Peter Lichter

Genetics of Tumor Viruses:
Prof. Dr. Hans-Christian Kaerner

Project Groups and their heads:

Human Retroviruses:
Prof. Dr. Rolf Flügel

7

7.1 Antisense RNA: A Tool for Selective Gene Inhibition Studied in an HIV Infection Model

by Michael Pawlita and Georg Sczakiel

During the past 10 years, developments in molecular biology and genetic engineering have introduced new concepts for the direct control of disturbed cell functions. These concepts are based on the use of nucleic acids, both as tools and as targets of intracellular intervention. With the aid of a model system, we investigated whether the "antisense principle" might be useful in the treatment of viral infections.

The Antisense Principle

All vital processes in a cell are based on the activity of a multitude of genes. They make up the chromosomes in the cell's nucleus and consist of deoxyribonucleic acid (DNA) chains, which are composed of four different components, the deoxyribonucleotides. One can think of the genetic information as a text written in a language that only has four letters. In order to have any effect a gene has to be active, which means that in the nucleus the genetic information is copied (transcribed) from the DNA sequence into a ribonucleic acid strand (messenger RNA, mRNA). After various maturation steps, the mRNA is moved from the nucleus to the cytoplasm; there it is the basis of information needed for the synthesis of proteins.

The nucleotides that compose DNA and RNA strands have the ability to form pairs. Nucleotide A pairs with nucleotide T (in the RNA, with nucleotide U), and nucleotide G with nucleotide C. As a consequence, two chains of nucleic acid can join if their sequences match, that is, if they are complementary. For example, a strand with the sequence 5'-GAATTGC-3' can join with a second, complementary strand having the sequence 3'-CTTAACG-5' to form a double strand. (By convention, the "head end" of a nucleic acid strand is labeled "5'-", the "rear end" is labelled "3'-".)

The mRNA coding for a protein is also called "sense" RNA; an RNA with the complementary sequence is called "antisense" RNA. If an antisense RNA (or a short synthetic single-stranded antisense DNA) with a sufficiently long

Fig. 92
Possible sites of action for antisense nucleic acids during gene expression. They make it possible to specifically inhibit the expression of a single gene.

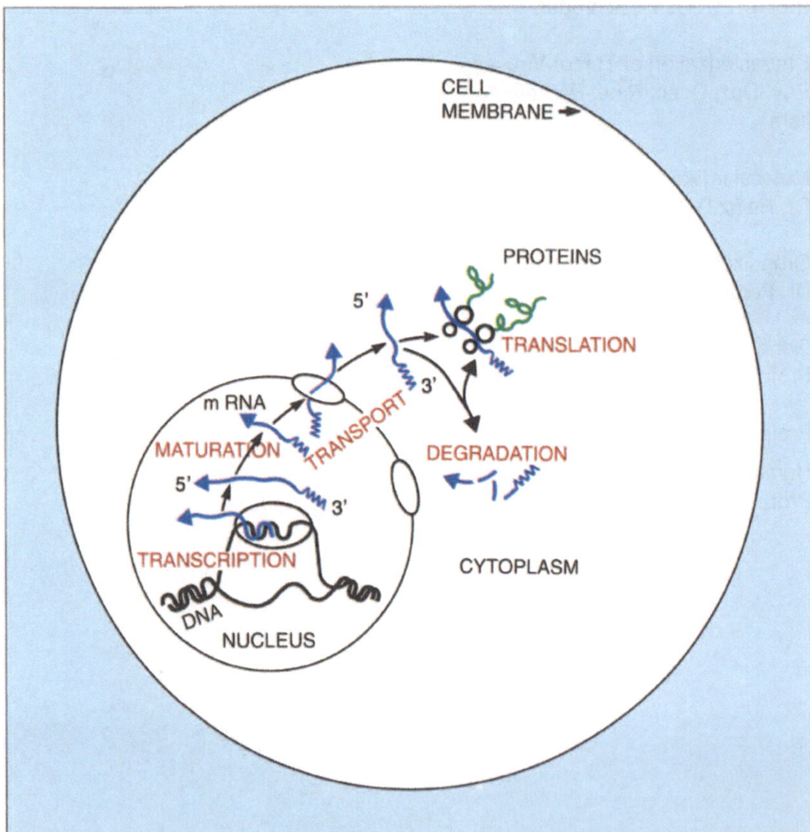

sequence that is complementary to the mRNA of a certain gene is experimentally introduced into cells, the single-stranded mRNA can be specifically complemented to form a double-stranded nucleic acid. In other words, the effect of this specific gene can be intentionally inhibited. Note that only the synthesis of the protein encoded by this one gene is inhibited, without any direct effect on the expression of other genes. The selectivity of this process is extremely high since the text (i.e. the nucleotide sequence) of a certain mRNA is unique in each cell. Even text sequences as short as about 15 letters (nucleotides) have a high probability of being unique within the entire active hereditary information of a cell.

Several mechanisms of action of antisense nucleic acids are at the moment being discussed; however, only in very few cases is the exact point of action known in detail. It should be possible, in principle, to inhibit every biological process that is based on the use of single-stranded RNA by initiating double strand formation with antisense RNA or antisense DNA.

The efficiency and the selectivity of the antisense principle have been shown experimentally in bacteria, in plants, as well as in animal cells. A Dutch working group has presented a particularly intriguing experiment on the petunia (Petunia hybrida). An artificial gene for antisense RNA directed against the chromogenic enzyme chalcon-synthase

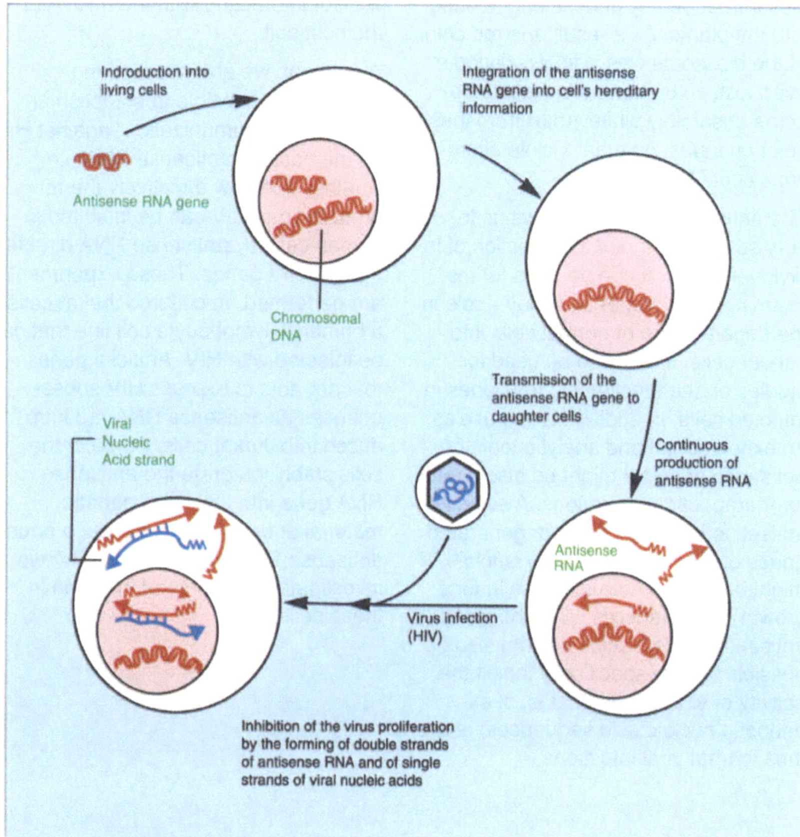

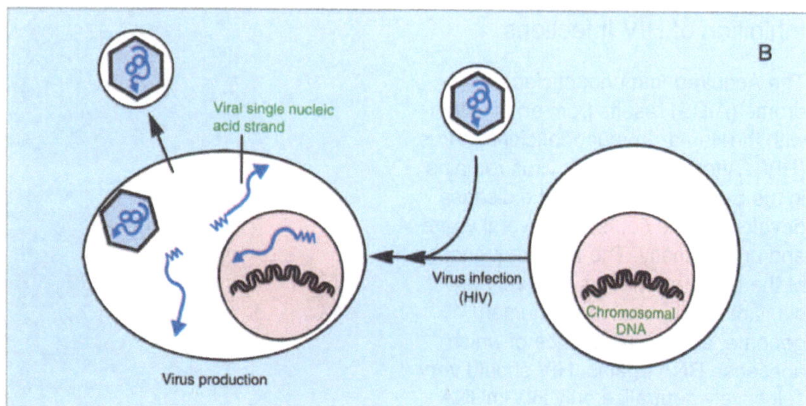

Figs. 93, 94
Antisense RNA, introduced into a cell, inhibits the multiplication of HIV viruses (A). For comparison, (B) shows how HIV viruses multiply in untreated cells.

was introduced by genetic engineering into the plants. As a result, the red color of the blossoms was visibly reduced or even lost, so that some blossoms became absolutely white. Apart from these color changes, no other visible alterations could be observed.

The antisense principle allows us to very selectively inhibit the function of individual genes. It can be used for the examination of genes that play a role in the degeneration of normal cells into cancer cells. It can also be used for studies on the function of viral genes in infected cells. In addition to the use as an experimental and analytic tool, the antisense principle might be also useful for therapeutic applications. A selective antisense inhibition of the degenerated genes of a cancer cell, for example, might be able to normalize the latter's growth characteristics. With the aid of antisense nucleic acids it might also be possible to very specifically inhibit the activity of viral genes (that is, of exogenous nucleic acid sequences) and thus to treat viral infections.

Use of Antisense RNA for the Inhibition of HIV Infections

The Acquired Immunodeficiency Syndrome (AIDS) results from an infection with the Human Immunodeficiency Virus (HIV). After infection, the virus remains in the body of the patient; the disease develops in the course of several years and ends lethally. The text (sequence) of the HIV genome has only very few similarities with that of the human genome, as a consequence of which antisense RNA against HIV should very selectively neutralize only HIV-mRNA without interacting with the mRNA of the host cell.

At present, we are investigating whether it is possible to establish an "intracellular immunization" against HIV on the basis of antisense RNA, i.e., whether and how effectively the reproduction of HIV can be inhibited in human cells by antisense RNA directed against HIV genes. These experiments are performed on cultured Jurkat cells, a human T-lymphocyte cell line that can be infected with HIV. Artificial genes that are able to express HIV subsequences as antisense RNA are introduced into Jurkat cells. Some of the cells stably integrate the antisense RNA gene into their own genetic material and thus continuously produce antisense RNA. After adding HIV, we investigate the course of infection in these cells.

Depending upon the selected target region, we observed an inhibition of 70-95% in the first days after infection, which, however, disappeared later. Even with comparatively high HIV infective doses (10^7 infectious particles per dish or 50 particles per cell) the number of HIV-infected cells was 5 to 20 times lower than in cultures that were free of antisense RNA. In addition, the antisense RNA cultures tested produced fewer mature, infectious viruses. This initial inhibiting effect diminished with time and could no longer be measured after 3 weeks. For infective doses smal-

Fig. 95
Multiplication of HIV viruses in cells with and without antisense RNA. In cells in which the HIV virus multiplies, virus protein can be detected with the help of fluorescent antibodies (yellow).

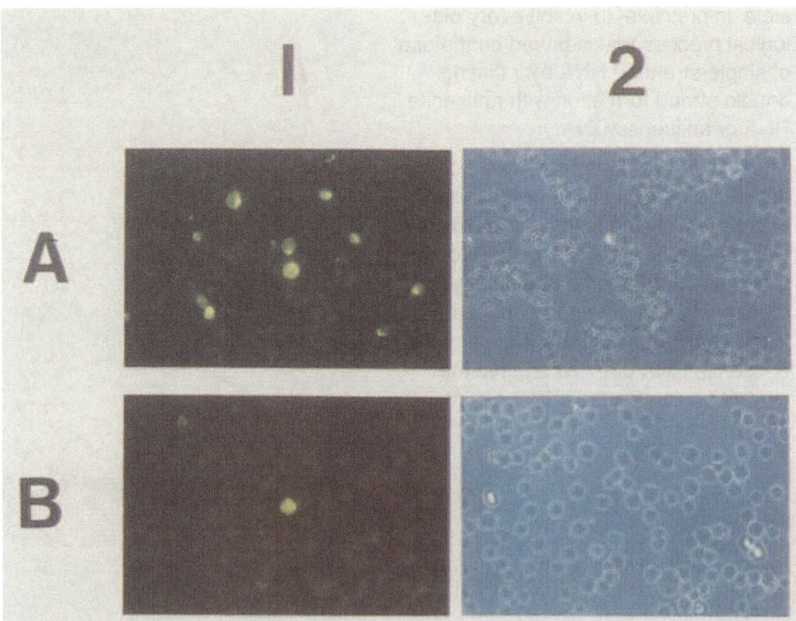

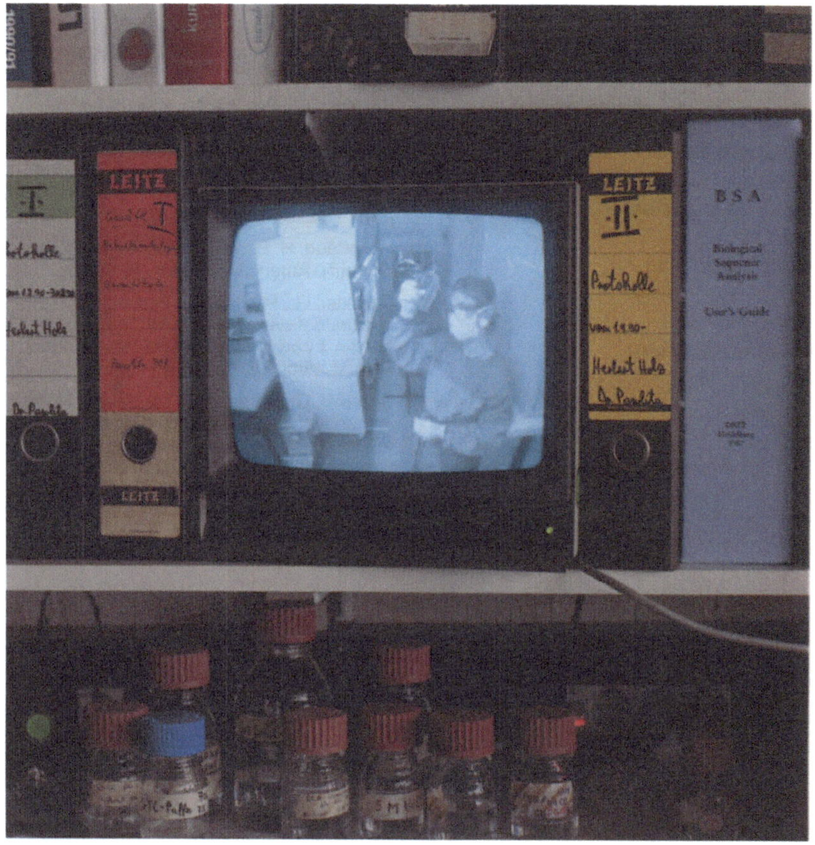

Fig. 96
Experiments with infectious HIV viruses are carried out in a specially secured laboratory. The researchers wear protective clothing and can be supervised from the outside via a video camera.

ler than 10^7 infectious particles per dish the inhibiting effect of the antisense RNA on the reproduction of HIV became ever more pronounced. Cells with HIV antisense RNA are completely protected against low infective doses that in cells without antisense RNA still suffice for a spread of the virus: no reproduction of the virus could be measured.

Prospects

Our experiments show that antisense RNA against HIV is able to reduce and, in the case of low infective doses, even to completely suppress HIV reproduction. These results indicate the power of the molecular-genetic principle of antisense RNA with respect to inhibiting viral infections in human tissue culture cells. At present, we are preparing experiments in which we plan to investigate whether the presently known results can be transferred to other experimental models (other cell lines, primary lymphocytes, animal experiments with immunosuppressed mice, and human blood cells).

Today, a therapeutic application of synthetic genes for the production of antisense RNA in man is theoretically possible. Prior to the clinical use, however, a host of problems still has to be resolved. It remains to be seen whether technological progress in general, and an assessment of the biological risks involved in particular, will allow a somatic genetic therapy with antisense RNA.

Dr. Michael Pawlita
Dr. Georg Szakiel
Division of Genome Modifications and Carcinogenesis

Participating staff

Karola Rittner
Andreas Kleinheinz

Selected publications

Baltimore, D.: Intracellular Immunization. Nature 335, 395–396 (1988).

Sczakiel, G., Pawlita, M., Kleinheinz, A.: Specific inhibition of human immunodeficiency virus type-1 replication by RNA transcribed in sense and antisense orientation from the 5'-leader/gag region. Biochem. Biophys. Res. Commun. 169, 643–651 (1990).

Weintraub, H. B. Antisense RNA and DNA. Scientific American 262, 34–40 (1990).

Sczakiel, G., Pawlita, M.: Inhibition of human immunodeficiency virus type-1 replication in human T cells stably expressing antisense RNA. J. Virol. 65, 468–472 (1991).

Sczakiel, G., Rittner, K., Pawlita, M.: Human immunodeficiency virus type-1 replication is reduced by intracellular antisense RNA expression. In: Prospects for antisense nucleic acid therapy of cancer and AIDS. Ed. E. Wickstrom, Wiley-Liss, New York, 179–193 (1991).

7.2 Fungi as Model Systems in Experimental Gerontology

by Heinz D. Osiewacz

Over the centuries, hardly any biological phenomenon has concerned mankind as much as the process of aging – understandably so, since the consequences, for the individual as well as for society, are numerous. For the individual, the number of diseases increases significantly with age, and the social position of older persons changes, maybe even dramatically. For society, a large number of retired persons inevitably causes economic and social burdens. In the future, the social factor in particular will become a serious problem in the industrial countries, in the next century, for example, one-third of the German population will be retired.

In view of these problems, the goals of modern gerontology have to be defined. Most gerontologists, when asked, would not answer that they want to prolong man's life span. After all, the average life expectancy in Germany has increased from some 36 years at the end of the 19th century to about 76 years today. Rather, today's goal of gerontology is to come to a fundamental understanding of the process of aging in order to give persons advanced in years a good chance of spending their lives as free from physical and mental infirmities as possible. Indeed, as many works of art from different cultural periods show, this has always been a desire of man.

A host of recent theories about aging, all of which try to explain the underlying biological processes, illustrate the increased interest in gerontology. None of the partly contradictory theories adequately explains the entirety of the processes taking place, and there is an urgent need for fundamental experimental research in order to clarify the biological basis of aging.

In past years a new branch of biology, molecular biology, has emerged and offers promising new insights for experimental gerontology, as well as for other disciplines. The use of recently developed methods has already led to some new findings about the molecular mechanisms that control the aging processes. In many cases, however, this knowledge does not result from studies of man; instead, it is, for different reasons, based on studies of mostly very simply organized model systems (for example, insects, nematodes, and fungi). However, there is reasonable hope that some of the findings gained from these organisms can be transferred to explain processes taking place in man.

Why use Fungi in Experimental Gerontology?

As a model organism for the examination of the genetic basis of aging we use, in our laboratory, the filamentous fungus Podospora anserina. This microorganism can be isolated naturally, e.g., from horse dung, and has been used intensively for the past 40 years. The reasons for this are manifold:

1) Cultures of this fungus are particularly simply organized and consist of long, highly branched “cells” (hyphae), which together form the vegetative body, the mycelium. Specialized cells and organs are formed only for sexual reproduction.

2) P. anserina can be cultured in the laboratory, both in liquid and on solid media.

3) The fungus has a short life span (i.e., 25 days for the wild strain race).

4) A complete reproductive cycle, i.e., the time between the hybridization of two strains and the development of mature progeny is 10 to 12 days.

5) P. anserina can be transformed, in the course of which isolated genetic information (desoxyribonucleic acid, DNA) can be introduced into prepared cells.

6) Cell organelles (e.g., mitochondria), nucleic acids and proteins can be isolated from P. anserina for molecular-biological studies.

These characteristics render the organism particularly attractive for genetic studies which depend on the possibility to perform defined hybridizations and to quickly isolate a maximum number of descendants. With other biological systems, these studies would either be significantly slower or not possible at all.

Several other fungi (for example, Neurospora intermedia) have characteristics similar to P. anserina; some of them are also used as model systems in experimental gerontology.

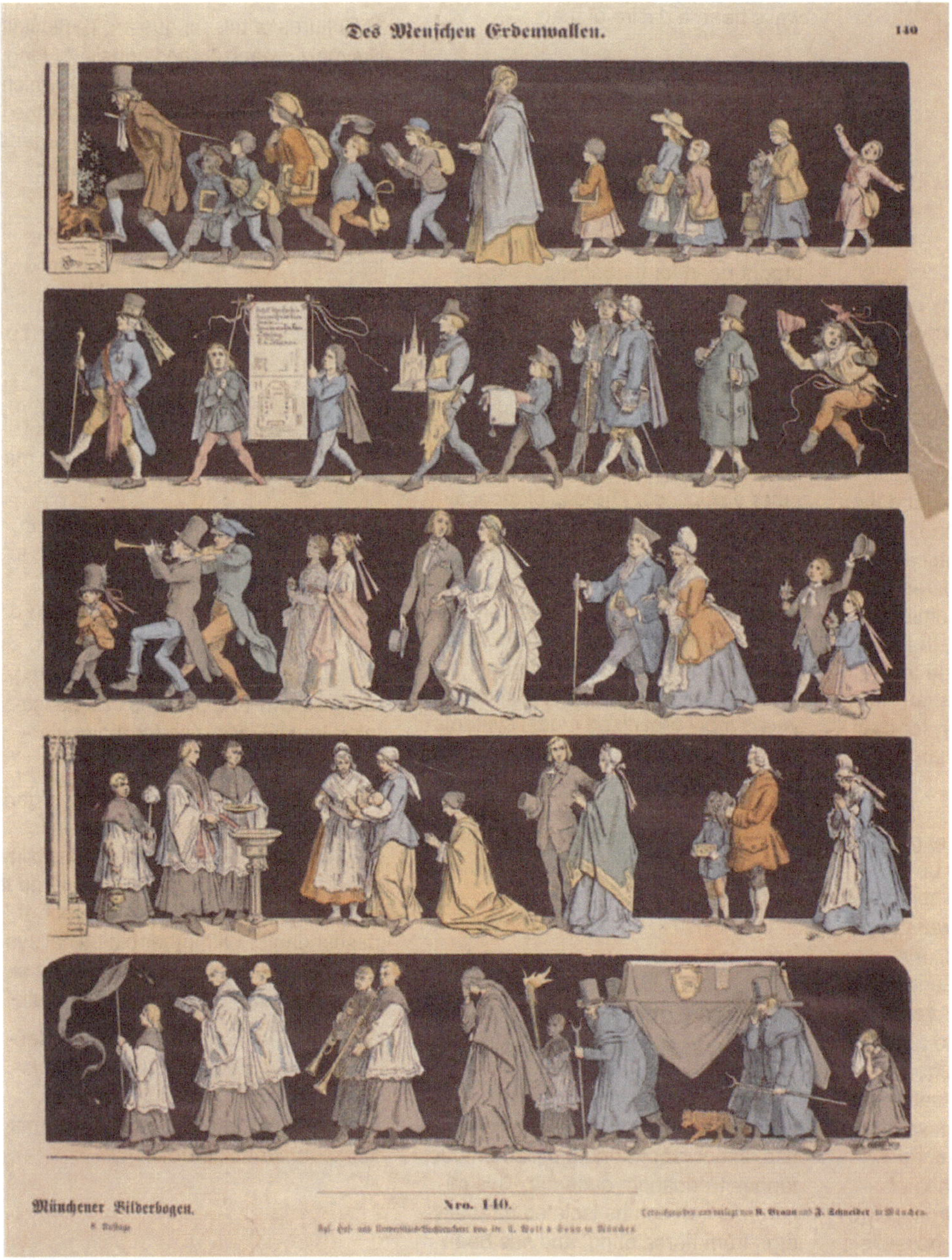

Fig. 97
"Man's earthly pilgrimage," a sheet of pictures from Munich, 1872. Living means aging. But how the process of aging is controlled genetically is not yet understood.

Genetic Control of Aging in Podospora Anserina

As early as the 1950s and 1960s, the involvement of genetic factors in the control of aging in P. anserina was demonstrated by the French scientists George Rizet and Denise Marcou; later, this work was continued by the group of the botanist Karl Esser (Bochum, FRG). These studies were mainly done with wild strains of P. anserina, which had been isolated from different regions in France and Germany, and mutants that had developed spontaneously in the laboratory (i.e., strains that genetically differ from the wild strain). In some cases, the genetic alterations (mutations) prolonged life; they could be localized by classical hybridization experiments on specific chromosomes in the nucleus of P. anserina. By hybridization of two mutants with slightly increased life span at a time, it was also possible to isolate two double mutants (i viv, gr viv), in which both mutations of the parent strains coexist. It is interesting to note that these strains do not show symptoms of aging; they have been growing in our laboratory for the past 15 and 10 years, respectively!

Along with the influence of these chromosomal hereditary factors (localized in the nucleus) on the life span, Marcou also demonstrated the existence of an "infectious principle," which later proved to be a circular DNA species, a plasmid (plDNA). If the conditions are such that a migration of the nuclei is impossible, this plasmid is transferred during the fusion of two Podospora cultures from the senescent culture to the juvenile one. There it spreads and, as a consequence, the juvenile culture stops growing and dies.

A molecular analysis of juvenile and senescent Podospora cultures showed that in juvenile cultures the Podospora plasmid is integrated into a larger circular molecule with high molecular weight, the mitochondrial DNA (mtDNA); there it acts as the first intron of a gene coding for a protein of the energy metabolism (subunit I of the cytochrome oxidase). In the course of aging, this sequence is liberated and amplified by a mechanism still unknown. At the same time, the mitochondrial DNA is rearranged, which leads to deficiencies in the mitochondria's enzyme supply.

The significance of the release and amplification of plDNA for senescence has been shown by experimental data. For example, in a molecular analysis of the immortal double mutants (i viv, gr viv) mentioned above, no excess of mitochondrial circular plasmid was found. This is an indication that the plasmid liberation and amplification is controlled by genes that are located in the nucleus of Podospora.

Apart from long-lived nuclear mutants, there are corresponding mutants in which the mutation is localized directly on the mitochondrial DNA. In two of these strains (ex1, ex2) a large part of the mitochondrial DNA is lost (deleted). Among the deleted parts is the sequence from which the Podospora plasmid is derived.

At present, we are analyzing another mutant whose life expectancy is 10 times longer than that of the wild strain. First molecular analyses have revealed that the circular plasmid (plDNA) is liberated or amplified with a delay. In senescent cultures, however, the number of copies of plDNA is increased again. It is interesting, to note that in this long-lived mutant, we have been able to show the existence of another plasmid, which to date could not be detected in any other Podospora strain, and which has a linear structure with sequences that resemble viral chromosomes. At present, our laboratory is intensively trying to elucidate the relation between the extended life span of this mutant and the molecular alterations in the mitochondria.

How can we explain the aging processes observed in Podospora anserina on the molecular level?

Let us sum up the most important experimental results. In juvenile cultures, the gene which encodes for the subunit I of the cytochrome oxidase (COI) – an essential component of the energy-producing system of the mitochondria – contains a piece of genetic information (intron) which, during aging, is released either by excision on the level of the DNA or by transcription of RNA (ribonucleic acid) into DNA (reverse transcription). After being released, it is amplified. This process is controlled by genes (i viv, gr viv) that are localized in the nucleus.

After a certain number of copies of the circular plasmid has been produced in senescent cultures, the plasmid might be able (this, however, is mere speculation) to integrate itself into essential sequences of mitochondrial DNA, which are thus inactivated (inactivation by insertion). This might block a vital metabolic process (e.g., energy metabolism), which would lead to the death of the culture from lack of energy.

Alternatively, it might be possible that the Podospora plasmid integrates one or more copies of itself into the circular

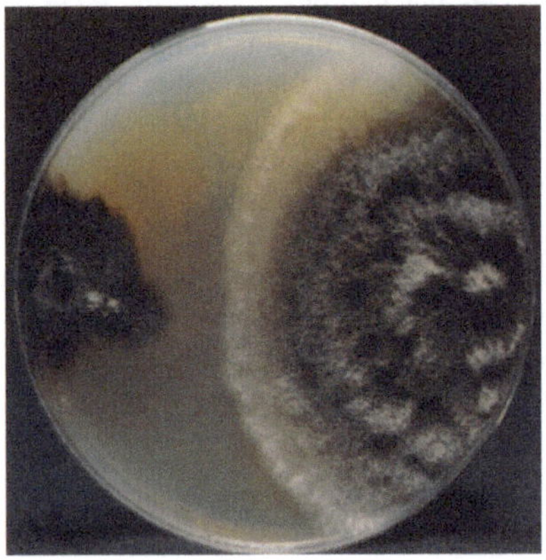

Fig. 98
In their quest for understanding the principles of aging, gerontologists study simple model organisms. The ascomycete, Podospora anserina, ages within 3 weeks. It is studied in order to find principles of regulation, which might also exist in more complicated being such as man.

mitochondrial DNA, which afterwards are reorganized. In the course of these processes, vital sequences might be lost, which would lead to the production of defective mtDNA molecules.

The same effect would be achieved if a protein encoded by the plasmid (a recombinase) caused a reorganization of the mitochondrial DNA, and if this reorganization were accompanied by a loss of essential nucleotide sequences. The analysis of the plasmid's sequence showed that it does indeed contain the genetic information for the coding of a protein (open reading frame, ORF). Recently, immunological experiments in senescent cultures have shown the presence of a protein encoded by Podospora's plasmid. The function of this protein, however, is still completely unknown.

In conclusion, the death of senescent Podospora cultures is due to defects in the energy metabolism which, in turn, is caused by the accumulation of defective mitochondrial DNA. Proof for this is the fact that, in the course of aging, the concentration of vital components (enzymes) of this metabolism, which are encoded by the mitochondrial genetic information, decreases to below the detection limit.

In spite of these, in part, very detailed conceptions about the molecular mechanisms of the aging of Podospora anserina, several questions remain to be answered. Some of the interesting problems are: How, in the course of aging, is the Podospora plasmid released in such a regular and exact way? Which function has a protein encoded by the Podospora plasmid? What is the role of the nuclear genes that influence the life span? Presently, we are trying to find the answers to these questions by means of a combination of classical genetic and molecular methods.

Are Molecular Alterations during Senescence in other Organisms Similar to those in P. Anserina?

During the past decade, it could indeed be proven that, in closely related fungi, genetic factors participate in the control of aging processes. In some cases, such as for P. anserina, it was possible to relate genetic elements (linear and circular plasmids) to aging. In Podospora curvicolla circular plasmids from mitochondrial DNA are released during senescence. The reverse process, the integration of circular plasmid DNA and the subsequent reorganization processes in the mitochondrial DNA was detected in certain strains of Neurospora intermedia and Neurospora crassa. It was also possible to identify linear mitochondrial plasmids in several wild strain isolates from the Hawaii is-

Fig. 99
In older ascomycete cultures, a specific sequence separates from the hereditary substance and forms independent rings, so-called plasmids. Mutated ascomycete cultures that do not develop these plasmids are considered immortal – a hint to the important role the DNA ring plays in aging.

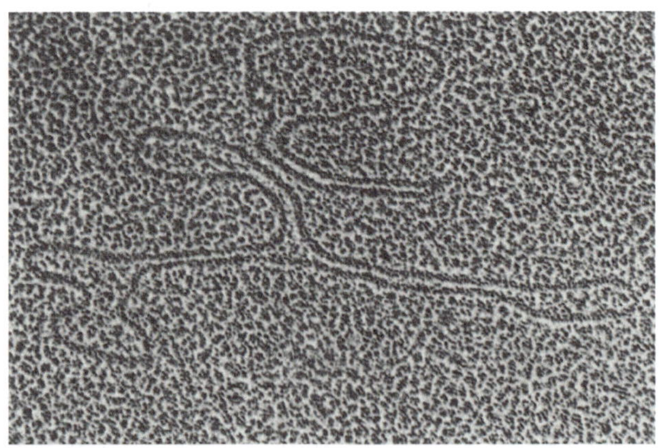

lands and from India of the same Neurospora species which, during aging, integrate into vital mitochondrial genes; this leads to a dysfunction of the affected organelles and, finally, to the death of the culture.

During recent years, alterations in the mitochondrial genetic information in certain tissues of man have also been found. With modern techniques of molecular biology it could be shown, for example, that in muscle tissue and in certain regions of the brain large sections of mitochondrial DNA are lost (deleted). In addition, it has been known for some time that certain diseases (such as mitochondrial myopathies) are caused by loss of genetic information in mitochondria.

The role of genetic elements in the aging of man, which has been shown in the case of several fungi, is not known to date. However, it cannot be expected that mitochondrial plasmids derived from intron sequences will be found, since it is known that the mitochondrial hereditary information of all mammals is structured extremely economically and is devoid of introns.

It is not clear yet if the nuclear genome (which in higher organisms is significantly more complex than in fungi) contains genetic information for mobile elements similar to those in the mitochondria of some fungi. Such nuclear elements could also lead to reorganizations of the genetic information and, thus, control senescence. Nevertheless, such processes have not been proven yet. In different tissues and in cell cultures of higher organisms, however, circular genes could be identified. Some of these elements display the typical characteristics of transposons, which are mobile genetic elements typically found in bacteria and in some higher organisms (such as plants).

Is it possible that reorganization processes similar to those in the mitochondria of some fungi take place in the nucleus of higher organisms? A positive answer to this would, of course, entail many more questions. Their answers might again be found in studies on more simply organized model systems, which then would have to be verified in higher organisms.

Dr. Heinz D. Osiewacz
Division of Molecular Biology of Aging

Participating staff

Anita Asseburg
Heike Böhli
Annette Clairmont
Josef Hermanns
Marion Huth
Klaus-P. Künkele
Dr. Rüdiger Ridder

In collaboration with

Prof. Dr. Thomas E. Elthon
University of Nebraska,
School of Biological Sciences,
Lincoln, Nebraska, USA

Prof. Dr. Karl Esser
Faculty of Biology,
Ruhr University, Bochum

Prof. Dr. Ulrich Kück
General Botany,
Ruhr University, Bochum

Selected publications

Esser, K., Kück, U., Lang-Hinrichs, C., Lemke, P., Osiewacz, H.D., Stahl, U., Tudzynski, P.: Plasmids of eukaryotes. Springer, Berlin (1986).

Kück, U.: Mitochondrial DNA rearrangements in Podospora anserina. Exp. Myocol 13, 111–120 (1989).

Osiewacz, H.D.: Molecular analysis of aging processes in fungi. Mutat. Res. 237, 1–8 (1990).

7.3 Analysis of Cancer Diseases by Molecular Cytogenetics

by Peter Lichter

Genetic diseases are the result of specific alterations (mutations) within the genetic material. In the case of classic hereditary diseases, all the cells of the organism (with rare exceptions) show the same alterations within their genetic material/genome. Cancer, on the other hand, results from specific mutations in the genetic material of an individual cell, which cause the alteration of specific genes (the oncogenes). The products of these genes normally have important control functions within the cell. If the normal functioning of the oncogenes is changes in a specific way, the cell begins to multiply excessively, i.e., to develop into a tumor. There are two kinds of oncogenes: dominant and recessive oncogenes. With only a few exceptions, each cell contains two identical copies of all genes. If oncogenicity is caused by an alteration in only one of the two copies of a specific oncogene, it is called dominant. If, on the other hand, a gene s function changes only if both of its copies are altered, or if one copy is altered and the unaltered copy is lost, the oncogene is called recessive.

As a rule, at least two different alterations in the genetic material having effect on the oncogene's function must have taken place in order to induce tumor growth. In the case of inherited cancers, all the cells of the body already have mutated oncogene. The probability that a second mutation occurs within a cell of the organism at some point of time during a person's life is considerably greater than the probability that two independent mutations occur within one and the same cell. Furthermore, in some families various types of cancer occur more often than others. In some of these cases there cases there is already one mutated oncogene; various changes in the genetic material of certain cell types may then cause different cancers within the family and even in one individual. The specific alterations in the genetic material leading to diseases may be identified with the help of the methods from the fields of molecular biology and cytogenetics. These methods are not only very useful for the causal analysis of the development and spread of certain tumors, they are also efficient tools for tumor diagnosis.

New Methods for the Diagnosis of Chromosomal Aberrations

Alterations of the genetic material that lead to changes in the function of oncogenes may be very small and thus may also be caused by chromosome alterations that are visible under the microscope. For example, the number of chromosome (numerical chromosome aberration) or their structure (structural chromosome aberration) may be specifically changed. These changes may be analyzed by conventional cytogenetic methods such as chromosomal banding. Numerical changes and chromosomal rearrangements can be investigated with in situ hybridization in a highly specific manner. In the case of non-isotopic in situ hybridization, a chemically modified DNA or RNA probe is hybridized to pretreated chromosome preparations. Due to the specific base pairing between the probe and the chromosomal DNA, the probe only binds on chromosome regions where a copy of the DNA to be detected occurs. The chemical modification then allows us to visualize the sample directly or indirectly, for example, via fluorescence. In order to make this localization method sufficiently efficient for any region of the human genome, complex DNA probes or probe sets are used. The presence of so-called repetitive DNA elements, which are ubiquitously distributed in the genome, cause serious problems. In collaboration with Thomas Cremer, we have therefore developed a method called chromosomal in situ suppression hybridization (CISS hybridization) which allows to use almost any genomic DNA probe for the specific detection of the corresponding sequence on chromosomes.

By selecting suitable DNA probes or probe sets, chromosomes and chromosomal subregions can be selectively stained. Combinations of various detections procedures can be used to stain different chromosomal regions on one and the same preparations with different colors. This development provides new tools to rapidly and precisely diagnose specific chromosomal alterations in genetic diseases. If, for example, three copies of one chromosome exist (trisomy), a suitable DNA probe will produce three signals on a set of chromosomes.

Chromosomal alterations that are particularly important for cancer diagnosis in humans are translocations (broken chromosomes which subsequently fuse with material of different

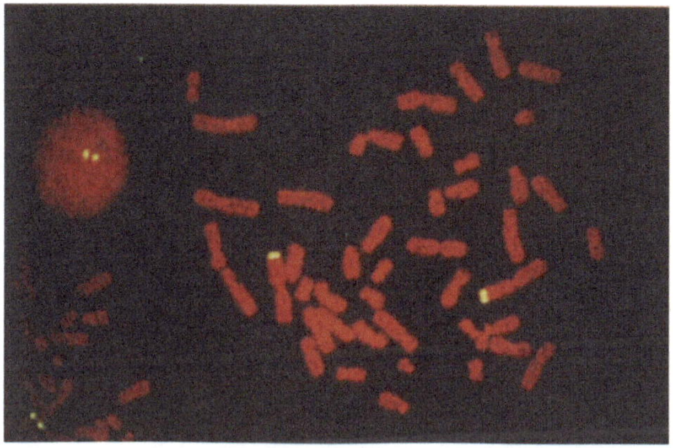

Fig. 100
A new method, the chromosomal in situ suppression hybridization, makes it possible to visualize chromosomes at various stages and to identify genetic defects faster and more easily.

chromosomal origin) and deletions (lose of chromosomal regions). Other chromosomal changes, such as duplications (of chromosomal regions) and inversions (inverted reintegration of chromosome sections), also play a role. In certain types, specific dominant oncogenes can be found in the breakpoint region of translocations typical for certain tumors. In these cases, the translocation either altered the oncogene itself or its regulation. CISS hybridization with suitable samples of the breakpoint region makes it possible to rapidly diagnose such specific translocations. The effect of recessive oncogenes can often be demonstrated by detecting deletions, which may be very small and thus are undetectable under the microscope. If a sufficiently large probe from the deleted region is available, it is possible to prove a deletion by the fact that after in situ hybridization there is only one signal (instead of two signals) on the chromosome set.

The detection of specific chromosomal alterations by in situ hybridization is not only possible on miotic chromosomes (the typical chromosomes are only visible during cell division (mitosis), but also in the nuclei of non-dividing cells,

Fig. 101
The bright yellow dye marks an oncogene which is related to the development of cancer.

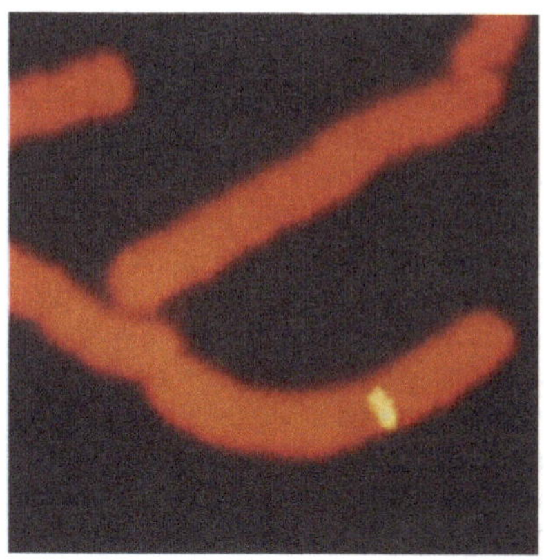

i.e., during the interphase. This is of particular importance in cases where dividing cells are difficult, or impossible to obtain, such as in many tumors. One example is the detection of numeric and structural chromosome aberrations in peripheral blood of patients with chronic lymphocytic leukemia. Together with Hartmut Döhner and Martin Bentz, we therefore initiated a collaborative study to investigate the incidence of certain chromosomal alterations in patients with chronic lymphocytic neoplasia by non-isotopic in situ hybridization to both miotic chromosomes as well as interphase nuclei.

The newly developed in situ hybridization methods and developments is the area of optical instrumentation and image processing also allow to investigate fundamental questions in cell biology regarding the specific order of chromatin regions in the nucleus. Our group is presently investigating the topographical organization of translocation breakpoint regions of certain tumors in the nucleus.

Rapid Mapping of Human DNA Fragments

The visualization of DNA fragments on chromosomes by in situ hybridization allows us to rapidly and precisely map DNA fragments along chromosomes. Thus, chromosome maps can be established showing the linear order of DNA fragments on the chromosome. Such maps are instrumental for identifying probes for further investigations of alterations in the genetic material by means of molecular biology. Regional

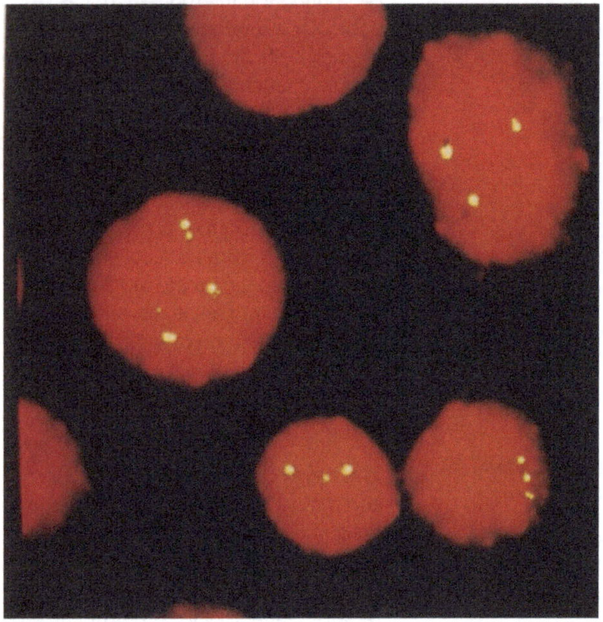

Fig. 102
In the cells of a child suffering from Down's syndrome, the yellow spots reveal that there are three instead of two copies of chromosome 21.

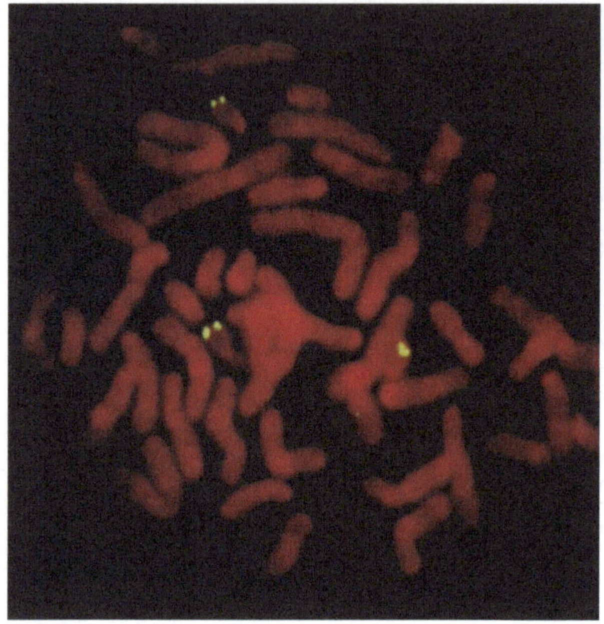

Fig. 103
The three revealing copies of chromosome 21 fluoresce at points that have been marked by a probe.

in situ hybridization chromosome maps are an important tool within the project to generate a complete map of all DNA fragments of the human genome. Our group contributes to this global goal by generating in situ hybridization maps of selected regions of the human genome. The resolution of in situ hybridization maps is in the order of one million base pairs. In order to further improve this resolution, we are also developing in situ hybridization protocol using differently prepared chromosome material.

The Significance of the Genome Project for Cancer Diagnosis

The ambitious project of decoding the complete human genetic information is of great importance for the analysis of genetic diseases. The information gained from this project will help us to understand hereditary diseases with simple and complex genetics as well as to identify many others oncogenes (their number being estimated to be several hundreds). Furthermore, the projects will be of great significance for cancer diagnosis. An intermediate goal of the genome project is the general availability of all DNA fragments of the human ordered along the chromosomes. Since this will allow us to select suitable probes for each chromosomal region, we will be able to diagnose all specific chromosomal alterations of the human genome detectable by in situ hybridization.

This project is supported by the Verein zur Förderung der Krebsforschung in Deutschland.

Dr. Peter Lichter
Division of Organization of Complex Genomes

Participating staff

Dr. Thomas Fink
Anette Kurz
Ulrike Mathieu
Sandra Weitz
Rebekka Zirbel

In collaboration with

Prof. Dr. Thomas Cremer
Institute of Human Genetics and Anthropology,
University of Heidelberg

Dr. Hartmut Döhner,
Dr. Martin Bentz
University Clinic and Outpatient Clinic,
University of Heidelberg

Prof. Dr. David Ward
Department of Human Genetics,
Yale University,
New Haven, Massachusetts, U.S.A.

Selected publications

Lichter, P., Cremer, T., Borden, J., Manuelidis, L., Ward, D.C.: Delineation of individual human chromosomes in metaphase and interphase cells by in situ suppression hybridization using chromosome specific library probes. Hum. Genet. 80, 224–234 (1988)

Cremer, T., Lichter, P., Borden, J., Ward, D.C., Manuelidis, L.: Detection of chromosome aberrations in metaphase and interphase tumor cells by in situ hybridization using chromosome specific library probes. Hum. Genet. 80, 235–246 (1988)

Lichter, P., Cremer, T., Tang, C.C., Watkins, P.C., Manuelidis, L., Ward, D.C.: Rapid detection of human chromosome 21 aberrations by in situ hybridization. Proc. Natl. Acad. Sci. USA 85, 9664–9668 (1988)

Lichter, P., Tang, C.C., Call, K., Hermanson, G., Evans, G.A., Housman, D., Ward, D.C.: High resolution mapping of human chromosome 11 by in situ hybridization with cosmid clones. Science 247, 64–69 (1990)

Lichter, P., Ward, D.C.: Is non-isotropic in situ hybridization finally coming of age? Nature 345, 93–95 (1990)

Lichter, P., Ledbetter, S.A., Ledbetter, D.H., Ward, D.C.: Fluorescence in situ hybridization with Alu and L1 polymerase chain reaction probes for rapid characterization of human chromosomes in hybrid cell lines. Proc. Natl. Acad. Sci. USA 87, 6634–6638 (1990)

Rowley, J.D., Diaz, M.O., Espinosa III, R., Patel, Y.D., van Melle, E., Ziemin, S., Taillon-Miller, P., Lichter, P., Evans. G.A., Kersey, J.H., Ward, D.C., Domer, P.H., Le Beau, M.M.: Mapping chromosome band 11q23 in human acute leukemia with biotinylated probes: Identification of 11q23 translocation breakpoints with a yeast artificial chromosome. Proc. Natl. Acad. Sci. USA 87, 9358–9362 (1990)

Lichter, P., Boyle, A.L., Cremer, T., Ward, D.C.: Analysis of genes and chromosomes by non-isotopic in situ hybridization. Genet. Anal. Techn. Appl. 8, 24–35 (1991)

7.4 Analysis of Genetic Diseases by Molecular Genetic Approaches

by Annemarie Poustka

The analysis of the human genome by molecular genetics is an essential step towards the understanding of many diseases with genetic components. This is especially the case for cancer research, since cancer is essentially a genetic disease of the somatic cell. In addition, the tendency to specific types of cancers is often found to be inherited, making the tendency to form tumors a genetic disease in the classical sense.

The genome contains the entire genetic information. This genetic information not only determines the obvious phenotypic features (e.g. eye color) of a human, but also controls development and behavior of each individual cell of the body. Since diseases are caused by the interaction between the environment with the genetically determined properties of the body and its individual cells, all diseases have genetic components. These become obvious if different forms of the genes involved in the disease process are found in the human population. Extreme examples of this are the classical genetic diseases (e.g., cystic fibrosis, Huntington's disease or fragile X), cases in which an essential gene is modified (a gene is the unit of the genome which contains the information for a specific genetic function, usually coding for a protein). Such a change in an essential gene usually leads to the formation of a changed (inactive or mis-acting) protein, causing disease and even death of the individual.

These inherited diseases also include a number of rare forms of tumors (e.g., retinoblastoma or Polyposis Coli), in which the tendency to form tumors is transmitted as a dominant trait in families. In this and other cases a change of a single base pair among the three billion bases of the human genome can therefore be the cause for a potentially lethal disease.

It can be shown that a number of common diseases (including some common cancers, e.g., breast cancer) also show an increased incidence in specific families. These common diseases are therefore also likely to have strong genetic components. In these cases it is, however, likely that multiple factors (both genetics and environment) are involved in the formation of these diseases, thus complicating the use of genetic analysis in identifying the major genes involved in these diseases. This represents one of the rationales for the planned complete mapping of the human genome, a major part of the human genome project, leading to an improvement in the analysis of complex genetic diseases.

Cancer is a Genetic Disease of the Somatic Cell

A tumor starts to form if the sequence of one of the genes controlling the growth of the cell is changed, either spontaneously, or caused by components of the environment (radiation, mutagenic chemicals). Such a cell escapes the control on its growth and, therefore, forms a tumor. Such a mutation can cause the formation of a dominantly acting oncogene, a gene which, in its mutatated form, causes uncontrolled growth. Alternatively, the function of a gene, which usually controls cell growth, can be disrupted, causing the cell to escape the normal growth regulation (recessive oncogenes).

Tumors can therefore be caused by minimal (single base) changes in the genome of a single cell of the body. Alternatively major changes in the genome of the single cell can similarly affect the structure (or presence) of specific genes involved in growth control, and can therefore trigger the formation of a tumor cell. Such changes (deletions, translocations, inversions, duplications) can therefore be used to predict the location of genes involved in tumour formation, since the genes involved will either be located within or at the border of the region affected by the rearrangement.

The Molecular Genetic Approach Offers Insight into the Causes of Human Diseases

To understand the mechanism causing diseases - in many cases this is a prerequisite for the ability to combat a disease - it is necessary to identify the genes involved in this process, and to understand their normal function.

The first step in identifying such a gene is its localization. In the case of inherited diseases this can often be achieved by linkage analysis, a process in which the region of the genome surrounding the mutated gene is found to be linked to the mutation through inheritance in families. In most cases this process of genetic mapping is able to localize a mutation to a region of a few centimorgan (one centimorgan corresponds to a distance giving rise to a 1% recombination probability, and corresponds roughly to a distance of one million basepairs).

Alternatively, it is possible to use major changes in the genome (e.g., cytogenetically visible deletions) correlated with mutations to identify the region of interest. Due to the limited resolution of these mapping techniques, it is, however, usually only possible to localize such disease genes to a region of, minimally, a few million base pairs.

From the Phenotype to the Gene

Biochemistry and molecular biology are inherently well suited to identify genes with known function, and especially genes with known gene product. Molecular genetics, the combination of genetic and molecular genetic analysis techniques offers the possibility to identify genes by observing the effect of mutations on the phenotype of the organisms.

Molecular genetic techniques have therefore been used successfully in identifying genes involved in, for example, essential steps of the development of the fruit fly Drosphila melanogaster. Though the analogous problems in mammalian genetics should therefore be accessible to a similar combination of genetic and molecular techniques, this proved difficult, due to the larger size of the mammalian genome, and the unavailability of many of the powerful genetic tools available for the analysis of the fruitfly genome. To allow a molecular analysis of such large regions of DNA, it was therefore necessary to extend the range of molecular cloning and analysis techniques from a few thousand to 10 thousand base pairs to millions of base pairs. Over the last 5 years this has triggered the explosive development of techniques designed to close this gap between distances accessible to standard molecular biological techniques and those resolved by genetic and cytogenetic analysis.

Development of Techniques for the Analysis of Large Genomes

To complement genetic and cytogenetic mapping techniques, we need, on one hand, a molecular mapping approach which allows the establishment of physical maps in the megabase range. This has been achieved by the development of pulsed field gel electrophoresis (PFGE), which is able to resolve DNA fragments of up to 7 megabases in agarose gels. In combination with the identification of restriction enzymes cutting sufficiently rarely in the mammalian genome this therefore allows the establishment of exact physical maps covering regions of a few megabases around a previously localized mutation. If the mutation is associated with a breakpoint in the DNA (e.g., breakpoints in chromosomes in leukemias), this analysis can also directly localize the position of the gene causing the mutation. Similarly, small deletions not identifiable by cytogenetic techniques can be used to localize the position of mutations, and serve as a diagnostic tool to identify the presence of a mutation.

Even if the position of the mutation cannot be directly localized, physical maps of the region surrounding the position of a mutation will improve the power of the genetic analysis techniques, and will simplify the design of appropriate cloning strategies to allow the cloning of the gene carrying the mutation.

To analyze larger regions in human chromosomes, we also need techniques to clone larger regions of DNA. Such cloning of long DNA regions was possible in the fruitfly genome by chromosome walking, a technique allowing the cloning of longer regions in steps, with a maximal step size of 40 kilobases. In the analysis of mammalian genomes this technique has been partly replaced by chromosome jumping, allowing a step size of up to 800 kilobases. This technique has for example allowed the identification of a number of genes, including the gene for Wilm's tumor, a kidney tumor occurring during childhood.

A second long range cloning approach, which has revolutionized mammalian molecular genetics is the development of yeast artificial chromosome vectors, allowing the cloning and analysis of DNA fragments of larger than one megabase in size.

These and other techniques have played an essential role in the identification of genes for a number of inherited diseases (Duchenne muscular dystrophy, cystic fibrosis, and one form of neurofibromatosis), as well as inherited tumors (Retinoblastoma, Wilm's tumor). Work on a number of other inherited diseases (Huntington's disease, polyposis coli) is advancing rapidly.

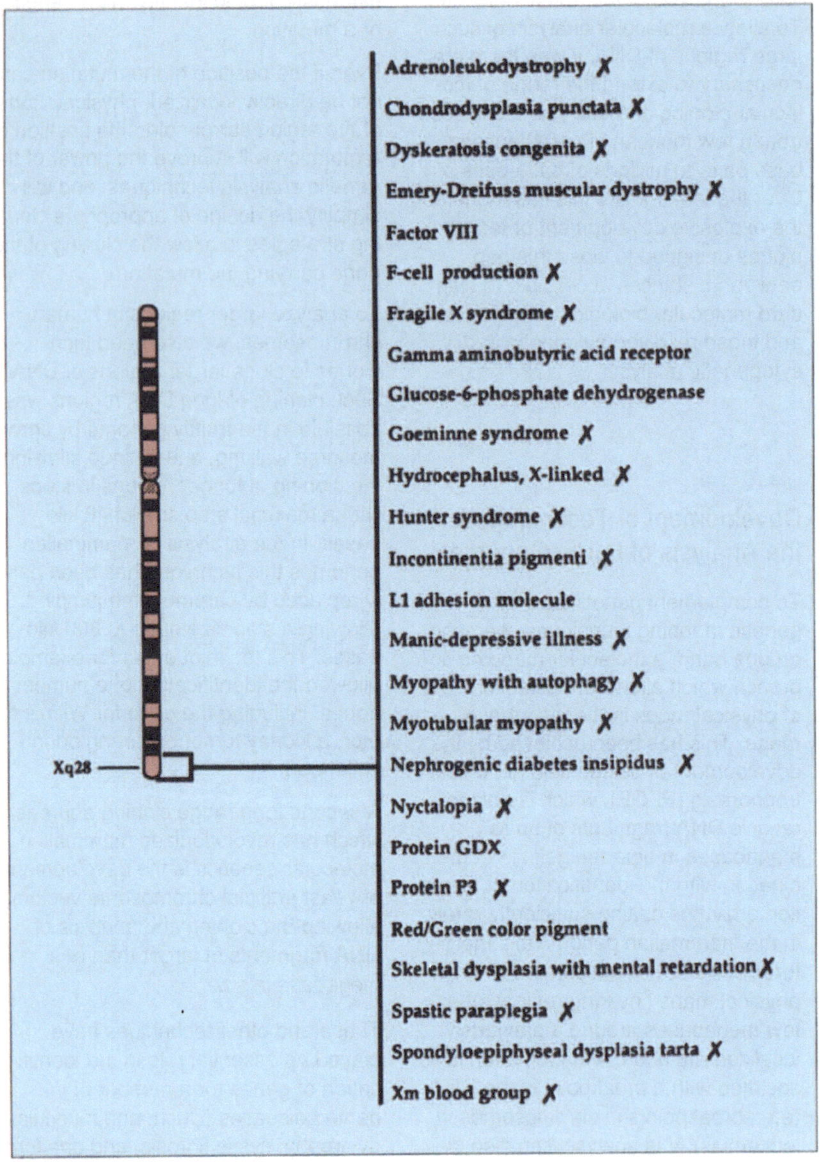

Fig. 104
Region Xq28, which comprises 8% of the human X chromosome, is one of the genetically richest regions in the human hereditary substance. Here, many genes causing hereditary diseases have been localized. Due to the advanced analysis and the high density of genes, this chromosome region is especially well suited as a model system for the advancement of methods of gene analysis.

Our laboratory has been especially interested in the analysis of the gene responsible for the fragile X syndrome. This mutation, the most common cause of inherited mental retardation, is defined cytogenetically by a fragile site close to the end of the long arm of the human X chomosome. In this work we have been able to clone the position of the fragility, and have isolated a candidate gene for causing the phenotype of the mutation. Based on this work, as well as the work of a number of other goups in this area, the mechanism of this mutation is therefore close to being understood.

The Human Genome Project

Since it can be expected that a large number of human genes will be involved in different diseases, a global effort to analyze the human genome has been proposed, and is being carried out in a number of countries. One of the goals of this analysis would therefore be to provide simplified access to genes of medical or biological importance. Our approach to the analysis of longer regions of human chromosomes (especially the Xq28 region of the human X chromosome therefore relies on the construction of ordered clone libraries, using a number of different vector systems (cosmids with 40 kb inserts, YACs with an average insert size of 600 kb). Such ordered clone libraries should also serve as the basis of a transcription map, which will allow us to establish the position of most or all genes, and could provide the substrate for the proposed sequence analysis of large regions of the human genome.

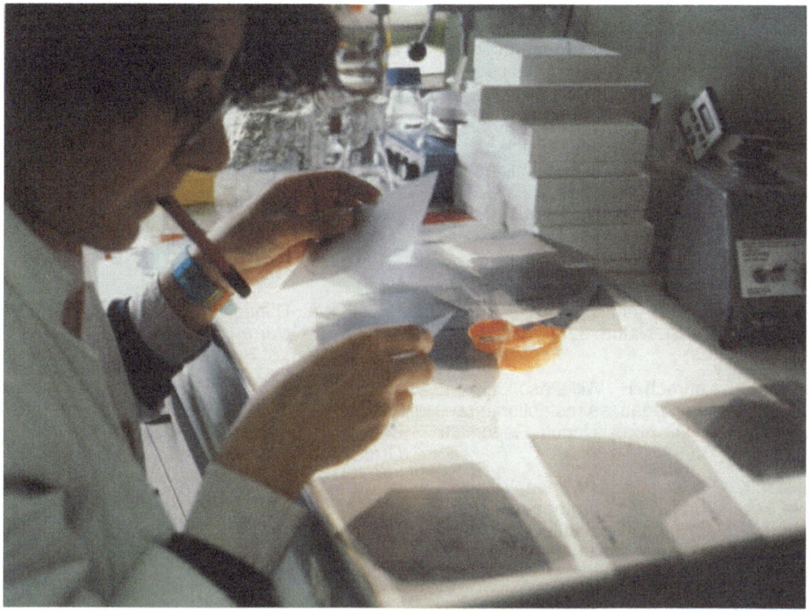

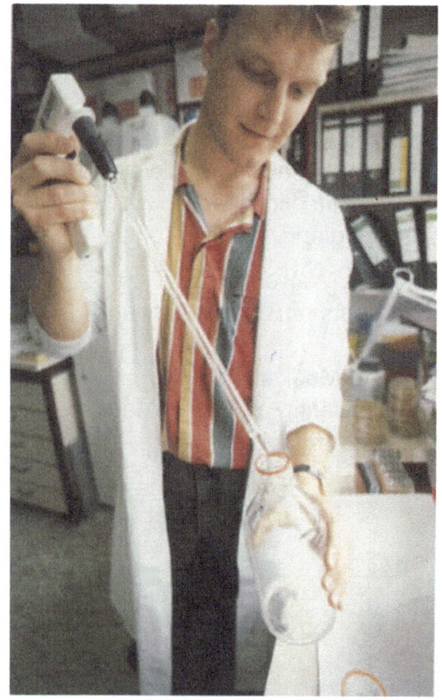

Fig. 105a, b
Searching for a needle in a haystack. Researchers use the most sophisticated molecular-biological methods to search for defective genetic elements that might cause hereditary diseases. Frequently, this means finding one such element among the three billion that describe the human hereditary information.

Our laboratory is especially involved in the analysis of the Xq28 region, a region of less than 10 megabases at the end of the human X chromosome, characterized by an especially high density of medically important mutations. The work on this region, which relies on a number of novel techniques, should contribute essentially to the isolation of the genes in the region (fragile X, Emery-Dreyfuss muscular dystrophy, adenoleukodystrophy, etc.), and should serve as a test for the analysis of larger genomic regions.

The Importance of the Human Genome Project for Cancer Research

This global analysis of the human genome is likely to be especially important for cancer research, since we expect that hundreds of genes will be able to mutate to give rise to cancer in one of the many cell types of the body. It has been estimated, that the identification of a single genetically defined gene (the gene mutated in cystic fibrosis) has involved costs of hundreds of millions of dollars. Identification of genes with more complex genetics will likely be even more difficult. Though a number of genes involved in carcinogenesis have been and will be isolated by the application of other techniques, it is nevertheless likely, that many of the genes involved in tumor formation will only be accessible by a molecular genetic analysis. This work will obviously be simplified or even made possible by the progress in the global analysis of the human genome, without which even the identification of a small number of genes would be considerably more expensive and slow.

Dr. Annemarie Poustka
Research Program Applied Tumor Virology

7

In collaboration with

Dr. Hans Lehrach
Imperial Cancer Research Fund,
London, England

Anthony P. Monaco
Institute for Molecular Medicine-ICRF,
John Radcliffe Hospital,
Oxford, England

Stephen T. Warren
Departments of Biochemistry and Pediatrics,
Division of Medical Genetics,
Emory University School of Medicine,
Atlanta, Georgia, U.S.A.

Selected publications

Poustka, A., Lehrach, H.: Jumping libraries and linking libraries: The next generation of molecular tools in mammalian genetics. Trends Genet. 2, 174–179 (1986)

Poustka, A., Pohl, T., Barlow, D.P., Zehetner, G., Craig, A., Michiels, F., Ehrich, E., Frischauf, A.-M., Lehrach, H.: Molecular approaches to mammalian genetics. Cold Spring Harbor Symp. Quant. Biol. LI (1), 131–139 (1986)

Poustka, A., Pohl, T.M., Barlow, D.P., Frischauf, A., Lehrach, H.: Construction and use of human chromosome jumping libraries from NotI digested DNA, Nature 325, 353–344 (1987)

Poustka, A., Lehrach, H., Williamson, R., Bates, G.: A five megabase restriction map spanning the cystic fibrosis locus. Genomics 2, 337–345 (1988)

Gessler, M., Poustka, A., Cavenee, W., Neve, R.L., Bruns, A.P.: Chromosome jumping in the WAGR region identifies CpG islands genes and deletions in Wilms tumors. Nature, 343, 774–778 (1990)

Herrman, B.G., Labeit, S., Poustka, A., King, T.R., Lehrach, H.: Cloning of T, a gene required in mesoderm formation in the mouse. Nature 343, 617–622 (1990)

Von Lindern, M., Poustka, A., Lehrach, H., Grosveld, G.: The (6;9) Chromosome Translocation, associated with a specific subtype af acute nonlymphocytic leukemia, leads to aberrant transciption of a target gene on 9q34. Mol. Cell. Biol., Vol. 10, 8, 8, 4016–4026 (1990)

Lehrach, H., Drmanac, R., Hoheisel, J., Larin, Z., Lennon, G., Nizetic, D., Monaco, A., Zehetner, G., Poustka, A.: Hybridisation Fingerprinting in Genome Mapping and Sequencing. In: Genome Analysis Volume 1, Ed. K. E. Davies, Cold Spring Harbor Laboratory Press, 39–81 (1990)

Poustka, A., Dietrich, A., Langenstein, G., Toniolo, D., Warren, S.T., Lehrach, H.: Physical Map of Human Xq27-qter Localising the Region of the Fragile X Mutation. PNAS 88, 8302–8306 (1991)

Dietrich, A., Kioschis, P., Monaco, A.P., Gross, B., Korn, B., Williams, S., Sheer, D., Heitz, D., Oberle, I., Toniolo, D., Warren, S.T., Lehrach, H., Poustka, A.: Molecular Cloning and Analysis of the Fragile X Region in Man. Nucleic Acids Research 19,10, 2567–2572 (1991)

7.5 Parvoviruses against Cancer?

by Jörg R. Schlehofer

Since the beginning of this century, it has been known that viruses can play a role in the development of tumors. The question arises, then, as to whether there are also viruses which can protect the organism from cancer.

In 1967, Helene Toolan from the Putnam Memorial Hospital in Bennington, Vermont, made an interesting observation: in a group of hamsters that had been infected with the virus H-1, a "parvovirus", the incidence of tumors was 95% lower than in the non-infected control group. In 1969, Victor Bergs from the Medical School of the University of Miami in Coral Gables, Florida, reported that leukemias, which in rats are caused by a certain oncogenic retrovirus, are suppressed by a rat parvovirus. Since then, various authors have published papers in which they showed that parvoviruses can suppress the development of tumors which in hamsters are caused by DNA-containing viruses. In addition, it has been reported that cancer which developed from tumor cells transplanted into hamsters can also be inhibited by parvoviruses.

Thus, in nature there are not only viruses that play an important part in the development of tumors, but also others that appear to help the organism in its fight against cancer cells.

What are Parvoviruses?

Parvoviruses are extremely small: they have a diameter of only 20 nanometers. (One nanometer is one millionth of a millimeter.) The genetic information they contain is a single-stranded deoxyribonucleic acid (DNA), in contrast to the two-stranded DNA (the well-known double helix), which carries the genetic information of most DNA-containing viruses and also of human chromosomes.

As is known, viruses by themselves are neither viable nor capable of proliferating: they need the cells of the host organism as a "culture medium". For replication, parvoviruses depend even more than other viruses on functions of their host cells. These functions appear to be related to cell division, because parvoviruses are only replicated in cells that divide (such as in cancer tissues). Moreover, some members of this class

Fig. 106a
Deep-frozen in liquid nitrogen, tissue culture cells can be preserved for many years.

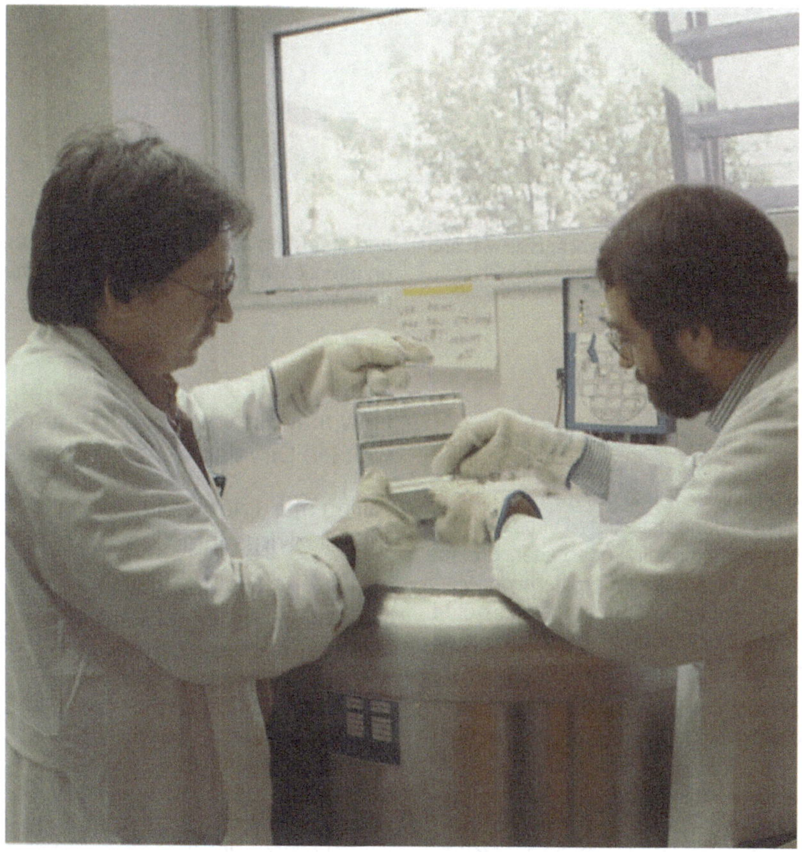

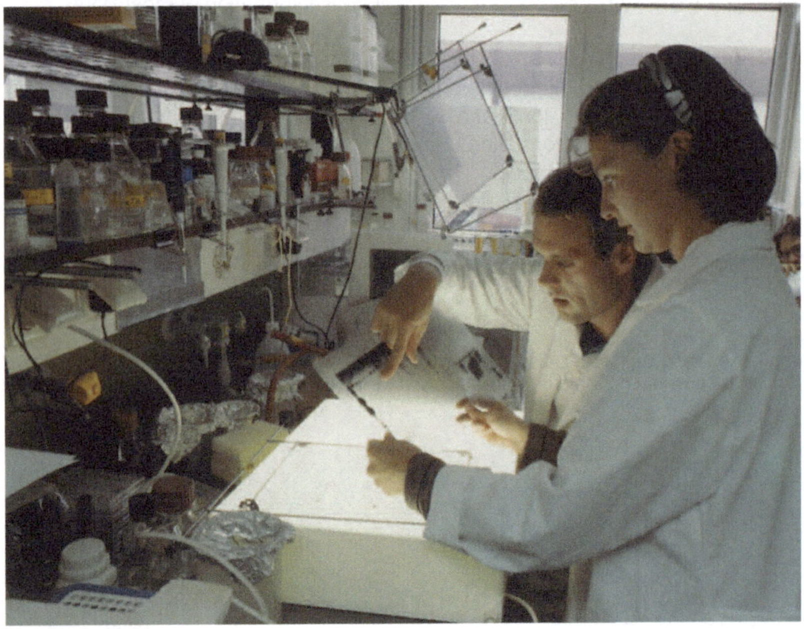

Fig. 106b
A comparison between cancer cells with and without parvovirus infection reveals differences in the specific patterns of the isolated DNA fragments.

of viruses can be propagated only if they are helped by another virus, a helper virus. These parvoviruses are called "adeno-associated viruses" (AAV) and (usually) need adenoviruses or herpes viruses for proliferation. Much of the research of our group is devoted to the investigation of the properties of these adeno-associated viruses.

The mentioned parvoviruses are not pathogenic in humans, in contrast to the B-19 virus, which causes the rather harmless "fifth disease" (erythema infectiosum). Only in exceptional cases, e.g., in patients with certain anaemias, and at certain stages of pregnancy, can an infection with the virus B-19 become dangerous.

How may Parvoviruses Interfere with the Development of Tumors?

Killing of Tumor Cells by Parvovirus Infection

In 1982, Jean Rommelaere and Suzanne Mousset, both from the Free University of Brussels, Belgium, showed that cells which had been transformed in vitro (in the tissue culture) into cancerous cells by a tumor virus (SV40) were killed by infection with the parvovirus MVM (minute virus of mice), whereas the non-cancerous cells survived. One year later, Regine Heilbronn of our research group obtained similar results. She showed that tissue culture cells, the genotype of which had been damaged by carcinogens, and which thus had only gone through the first step towards becoming a cancer cell, died when infected with adeno-associated viruses.

Another finding indicating one of the possible mechanisms of cancer inhibition by parvoviruses again resulted from experiments of Rommelaere's group. It was shown that the abovementioned parvovirus H-1 does not kill normal human cells but only cells that have become malignant by infection with the well-studied SV40 (tumor) virus. Our group and Rommelaere's were in close contact with each other. In the past years, Steffen Faisst of our group confirmed the result of the Brussels group, and also showed that parvoviruses, without affecting normal cells, do not only selectively kill SV40-transformed cells, but almost all human tumor cells. Preferred "victims" of parvovirus H-1 are those cells whose "transformed phenotype" (cancerous growing behavior) is related to the presence of a tumor virus (such as the SV40, the papilloma, or the Epstein-Barr viruses).

These characteristics of parvovirus H-1 were also confirmed in animal experiments: fast-growing tumors develop after injection of HeLa cells (established 40 years ago from human cervix uteri cancer tissue) into mice. The growth of these tumors can be slowed down by infecting the animals with par-

Fig. 107
The computer model shows the spatial structure of a parvovirus.

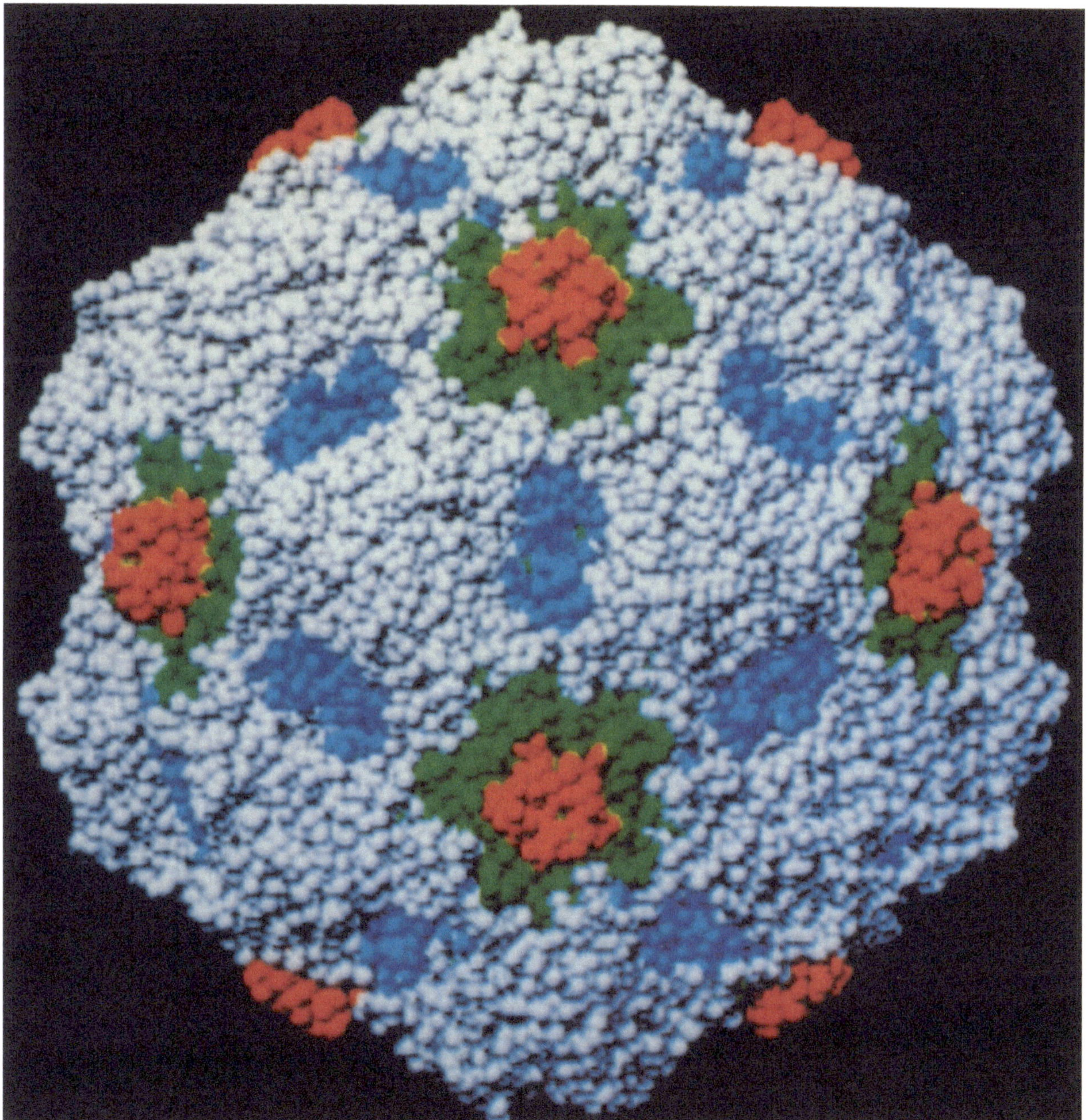

vovirus H-1 (and also with adeno-associated viruses); in some cases it was possible to almost completely suppress tumor growth. The parvovirus infection itself does not affect the animals. Thierry Dupressoir (of Rommelaere's group at the Pasteur Institute in Lille, France) confirmed these studies for the suppression of the growth of human mammary cancer cells in mice.

Thus, parvovirus infections may be a natural "defense" against cancer. Since many parvoviruses proliferate almost exclusively in tumor cells and not in healthy cells, the described findings suggest that parvoviruses might act by preferentially killing tumor cells.

The Influence of Parvovirus Infections on Molecular-Genetic Events in the Early Period of the Development of Malignancy

Some years ago, it was shown that not only mutagenic events (direct damage or alteration of genetic material), but also selective DNA amplification plays a part in the very early stages of tumor development. DNA amplification, as well as mutations, can be caused by carcinogenic substances (such as benzo(a)pyrene or dimethylbenz(a)-anthracene), and also by radiation.

Experiments on cells treated with carcinogens (in vitro) showed that DNA amplification is prevented by infection with adeno-associated viruses and that mutations occur less frequently. Parvoviruses thus may be able to prevent genetic alterations that contribute significantly and at very early stages to the development of cancers.

Influence of Parvovirus Infections on Molecular and Cytological Processes

Recent findings indicate that parvoviruses control the activity of certain genes, i.e., they can change the amount of gene products that are involved in specific cell functions. Kenneth Berns and his New York group observed that, for instance, certain genes of adeno-associated viruses may suppress the expression of "foreign" DNA introduced into cells. We have shown that parvovirus H-1 and adeno-associated virus alter the expression of tumor virus DNA in tumor cells, the development of which involved (tumor) viruses. At present, Jürgen Kleinschmidt and his group are investigating this parvovirus function with regard to the influence of adeno-associated viruses on the expression of human papilloma virus genes. (Faisst of Rommelaere's group at the Pasteur Institute in Lille is doing this for parvovirus H-1.)

Parvoviruses also alter "normal" cellular genes. Petra Klein-Bauernschmitt and Valérie Botquin of our group have demonstrated that genes which are important for cellular differentiation are activated by infection with adeno-associated viruses. Differentiation means that "immature" precursor cells proceed to specialized stages in which they take on their actual task without further dividing. One characteristic of cancer cells is their "immaturity", in particular, their unlimited capacity to divide. Thus, if differentiation genes are activated by parvovirus infection, the cell will mature and will no longer be able to divide; it will thus no longer be malignantly transformed. The observed inhibition of tumor development by parvoviruses might therefore also be caused by a promotion of the differentiation of "transformed" cells.

It has been known for some time from cell culture experiments that after infection with adeno-associated viruses the viral DNA is integrated into the genome of the host cells. It is still not known whether such integration also takes place in humans and if certain tissues may be preferentially affected by this "permanent" infection. Since this appears to be very likely, we studied the effects of such integration on human tumor cells (in the tissue culture). Christian Walz of our group infected HeLa cells with adeno-associated viruses and analyzed in more detail the cells that had integrated the viral DNA. It turned out that these cells divided much slower than the uninfected cells. In addition, cells containing the parvovirus DNA were more sensitive to radiation and toxic substances such as those used in cancer therapy. Decelerated growth and higher radiosensitivity also became evident in animal experiments: tumors of HeLa cells with integrated parvovirus DNA grew slower and regressed faster after irradiation than uninfected tumors. At present, Christian Walz is investigating which parvovirus functions may be responsible for these changes. So far, he has discovered that the integration of the parvovirus DNA takes place in the HeLa cell's chromosome 17. Now, he is trying to determine if a gene linked to tumor growth is affected by this integration of viral DNA.

For melanoma cells and vaginal carcinoma cells, Ursula Bantel-Schaal of our division has demonstrated (in vitro) the growth-inhibiting and eventually cytocidal influence of adeno-associated viruses. She has also observed an increased sensitivity of SV40-transformed hamster cell cultures (cell cultures that had been cancerously altered by the SV40 tumor virus) to "genotoxic stress" (such as carcinogens and radiation) if the cells were infected with adeno-associated viruses.

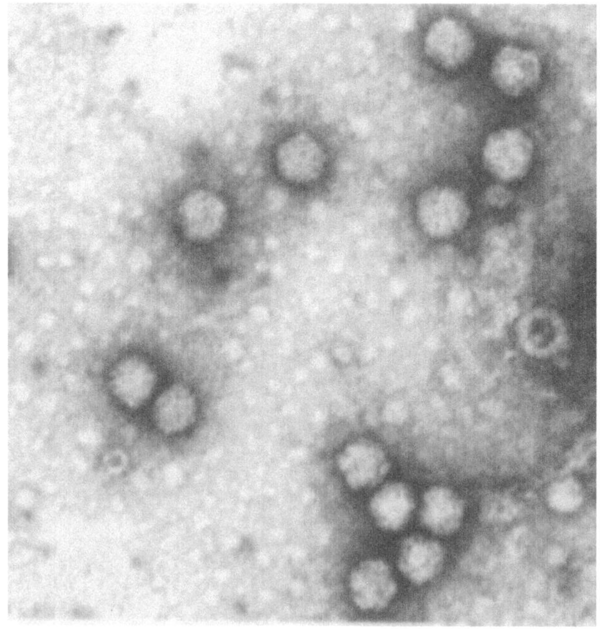

Fig. 108
Parvoviruses are so small that for decades they simply escaped notice. Only by using an electron microscope can they be seen.

Applicability and Problems of Tumor Therapy

Observations in cell culture and in animal experiments raise the question of whether there are also examples for tumor inhibition by parvoviruses in humans.

In the 1970s, Heather Mayor from Texas, Suzanne Sprecher-Goldberger of the Brussels group and, in the early 1980s, Brigitte Georg-Fries from Freiburg showed that the incidence of certain cancers (in particular, cervical carcinoma) is lower in persons who have a strong immunologic response to parvovirus (AAV) infection than in persons whose organism has had no contact with AAV. The group of John R. Pattison of the Department of Medical Virology of University College, London, recently reported that certain tumors are observed less frequently in persons who have been infected by parvovirus B-19. It thus appears that there is an influence of parvovirus infection on tumor development in humans, too.

It may be possible to make direct use of the property of parvoviruses to preferentially destroy tumor cells. We have already started to investigate this problem with animal experiments. Prior to seriously considering therapeutic application, however, it must be proven that such parvoviruses (H-1) really do not cause any diseases. To this end, we conduct epidemiologic and serologic studies in which we measure the blood (serum) antibodies (i.e., an immunologic response) to parvoviruses (H-1, AAV, and B-19) in humans. (We can determine the incidence of parvovirus infections from the rate of healthy persons and patients with various symptoms having parvovirus antibodies in the blood, and from this we might draw conclusions regarding the symptoms caused by these infections.) Infections with parvovirus H-1 seem to occur relatively frequently in humans without causing any disease. The significance of such infections is presently being studied by Karsten Geletneky of our group and Brigitte Schlehofer of the Division of Epidemiology in an extensive sero-epidemiologic study. They are attempting to find out whether the presence of antibodies against parvovirus H-1 is related to a reduced "cancer predisposition" (as is the case in the aforementioned studies with adeno-associated viruses).

In cooperation with Michael Flentje of the Radiologic Clinic of the University of Heidelberg and Christian Walz of our group, we have shown that an infection of HeLa and other tumor cells with adeno-associated viruses increases the cells' radiosensitivity. On the basis of these investigations, we have developed a research project in which we

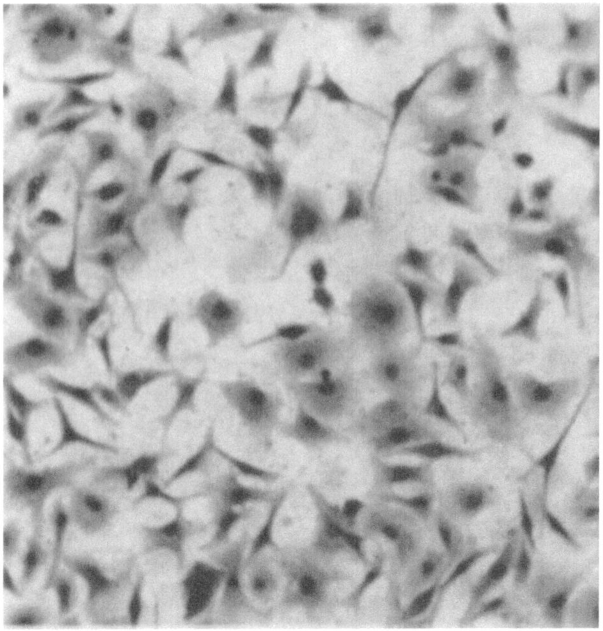

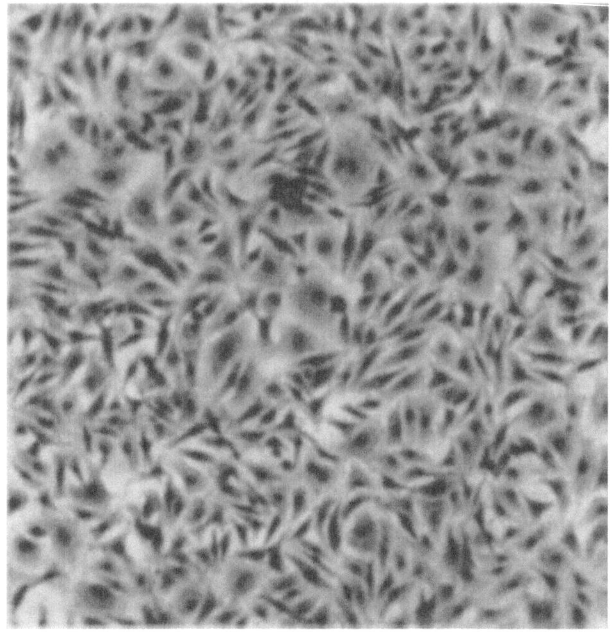

Figs. 109, 110
The growth of human melanoma cells is inhibited by infection with adeno-associated parvoviruses (Fig. 109). Figure 110 shows a non-infected control culture.

want to establish whether and how parvovirus infections can be used in therapy to increase radiosensitivity, e.g., to allow tumor treatment with lowered doses of radiation.

It might also be possible to exploit the preference of most parvoviruses for proliferating tissue (such as tumor tissue) for using them as a vehicle to channel anti-tumor agents into cancer cells. Jürgen Kleinschmidt and his group are presently trying to produce artificial parvovirus particles for this purpose. This might be another possible basis for new forms of cancer therapy.

It is obvious that the mechanisms of tumor inhibition by parvoviruses are extremely complex. So far, very little is known about the underlying molecular biological mechanisms, and many investigations still have to be performed. Once the underlying mechanisms are known, we might have a new concept of tumor therapy which would be based on the use of naturally existing antitumor principles.

Our work has been sponsored by the German Society for the Advancement of Scientific Research (Deutsche Forschungsgemeinschaft), by the cooperation between the Deutsches Krebsforschungszentrum and the National Council of Research and Development (Israel), as well as by the program for the promotion of young scientists by the Major Science Research Institutions (Arbeitsgemeinschaft der Großforschungseinrichtungen).

Priv.-Doz. Dr. Jörg Schlehofer
Division of Tumor Virology

Participating scientists

Dr. Ursula Bantel-Schaal
Valérie Botquin
Matthias Ehrbar
Karsten Geletneky
Dr. Petra Klein-Bauernschmitt
Dipl.-Biol. Christian Walz
Ilona Wesch
Prof. Dr. Harald zur Hausen

In collaboration with

Dr. Regine Heilbronn
Dr. Jürgen Kleinschmidt
Division of Tumor Virology,
Deutsches Krebsforschungszentrum

Dr. Volker Rudat
Division of Oncological Diagnostics and Therapy,
Deutsches Krebsforschungszentrum

Dr. Brigitte Schlehofer
Dr. Jürgen Wahrendorf
Division of Epidemiology,
Deutsches Krebsforschungszentrum

Dr. Michael Flentje
Radiologic Clinic of the University of Heidelberg

Prof. Dr. Jörg Michaelis
Institute for Medical Statistics and Documentation, University of Mainz

Prof. Dr. Hans-Jörg Riehm
Pediatric Clinic of the Medical University Hannover

Dr. Tino F. Schwarz
Max von Pettenkoffer Institute for Hygienics and Medical Microbiology,
University of Munich

Dr. Steffen Faisst
Institut Pasteur,
Lille, France

Prof. Dr. Jean Rommelaere
Unité d'oncologie moléculaire,
Institut Pasteur,
Lille, France
Département de biologie moléculaire,
Université Libre de Bruxelles,
Rhode-St.-Genèse, Belgium
Now: Division of Tumor Virology,
Deutsches Krebsforschungszentrum

Dr. Jacov Tal
Ben-Gurion-Universität,
Beer-Sheva, Israel

Selected publications

Rommelaere, J., Tattersall, P.: Oncosuppression by parvoviruses. In: Handbook of parvoviruses, Vol. II, Ed. P. Tijssen, CRC Press Inc., Boca Raton, Fla., pp. 41–57 (1990) (Übersicht)

Schlehofer, J.R., Heilbronn, R., Georg-Fries, B., zur Hausen, H.: Inhibition of initiator-induced SV40 gene amplification in SV40-transirmed Chinese hamster cells by infection with a defective parovirus. Int. J. Cancer 32, 591–595 (1983)

Heilbronn, R., Schlehofer, J.R., zur Hausen, H.: Selective killing of carcinogen-treated SV40-transformed Chinese hamster cells by a defective parvovirus. Virology 136, 349–441 (1984)

Faißt, S., Schlehofer, J.R., zur Hausen, H.: Transformation of human cells by oncogenic viruses supports permissiveness for parvovirus H-1 propagation. J. Virol. 63, 2152–2158 (1989)

Bantel-Schaal, U.: Adeno-associated parvoviruses inhibit growth of cells derived from malignant human tumors. Int. J. Cancer 45, 190–194 (1990)

Schlehofer, J.R., Heilbronn, R.: Infection with adeno-associated virus type 5 inhibits mutagenicity of herpes simplex virus type 1 or 4-nitroquinoline-1-oxide. Mut. Res. 244, 317–320 (1990)

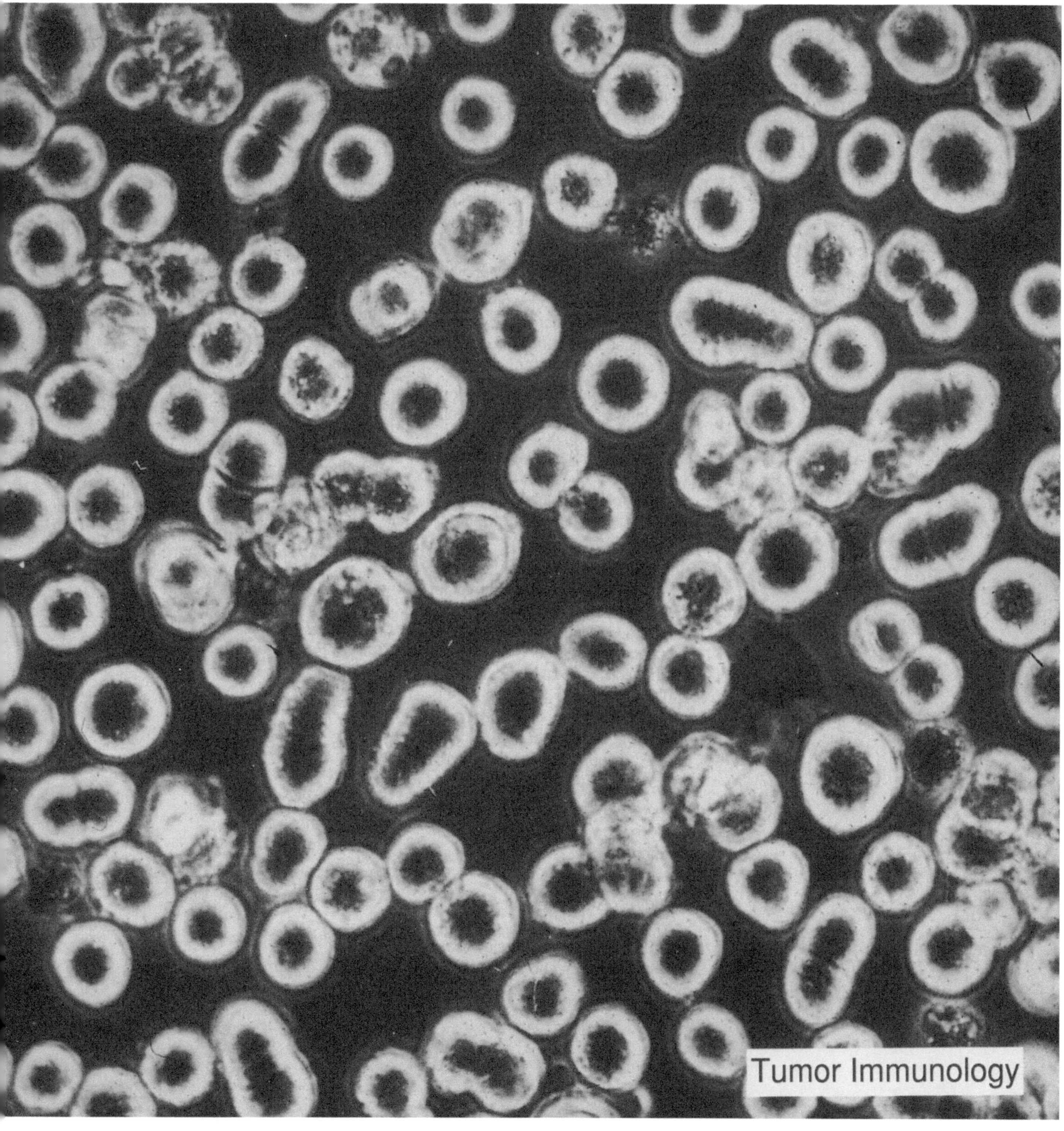
Tumor Immunology

8

Tumor Immunology

The work of the Research Program is concentrated on new immunological methods of tumor diagnostics as well as on immunological concepts for tumor therapy and the investigation of the biological mechanisms underlying processes of cellular interaction and metastatic spreading.

The priorities are in the following fields:

- Manufacturing of monoclonal antibodies against tumor-associated antigens and differentiation antigens for diagnosis and therapy of tumors.
- Expression of membrane antigens on cells. In this context, not only tumor-specific antigens, but also viral antigens and mainly histocompatibility genes are investigated. In particular, their role is being explored in the immunological struggle between the host and the tumor.
- Regulation of the immune system. This includes the investigation of immunoregulatory products of tumor cells, the identification and biochemical characterization of lymphokines, biochemical aspects of the activation and regulation of T-lymphocytes under normal and pathological conditions, investigations of mutagenized tumor cell lines as well as the structure of antigens and lymphokine receptors.
- Analysis of the immuno-pathogenetic mechanisms for cancer and HIV infection.
- In addition, the research program investigates the programmed cell death (apoptosis) and its significance in tumor research and in the immune system.
- More recently, auto-immune disease models and immunological tumor models have been established in transgenic mice with histocompatible and other genes. These give important insights into the mechanisms of regulation and pathogenesis.
- Another focus of research is concerned with the mechanisms of tumor invasion and the development of metastases.

The development of new therapeutic concepts with an immunological basis is an important objective of research which is being worked on along various lines in all divisions. These investigations take into account that tumor cells are recognized by the immune system in many cases and also that they can potentially be eliminated. On the other hand, currently unknown regulatory mechanisms prevent resistance in terms of transplant rejection.

Coordinator of the Research Program:
Prof. Dr. Peter Krammer

Divisions and their heads:

Cellular Immunology:
Prof. Dr. Volker Schirrmacher

Immunochemistry:
Prof. Dr. Wulf Dröge

Immunogenetics:
Prof. Dr. Peter Krammer

Somatic Cell Genetics:
Prof. Dr. Günter Hämmerling

Project groups and their heads:

Tolerance and Immune Response:
Priv.-Doz. Dr. Margot Zöller

8.1 Influence of Cysteine on Gene Expression and Lymphocyte Functions – A Cellular Cysteine Deficiency as a Common Pathogenetic Factor of AIDS and of Certain Types of Cancer

by Wulf Dröge

Introduction

Patients with advanced malignancies frequently suffer from a reduced immunological reactivity that is associated with a decreased resistance to life-threatening infections. Many patients also suffer from severe weight loss (cachexia). This combination of symptoms is reminiscent of the acquired immunodeficiency syndrome (AIDS). The decreased immunological reactivity of cancer patients may also be seen in the context of the old question: Why is the immune system not capable of rejecting cancer cells? There are several recent reports claiming that certain types of human cancer cells can be recognized and killed by autologous cytotoxic T cells (killer cells). Several laboratories have succeeded in isolating tumor specific cytotoxic T cell clones from patients with melanoma. Moreover, the successful treatment of patients with advanced cancer by tumor infiltrating lymphocytes in the laboratory of Steven Rosenberg (National Institute of Health, USA) has also shown that activated cytotoxic T cells can express substantial therapeutic efficacy. But why are these cytotoxic T cells not normally sufficiently activated in the patient to defend the host against its own tumor?

Recent clinical studies in the division of immunochemistry in collaboration with several hospitals in the Heidelberg area have shown that there is a link between the decreased immunological reactivity and a tumor-induced dysregulation of plasma amino acid levels. The hallmark of this dysregulation is a strongly increased glutamate level in the blood plasma. An even more extreme increase of plasma glutamate levels has been observed in HIV infected patients. Glutamate (the salt of glutamic acid) is an amino acid and thus a component of all protein molecules. It is transported into the cell with the help of a specific membrane transport system (system xc-) which also transports the amino acid cystine. As a consequence of this competition between the two amino acids for the same membrane transport system, an elevation of the extracellular glutamate concentration causes an increased influx of glutamate and a decreased influx of cystine into the cell. Since each molecule of cystine is split within the cell into two molecules of the small amino acid cysteine, the inhibition of the cystine transport leads ultimately to an intracellular deficiency of cysteine.

The Importance of Cysteine for the Regulation of Gene Expression and Lymphocyte Functions.

The regulatory role of oxidizing and antioxidative conditions

The transcription factor NFkB regulates the activity of several immunologically relevant genes, including the gene for the IL-2 receptor and tumor necrosis factor (TNF-a). In experiments with a human T cell line (Molt 4) and a promonocytic line (U937), we have shown that increased extracellular cysteine concentrations inhibit the activation of this transcription factor. Subsequent experiments by Patrick Baeuerle (Max-Planck-Institute of Biochemistry, Munich-Martinsried) have indicated that this transcription factor is stimulated by active oxygen derivatives such as hydrogen peroxide and inhibited by antioxidants such as cysteine or cysteine derivatives. A similar antagonistic regulation by hydrogen peroxide and antioxidants has been demonstrated in our department by Steffen Roth for the production of interleukin 2 and for IL-2 gene expression. IL-2 production was shown to be stimulated by hydrogen peroxide and inhibited by the cysteine derivative glutathione.

In order for these immunologically relevant genes to be activated, it is obviously important that the lymphocytes should normally have a relatively low intracellular cysteine concentration. Our analysis of a large series of human and murine T cell preparations, T cell clones, and T cell tumors revealed that T cells do generally have a relatively low membrane transport activity for cystine and, therefore, normally a relatively low cysteine supply.

If the cysteine supply to the T cells is further decreased (for example, as a consequence of increased extracellular glutamate levels) negative consequences, such as oxidative damage and an unphysiological over-expression of certain genes, have to be expected. An over-expression of NFkB-dependent gene products has indeed been observed in HIV-infected patients, as will later be discussed. Moreover, a decreased supply of cysteine can also lead to a decreased intracellular concentration of glutathione. This is a substance that consists of the three amino acids cysteine, glutamate, and glycin, and which plays an important role in many biochemical processes within the cell. Studies in cell cultures with approximately physiological amino acid concentrations have shown that a decrease of the intracellular glutathione level inhibits two particular important functions, i.e., the activation of cytotoxic T cells and the IL-2 dependent proliferation of T cells. These functions are greatly inhibited even by a relatively moderate decrease of the extracellular cysteine supply. In such cell culture experiments we have also been able to show that the elevation of extracellular glutamate levels causes a decreased intracellular cysteine level and inhibits lymphocyte functions.

Taken together, these studies indicate that certain aspects of T cell-mediated immune responses require oxidizing conditions, whereas other aspects require antioxidative conditions. Accordingly, the immune system can only function well if oxidizing and antioxidative conditions are properly balanced.

The Macrophage as a "Cysteine Pump"

The disulfide cystine accounts for approximately 90% of the low molecular weight cysteine in the blood plasma. The plasma concentration of reduced cysteine is only 15 micromolar and, therefore, extremely small in comparison to virtually all other protein-forming amino acids, whereas cystine occurs in the blood plasma at a concentration of about 60–80 micromolar, corresponding to a concentration of 120–160 micromolar cysteine equivalents. Since T cells generally only have relatively weak membrane transport activity for cystine, they can barely utilize this rela-

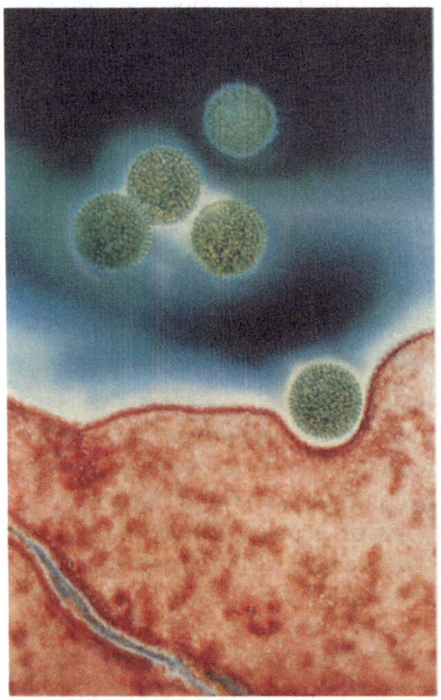

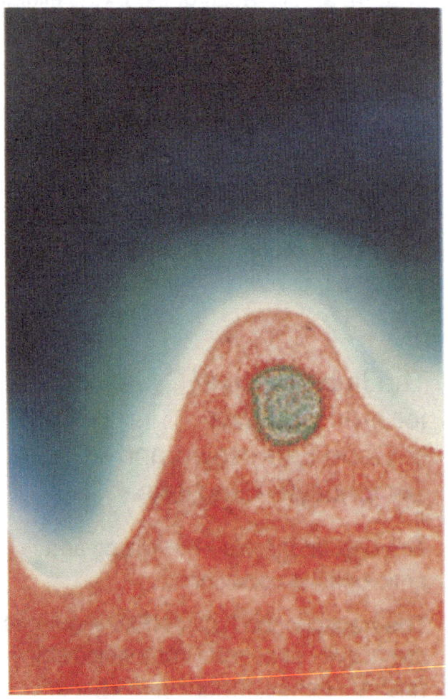

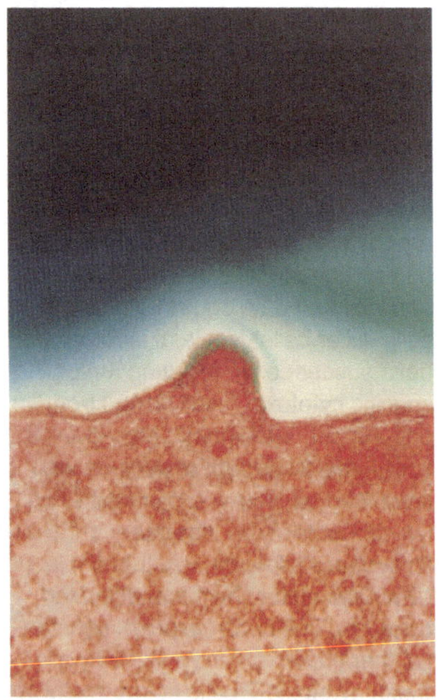

Figs. 111–114
The figures show how HIV viruses in the body establish close contact with defense cells and are imported into their interior. There, the hereditary material is replicated and new virus particles are formed. They arrange themselves into complete virus particles which leave the infected cell. The mechanism which ultimately leads to the destruction of the immune system of the HIV-infected individual is not yet understood in detail and is the subject of ongoing research.

tively high extracellular cystine concentration. T cells, therefore, depend to a great extent on the extracellular cysteine concentration which is relatively low in the blood plasma. However, in the course of the immune response T cells come into intimate contact with macrophage-like cells that have a relatively strong membrane transport for cystine and are therefore capable of releasing large amounts of reduced cysteine into the extracellular space. The cysteine export can be further increased by stimulation of the macrophages with various agents. T cells that are binding to processed antigens on the surface of the macrophages and which therefore come into intimate contact with these cells are exposed to relatively high extracellular concentrations of cysteine. In double chamber experiments we have been able to show that macrophages can provide T cells with cysteine and elevate the intracellular glutathione level and the proliferative activity of stimulated lymphocytes even if the two types of cells are separated by a permeable membrane. Cysteine, therefore, appears to have a regulatory role in the immune system analogous to the role of the hormone-like cytokines and lymphokines. Cysteine is released by immunologically relevant cells (macrophages) at a variable and regulated rate and regulates immunologically relevant functions of lymphocytes. The physiological "purpose" of the low cystine membrane transport of T cells in combination with this cysteine pumping function of the macrophages seems to be that T cells can be switched by the macrophages from relatively oxidative conditions to more antioxidative conditions. Since elevated extracellular concentrations of glutamate inhibit the membrane transport of cystine into the macrophage, this cysteine pumping function of the macrophages is greatly inhibited by elevated extracellular glutamate.

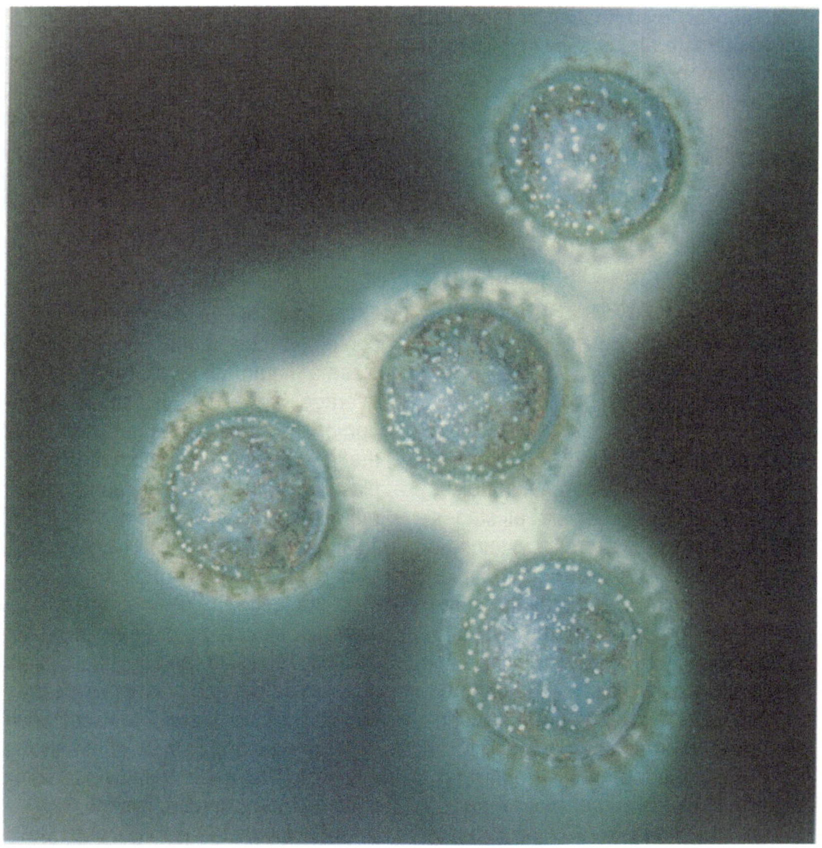

The Link between the Cellular Cysteine Supply and the Number of CD4+ T Cells in Healthy Human Individuals

Studies on healthy human individuals have indicated that the transport of cystine into the cells also plays a limiting role in the immune system of healthy living organisms. In one of these studies, we investigated the correlation between individual CD4+ T cell counts and individual serum glutamate and cystine levels. When the persons were divided into four groups of about equal size on the basis of their median glutamate and cystine levels (represented by four segments in Figure 116), it was found that the group with the low gluta-

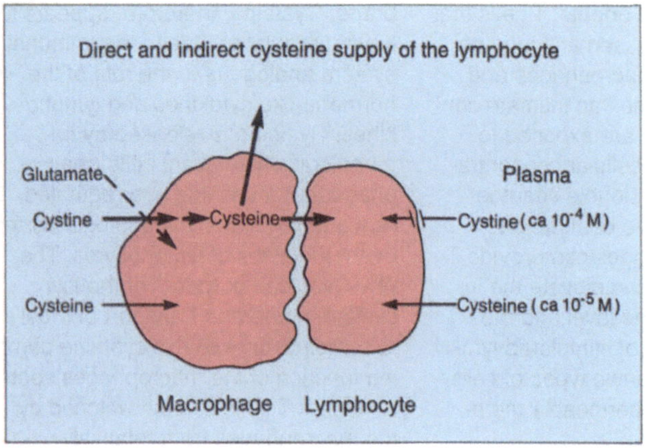

Fig. 115
The T-cell mediated immunoreaction is in part controlled by the intracellular cysteine concentration. In the plasma, the amino acid exists mostly in its oxidized form, called cystine. Macrophages can take up larger amounts of cystine and metabolize it to cysteine, which is passed on to the lymphocytes. If the glutamate concentration outside of the cells is increased, the membrane transport of cystine into the macrophages is inhibited and the "cysteine pump effect" is suppressed.

mate and high cystine levels (i.e., segment 1) had a significantly higher CD4+ T cell count than the other three groups. In a second study, we analyzed the correlation between lymphocyte function (mitogenic response) and glutamate and cystine levels. In analogy to the first study, the results showed that the group with low glutamate and high cystine levels had a significantly higher lymphocyte reactivity than the other three groups.

Since our experiments with cell cultures had shown already a causative influence of the extracellular glutamate levels on the intracellular cysteine level, and since the in vivo studies showed simultaneously a correlation of T4 counts with glutamate and cystine levels, these findings strongly suggest that glutamate and cystine levels may have a causative influence on the immune system in healthy human individuals as well.

Elevated Plasma Glutamate and Decreased Cysteine and Cystine Levels as Pathogenetic Factors in the Acquired Immunodeficiency Syndrome (AIDS)

Several years ago, we observed in two consecutive and independent studies that HIV-infected patients of all stages of the disease suffer from a cysteine and cystine deficiency that is accompanied by markedly elevated mean glutamate levels. We proposed that this cysteine deficiency may be responsible for the progressive destruction of the immune system in these patients. Some of the HIV-infected persons were found to have less than one-fifth of the normal value of cysteine and/or more than fivefold the normal level of plasma glutamate. The cysteine deficiency was associated with a significant decrease of intracellular glutathione levels. These results were confirmed later by other laboratories, among others at the National Institute of Health, and at Stanford University in the USA. It is important to note that the decreased cysteine level and the elevated plasma glutamate concentrations have been observed already in asymptomatic HIV-infected persons, i.e., in the very early phase of the disease. In collaboration with scientists of the German Primate Center in Göttingen, we have also shown that the cysteine level starts to decrease and the glutamate level starts to increase in rhesus macaques within 1 week after infection with the simian immunodeficiency virus (SIV). This indicates that the virus-induced dysregulation of the plasma amino acid levels precedes the destruction of the immune system and may also be the causative factor in this closely related animal model of AIDS.

Our studies of HIV-infected patients confirmed the rule that persons with low plasma glutamate levels have, on the average, higher T4+ cell counts than persons with high glutamate levels and that persons with a combination of high plasma cystine and low plasma glutamate levels, (i.e., segment 1 in Figure 116) have the highest T4+ cell count. Moreover, since HIV-infected persons of all stages of the disease have, on the average, elevated glutamate levels and decreased cystine and cysteine levels, our studies provide a simple explanation for the decreased T4+ T cell counts in these patients. In view of the strong interindividual and intraindividual variations of the glutamate, cystine, and cysteine levels in these patients, our results are best compatible with the interpretation that the damaging immunological consequences of the occasional episodes with extremely high glutamate and/or low cysteine and cystine levels may be essentially irreversible and that they accumulate over many years. This assumption would explain the slow but progressive decline of the T4+ counts that leads ultimately to the typical symptoms of AIDS.

As expected from the cysteine deficiency, HIV-infected persons were indeed found to over-express certain NFkB-dependent gene products. For example, these patients were shown to have an over-expression of IL-2 receptors and relatively high concentrations of tumor necrosis factor-a (TNF-a). The elevated TNF-a levels are generally believed to contribute to the weight loss (cachexia) of these patients. It is also important to note that the genome of the immunodeficiency virus (HIV) itself is also under the control of the transcription factor NFkB and, therefore is, expected to benefit from the cysteine deficiency in these patients. Cysteine and N-acetylcysteine were found to inhibit HIV replication. The detailed analysis of the role of cysteine in the regulation of gene expression is the subject of ongoing research.

Treatment of HIV-Infection with N-Acetyl-Cysteine (NAC)

In view of the cysteine deficiency in HIV-infected patients, we proposed as early as in 1988 that cysteine, cysteine derivatives or methionine should be considered for the treatment of HIV-infected patients. N-acetyl-cysteine (NAC) was favoured by us since it is a well established drug for the treatment of chronic bronchitis in many western countries and is known as a relatively safe drug with virtually no serious side-effects.

We expect that treatment of HIV-infected patients in the early stages of the disease with N-acetyl-cysteine may help to prevent the progression to full-blown AIDS, i.e., the typical late stage of this disease. Since about 90% of the HIV-infected persons are still in the pre-AIDS stages, we would consider it as a great success if the progression to full-blown AIDS could be prevented in these patients. However, once the patients have reached this late stage of the disease, they suffer from numerous additional metabolic and immunological deficiencies. Unfortunately, we therefore have no optimistic expectations for this group of patients. We have also seen a substantial improvement after treatment with NAC in anecdotal cases of manifest AIDS. However, the many deficiencies of the late stage may be too overwhelming and too irreversible to be corrected by a single substance. On the basis of our investigations and recommendations, clinical studies have been initiated. But there are no published results yet.

Fig. 116
The mortality among patients with lung cancer strongly depends on their plasma glutamate and cystine concentrations. In a study, all patients with a survival time of more than 8 months had high cystine and low glutamate levels (group 1). Patients in the remaining three groups, group 2 – high cystine and glutamate levels, group 3 – low cystine and glutamate levels, and group 4 – low cystine and high glutamate levels, died in less than 9 months.

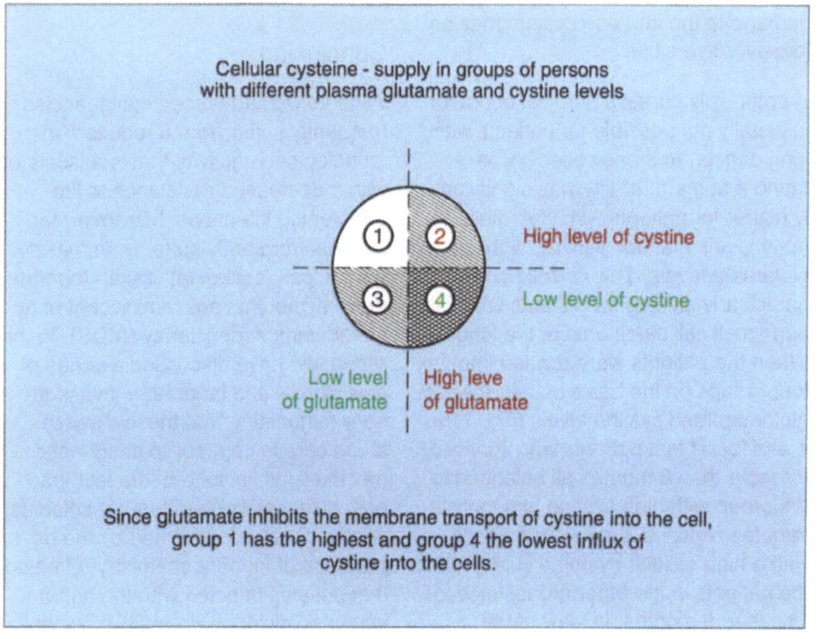

Elevated Glutamate Level as a Pathogenetic Factor for the Decreased Immunological Reactivity in Cancer Patients

Patients with advanced malignancies are also known to have elevated plasma glutamate levels and a strongly decreased lymphocyte reactivity. A study performed in collaboration with several hospitals in the Heidelberg area and altogether 134 persons with different types of cancers revealed a statistically highly significant inverse correlation between the individual glutamate level and the individual lymphocyte reactivity. Plasma glutamate levels of patients with colorectal carcinoma were found to return to approximately normal levels within 1 week after a potentially curative surgical operation. The lymphocyte reactivity, however, was found to remain low for several months, suggesting that the metabolically induced damage to the immune system may be largely irreversible.

A potentially curative surgical operation is usually not possible for patients with lung cancer. In these cases it was found that the mortality was significantly higher for patients with high glutamate levels than for patients with low glutamate levels. This correlation was particularly striking for patients with non-small cell carcinoma of the lung. When the patients were divided into four groups on the basis of their median glutamate and cystine levels (Fig. 116), it was found that patients who survived for more than 8 months all belonged to the group with high cystine and low glutamate levels, i.e. they were patients with a high cellular cysteine supply. All the patients in the other groups died in less than 9 months. In view of the causative effects of the extracellular glutamate concentrations on the intracellular cysteine level and lymphocyte functions, these findings clearly suggest the possibility that the cellular cysteine supply may also play a causative role in the disease progression of patients with non-small cell carcinoma. Of course, this does not necessarily mean that the immune system is protective against cancer. It is quite conceivable that the decreased cysteine supply may cause an over-expression of certain cytokine genes which, in turn, may either stimulate the growth of lung cancer cells or (as in the case of TNF-a) contribute to the development of cachexia. There is also the possibility that the individual glutamate and cystine concentrations of lung cancer patients may be a useful diagnostic tool with high prognostic value.

Conclusion

Patients with advanced malignancies frequently suffer from a reduced immunological reactivity that is associated with a decreased resistance to life-threatening infections. Moreover, the patients frequently suffer from massive weight loss (cachexia). Taken together, these symptoms are reminiscent of acquired immunodeficiency (AIDS). In this report, we have discussed a series of new clinical and laboratory investigations suggesting that these diseases share certain common pathogenetic mechanisms, in spite of the fact that both diseases have different etiological origins. Studies performed by the department of immunochemistry revealed that patients infected with the human immunodeficiency virus (HIV), as well as patients with (certain types of) cancer suffer from a cellular deficiency of cysteine. And additional laboratory studies have shown that the cellular supply of cysteine has a strong influence on gene expression and lymphocyte functions. The results of these studies may have important implications with respect to the development of new therapeutic strategies for HIV-infection and (certain types of) cancer.

In order to replenish the cysteine deficiency of HIV-infected patients, we have proposed to treat these patients with the cysteine derivative N-acetylcysteine (NAC). This substance is a well established drug in clinical medicine with well-documented pharmacokinetic and safety records.

Our projects have been supported in part by the Federal Department of Health, Berlin, within the research program on AIDS, by the Tumor Center Heidelberg/Mannheim, and by Inpharzam Corp.

Prof. Dr. Wulf Dröge
Division of Immunochemistry

Participating scientists

Dr. Hans-Peter Eck
Dr. Sabine Mihm
Dipl.-Biol. Helmut Gmünder
Dr. Steffen Roth
Jong-Seok Lim

In collaboration with

Dr. Helmut Näher
Dr. Ursula Pekar
Dr. Martin Hartmann
Prof. Dr. Detlef Petzoldt
Dermatological Clinics, University of Heidelberg

Dr. Volker Daniel
Institute of Immunology and Serology, University of Heidelberg

Prof. Dr. Thomas Mertens
Institute of Virology, University of Cologne

Dr. Heinrich Rasokat
Dermatological Clinics, University of Cologne

Dr. Gerd Fätkenheuer
II. Clinics and Polyclinics of Internal Medicine, University of Cologne

Dr. Christoph Pohl
I. Clinics of Internal Medicine, University of Cologne

Prof. Dr. Michael Betzler
Prof. Dr. Peter Schlag
Surgical Clinics,
University of Heidelberg

Prof. Dr. Peter Drings
Prof. Dr. Werner Ebert
Thorax Clinics, Heidelberg

Selected publications

Dröge, W., Eck, H.-P., Näher, H., Pekar., U., Daniel, V.: Abnormal amino acid concentrations in the blood of patients with acquired immune deficiency syndrome (AIDS) may contribute to the immunological defect. Biol. Chem. Hoppe-Seyler 369, 143–148 (1988)

Eck, H.-P., Dröge, W.: Influence of the extracellular glutamate concentration on the intracellular cyst(e)ine concentration in macrophages and on the capacity to release cysteine. Biol. Chem. Hoppe-Seyler 370, 109–113 (1989)

Eck, H.-P., Gmünder, H., Hartmann, M., Petzold, D., Daniel, V., Dröge, W.: Low concentrations of acid-soluble thiol (cysteine) in blood plasma of HIV-1 infected patients. Biol. Chem. Hoppe-Seyler 370, 101–108 (1989)

Eck, H.-P., Drings, P., Dröge, W.: Plasma levels, lymphocyte reactivity and death rate in patients with bronchial carcinoma. J. Cancer Res. Clin. Oncol. 115, 571–574 (1989)

Gmünder, H., Eck, H.-P. Benninghoff, B., Roth, S., Dröge, W.: Macrophages regulate intracellular gluthatione levels of lymphocytes. Evidence for an immunoregulatory role of cysteine. Cell. Immunol. 129, 32–46 (1990)

Eck, H.-P., Betzler, M., Schlag, P., Dröge, W.: Partial recovery of lymphocyte activity in patients with colorectal carcinoma after curative surgical treatment and return of plasma glutamate concentrations to normal levels. J. Cancer Res. Clin. Oncol. 116, 648–650 (1990)

Gmünder, H., Roth, S., Eck, H.-P., Gallas, H., Mihm, S., Dröge, W.: Interleukin-2mRNA expression, lymphokine production and DNA synthesis in gluthathione depleted T cells. Cell. Immunol. 130, 520–528 (1990)

Dröge, W., Eck, H.-P., Gmünder, H., Mihm, S.: Modulation of lymphocyte functions and immune reponses by cysteine and cysteine derivates. Am. J. Med. 91 (Suppl. 3C), 140S–144S (1991)

Eck, H.-P., Stahl-Hennig, C., Hunsmann, G., Dröge, W.: Metabolic disorder as early consequence of simian immunodeficiency virus infection in rhesus macaques. Lancet 338, 346–347 (1991)

Mihm, S., Ennen, J., Pessara, U., Kurth, R., Dröge, W.: Inhibition of HIV-1 replication and NF-kB activity by cysteine and cysteine derivates. AIDS 5, 497–503 (1991)

8.2 Adherent Molecules and Formation of Metastases

by Margot Zöller

In general, locally growing tumors can be treated curatively. It is the ability of a tumor cell to form metastases that makes it potentially life-threatening. The development of metastases is a complex process: a tumor cell separates from the primary tumor, enters the blood stream or the lymph, attaches itself to capillary endothelium cells, and from there invades the surrounding tissue and displaces it. In order to successfully metastasize, a tumor cell thus has to have specific characteristics:

1) It must possess certain factors that allow the cell to separate from the primary tissue;
2) It must be capable of moving directedly;
3) It must have adherent properties;
4) It must have enzymes that enable the cell to invade secondary tissue.

Although these characteristics of metastasizing tumor cells can be listed, the corresponding structures are still largely unknown. This has two main reasons: During tumor progression, the characteristics of tumor cells change constantly. Thus, the tumor tissue of a given cancer patient contains cells at different stages of progression. Consequently, the characterization of a specific molecule on individual tumor cells does not indicate whether or not it is of importance for the formation of metastases. On the other hand, there is only a limited number of experimental tumor models that spontaneously form metastases, as has generally been observed in tumor patients.

In order to gain information on the characteristics that allow a tumor cell to metastasize, one needs a tumor model in which some of the cells are able to metastasize, whereas other cells are not able to do so. In addition, the ability or inability of the tumor cells' subpopulations to form metastases should be a stable characteristic. By cloning these subpopulations, it might be possible to obtain information on the molecules that is relevant for metastatic spread on the basis of differences among the intracytoplasmic structures or among the antigens expressed on the cell's surface.

Requirements of a Tumor Model for the Examination of Metastatic Progression

Such a model has been developed from a rat carcinoma of the pancreas (BSp73). One part of its cells grows locally, whereas the other part metastasizes via the lymph into the lung. The locally growing subpopulation differs both morphologically in vivo and in vitro from the metastasizing subpopulation. The metastasizing cells (BSp73ASML) grow spherically and do not adhere to the culture dishes nor to each other. In contrast to this, the non-metastasizing subpopulation (BSp73AS) spreads on the culture dishes, and the cells adhere to each other.

In vivo, the two subpopulations develop quite differently. We implanted cultures of both subpopulations into rats. If the tissue around the implantation site was excised some time later, the rats that had received BSp73AS cells survived. However, animals that had received BSp73ASML cells died within 5 to 7 weeks of metastases in the lymphatic nodes and in the lung.

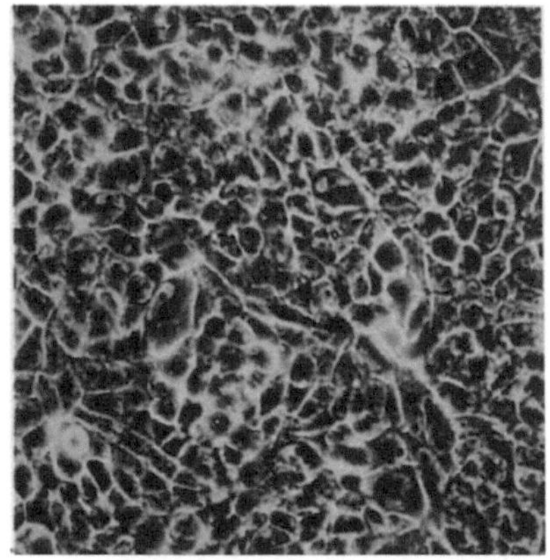

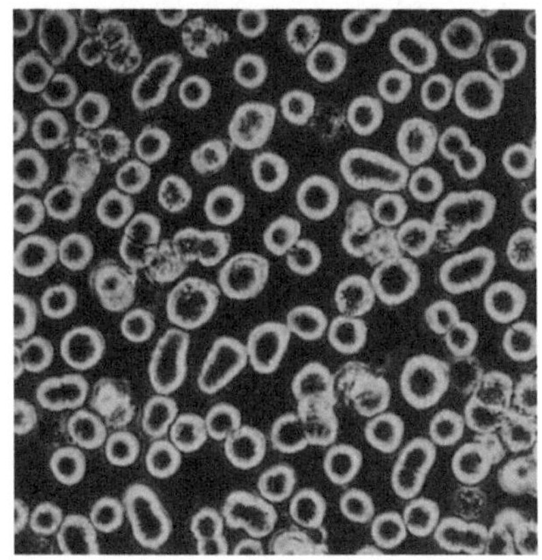

Figs. 117, 118
Two sub-groups of pancreas tumors in the tissue culture. Figure 117 shows non-metastasizing cells adhering to the culture medium.
Figure 118 shows metastasizing cells that do not adhere to the culture medium.

This tumor model is thus particularly well suited for investigation of the factors that make a tumor cell capable of metastasizing.

Metastatic Progression as a Consequence of a Loss of Cytoskeleton Proteins

Because of the morphological differences, and since the construction of the cytoskeleton determines whether and how cells adhere to one another and to the extracellular matrix, it seemed likely that the cytoskeleton might be the distinctive characteristic of the two subpopulations. Indeed, our investigations showed significant differences in the expression and organisation of most of the known cytoskeleton proteins. Only one of the differences will be mentioned here. Vinculin is a cytoskeleton protein that might play an important part in wound healing. BSp73AS cells express vinculin, whereas in BSp73ASML cells no vinculin could be detected. When the gene for vinculin was introduced into BSp73ASML cells, which were then implanted into rats, the animals survived significantly longer than others that had received non-transfected BSp73ASML cells.

These studies are the beginning of a series of experiments which we will carry out in order to find out whether the loss of certain (intracellular) proteins enables a cell to metastasize. Since the transduction of vinculin alone significantly reduces the ability to metastasize, we are now looking for one or several additional intracellular proteins that are absent in the metastasizing subpopulation. Our working hypothesis is that the first step of metastatic progression, the separation from the primary tissue, is not necessarily due to new capabilities of the metastasizing cell, but possibly due only to a loss of adhesiveness.

Metastatic Progression by Reactivation of Genes

Though it is disputable whether the separation of a tumor cell from the primary tissue is due to a loss of certain adhesive characteristics (that is, a passive process), it is indisputable that the immigration and embedding of a metastasizing tumor cell into the secondary tissue are active processes. Thus, these capabilities probably require the expression of suitable structures. Since the metastasizing cell has to establish contact with the extracellular matrix and possibly with other cells, it is likely that the necessary structures are (also) expressed on its surface. In order to find these surface markers, which are expressed exclusively on the metastasizing subpopulation, we immunized mice with BSp73ASML cells, thus producing monoclonal antibodies, and investigated which antibodies bind to the metastasizing, but not to the non-metastasizing subpopulation. We have found several such antibodies, which proves that the metastasizing subpopulation does indeed have a specific surface structure.

With the help of monoclonal antibodies it is possible to identify RNA and DNA sequences that encode for certain proteins. We discovered that the monoclonal antibody specific to ASML cells recognizes a molecule which is similar to one that exists primarily on lymphocytes (CD44). It is known that CD44 plays a part in the homing of lymphocytes, which means that, with the help of this molecule, lymphocytes from the blood stream attach to specific structures of the vessel wall, then leave the vessel and settle in the lymphatic nodes. Those parts of the molecule that are very similar to CD44 are also present in the non-metastasizing subpopulation. However, in the metastasizing tumor cells this molecule has an additional domain, which up to now has never been found on non-metastasizing tumor cells.

Since variant CD44 (vCD44) has been found only on metastasizing tumors, we proposed that the variant region of the CD44 molecule is somehow responsible for metastatic spread. In order to verify our hypothesis, the molecule was introduced into metastasizing BSp73AS cells.

We had already shown that rats, after application of BSp73ASML and excision of the tumor, develop lung metastases, whereas no metastatic spread was observed after application and excision of BSp73AS. However, after application of transfected BSp73AS cells (which express the vCD44 molecule on their surface) to rats and subsequent excision of the local tumor we found a metastatic colonization of the lymphatic nodes and of the lung in all animals. This is proof that the variant region of the CD44 molecule is indeed of significant importance for metastatic progression and suffices to initiate metastatic progression in non-metastasizing tumors.

We therefore conclude that vCD44 is of significant importance for at least one

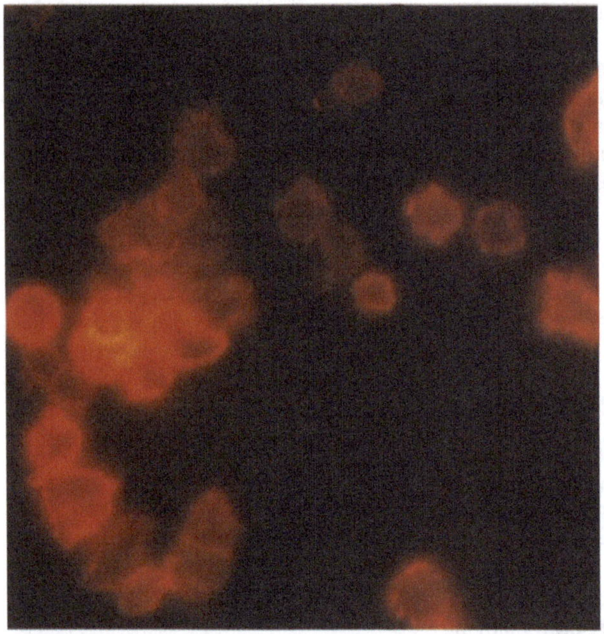

Fig. 119

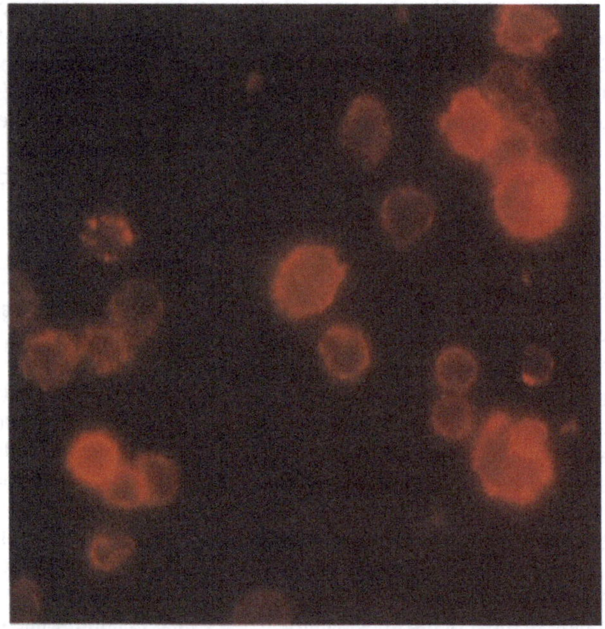

Fig. 120

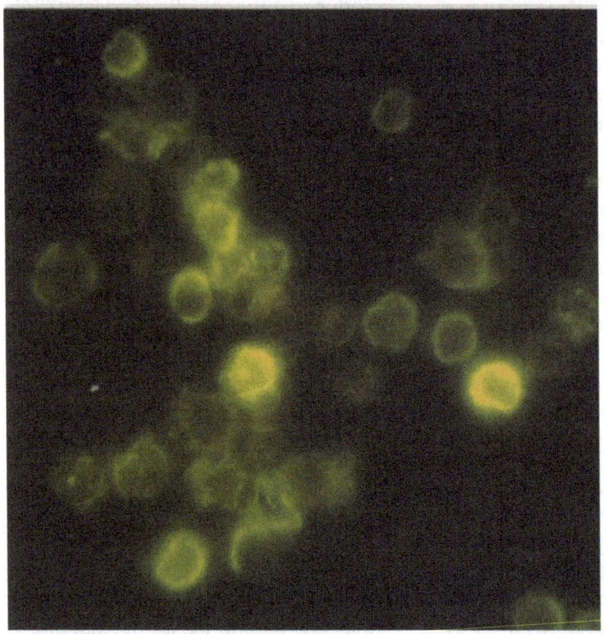

Fig. 121

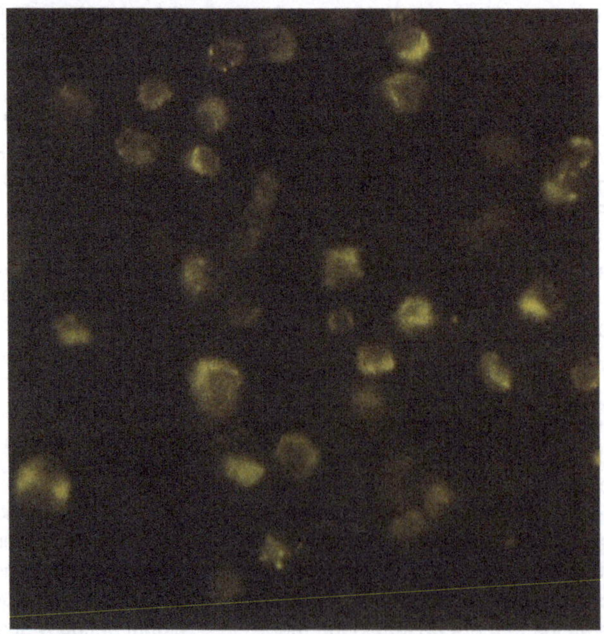

Fig. 122

step in the cascade of metastatic progression. For therapeutic approaches it is very important to know not only which structure within the cell can initiate metastatic spread, but also to know the function of this structure. Thus, we are presently trying to define the function of the vCD44 molecule. As mentioned in the beginning, this could be one of three functions of metastasizing tumor cells: separation from the primary tissue, invasion into the secondary tissue, and colonization within the secondary tissue. First indications for the role of vCD44 in the process of metastatic spread may be obtained by blocking the molecule with antibodies.

The simultaneous administration of metastasizing tumor cells together with the vCD44-specific antibody 1.1ASML leads to a delayed colonization of the draining lymphatic nodes. After a single administration of 1.1ASML, this effect is only temporary and is followed by an accelerated increase in the number of metastatic cells compared to untreated animals. Thus, it appears possible that 1.1ASML does not block the invasion of tumor cells into the secondary tissue, but that vCD44 might be necessary for the growth of tumor cells in the secondary tissue.

Figs. 119–122
Surface molecules (CD44) of pancreas tumor cells are stained with dye-coupled antibodies. The staining with the antibody, which is directed against "standard" CD44, reveals that both metastasizing (Fig. 119) and non-metastasizing (Fig. 120) cells contain the surface marker. The antibody which is directed against the "metastasis-specific" variant CD44 only stains the metastasizing cells (Fig. 121). After identical treatment, the locally growing cells, which only carry the "standard" CD44 on their surface, do not fluoresce under the fluorescence microscope (Fig. 122).

If the blocking of vCD44 inhibits the growth of metastasizing tumor cells in the secondary tissue, continuous application of the antibody should lead to a decrease in the number of established metastases and to a significantly extended survival time. Whereas in untreated animals the draining lymphatic nodes began to grow significantly and continuously from the 10th day after tumor application, no such growth could be observed in animals that received 1.1ASML twice a week. In addition, all untreated rats died 52 to 70 days after tumor application, whereas the treated animals survived between 70 to 162 days. The macroscopic autopsy findings showed that all draining lymphatic nodes of the untreated animals were massively infiltrated by tumor tissue and that the lungs were colonized by multiple metastases (numbering 10 to 50). Autopsy findings showed that, in the animals treated with 1.1ASML, all lymphatic nodes were macroscopically and histologically free from tumor tissue. The animals died of individual (one to three) large metastases which developed in the lung tissue. This proves that metastasizing tumor cells rely on the expression of vCD44 for their growth in secondary tissue, and that monoclonal antibodies that block this structure can significantly delay metastatic spread.

Our experiments demonstrate that, with the aid of a tumor model, it is possible to analyze the individual steps of the metastatic process. In addition, the presently available data indicate that highly complex biological processes, such as metastatic progression, are not based on a single alteration of the cell. In order to progress from phenomenology to the definition of the molecule and its function, there is a need for concerted research in different scientific fields. However, our findings indicate that the knowledge of only one of these many mechanisms that promote the metastatic spread of tumor cells can supply important information for the improvement of therapeutic approaches.

Priv.-Doz. Dr. Margot Zöller
Project group Tolerance
and Immune Response

Participating staff

Robert Arch
Dr. Sonja Reber-Kalthoff
Simone Seiter
Karin Wirth

In collaboration with

Prof. Dr. Peter Herrlich
Prof. Dr. Helmut Ponta
Dr. Ulla Günthert
Martin Hofmann
Institute for Genetics and Toxicology of Nuclear Fuels, Nuclear Research Center (KFK), Karlsruhe

Priv.-Doz. Dr. Siegfried Matzku
E. Merck, Darmstadt

Prof. Avri BenZe'ev
Department of Molecular Genetics and Virology,
The Weizmann Institute of Science, Rehovot, Israel

Selected publications

Matzku, S., Komitowski, D., Miltenberger, M., Zöller, M.: Characterization of BSp73, a spontaneous rat tumor and its in vivo selected variants showing different metastasizing capacities. Invas. Metast. 3, 109–123 (1983)

Ben-Ze'ev, A., Zöller, M., Raz, A.: Differential expression of intermediate filament proteins in metastatic and nonmetastatic variants of the BSp73 tumor. Cancer Res. 46, 785–790 (1986)

Matzku, S., Wenzel, A., Liu, S., Zöller, M.: Antigenic differences between metastatic and nonmetastatic BSp73 rat tumor variants characterized by monoclonal antibodies. Cancer Res. 49, 1294–1299 (1989)

Aruffo, A., Stamenkovic, I., Melnick, M., Underhill, C.B., Seed, B.: CD44 is the principal cell surface receptor for hyaluronate. Cell 61, 1303–1313 (1990)

Dehar, S.,: Integrins and tumor invasion. Bio Essays 12, 583–590 (1990)

John, T.S., Meyer, J., Idzerda, R., Gallatin, W., M.: Expression of CD44 confers a new adhesive phenotype on transfected cells. Cell 60, 45–52 (1990)

Reber, S., Matzku, S., Günther, U., Ponta, H., Herrlich, P., Zöller, M.: Retardation of metastatic tumor growth after immunization with metastasis-specific monoclonal antibodies. Int. J. Cancer 46, 919–927 (1990)

Günther, U., Hofmann, M., Rudy, W., Reber, S., Zöller, M., Haußmann, I., Matzku, S., Wenzel., Ponta, H., Herrlich, P.: A new variant of glycoprotein CD44 confers metastatic potential to rat carcinoma cells. Cell 92, 13–24 (1991)

Arch, R., Wirth, K., Hofmann, M., Ponta, H., Matzku, S., Herrlich, P., Zöller, M.: Participation in normal immune responses of a metastasis-inducing splice variant of CD 44. Science 257, 682–685 (1992)

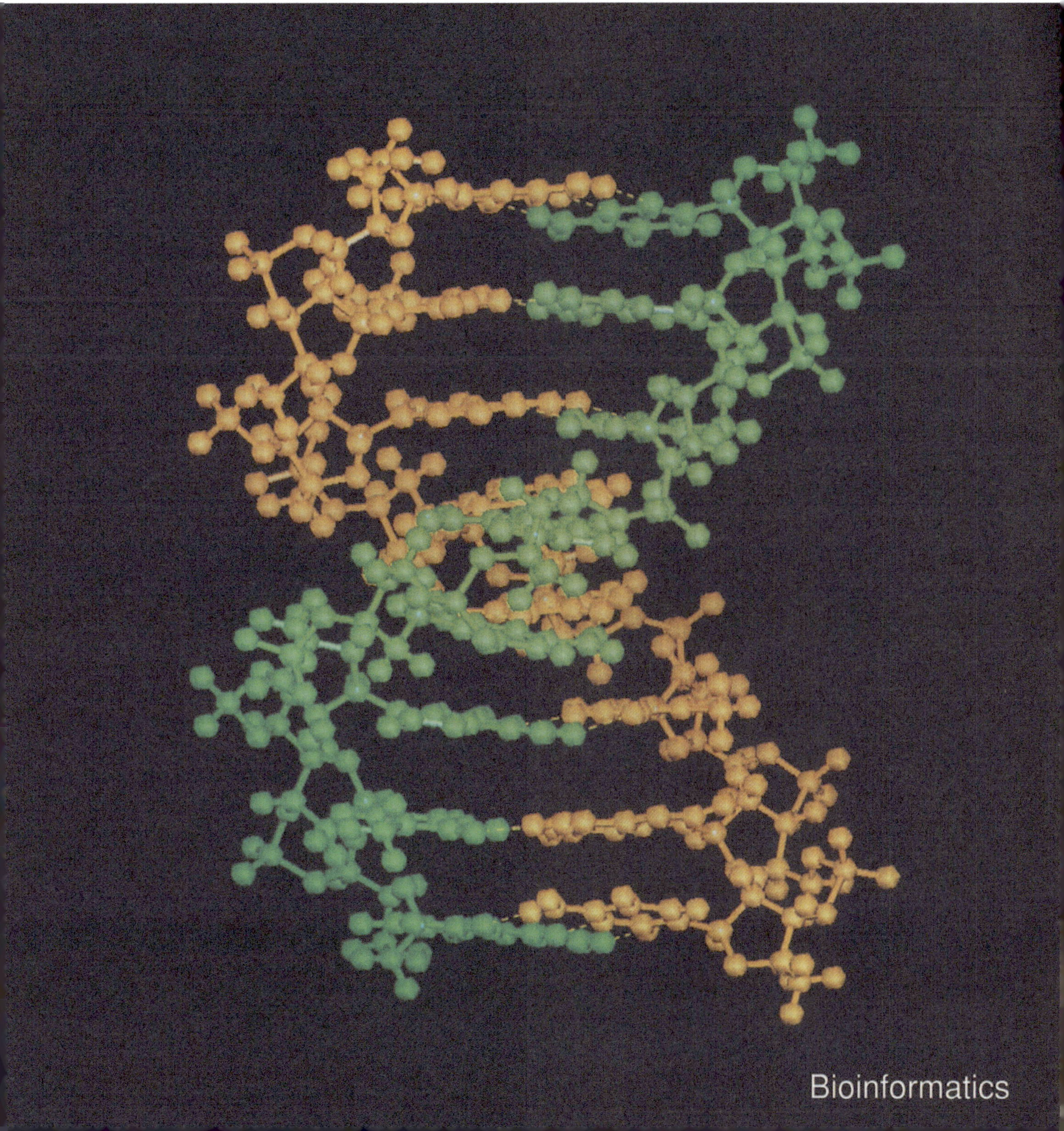

Bioinformatics

9

Bioinformatics

Although the term "informatics" (equivalent to "computer science") was coined more than 30 years ago, a definition in due logical form still does not exist. For some scientists informatics is "a fuzzy semantic construct whose origin is intuitive usage which fills a communication need," whereas for many others an operational definition may be sufficient: informatics encompasses numerous different disciplines which are in some way concerned with the analysis, application, acquisition and accessibility of information.

Bioinformatics at the Deutsches Krebsforschungszentrum has a broad spectrum, comprising the activity of four basic domains of research, namely, biomedical informatics, biophysics, biostatistics, and mathematical biology. In all four disciplines there is a "continuum" between the fundamental research for new knowledge and the application of current knowledge to a specific practical problem ("application research" or, in technical language, "engineering"). For example, the "engineering" aspects of bioinformatics would involve the design, creation, and development of new information methods and systems in biology and medicine.

One example for application research included in the Program "Bioinformatics" is computational statistics, which aims to improve the existing statistical software, to explore new algorithms for complicated statistical problems and to include the "expert knowledge" in the analysis of collected data.

Another "engineering" work in the Program will be the "scientific visualization": it designates the application of graphic and imaging techniques to computational science and will encompass all our research domains, from molecular structural design to medical imaging and spatial reconstruction.

Perhaps the best recent example of the continuum between application and fundamental research is given by the activity in genome informatics. In the Deutsches Krebsforschungszentrum there exist different experimental groups doing molecular research, and they require information about homologous DNA and protein sequences. The quantity (there is a "deluge" of sequence information) and importance of such data make it essential that the data be collected in easily accessible and current databases. The database work (data collection, handling, data distribution) is (and remains) the primary practical aim of the applied research in genome informatics at the Center. Within GENIUSnet at the Deutsches Krebsforschungszentrum there has been established the German base of a European network for the distribution of molecular biology data. In addition, the research group dealing with molecular biophysics has also actively participated in the creation of an integrated genetic database management system.

In quite a rough and general formulation, the research themes of the Program Bioinformatics at the Deutsches Krebsforschungszentrum would include:

1) dynamics of genes and molecules,
2) cell population dynamics, and
3) clinical informatics.

In short, the unifying concept is modeling processes and structures.

Indeed, one part of the first topic is devoted to the study of molecular dynamics of macromolecules of biological interest: it has practical applications in problems related to, e.g., mutagenesis and drug design. Molecular dynamics simulation represents the most informative method for obtaining detailed descriptions of atom fluctuations in biopolymers and of the variation with time of their structural parameters. Other methods are used to predict three-dimensional protein structures.

The second topic of the Program Bioinformatics consists of a variety of mathematical, statistical, and computer models trying to describe (and to understand) the growth of normal and malignant cell populations. This aim is related to the investigation of the cell cycle and its control, as well as of other significant events throughout the cell's life, e.g., differentiation, adaptation and survival. In the framework of probability theory, the above cell populations can be considered as large random systems, specifically "spatial random systems with interactions," an interpretation which introduces new concepts (interaction, cooperative phenomena, stability and metastability, complexity, etc.) and allows to re-formulate some biological questions about the heterogeneity of cell populations, the effect of small random perturbations, the existence of different biological time scales, the influence of spatial dimension on the qualitative behavior of cell systems, etc. As it is known, this analysis of large stochastic systems requires the extrapolation from the microscopic level at which the systems are defined, to a macroscopic level at which the laws governing the behavior of interacting cell systems are formulated. Actually, the problem of the integration of local mechanisms into a global structure is the central problem of biology: morphogenesis as well as carcinogenesis are the best, but most complex examples.

A special class of models deserves mention in view of their correlation to current experiments in chemical carcinogenesis and risk assessment. These models may be divided into three groups:

1) "physiologically based" pharmacokinetic models describing the biotransformation of a putative carcinogen,

2) compartment models for tumor incidence and mortality, and

3) "tumor incidence models" that describe the apparition of a malignan clone through a directed chain of events (including such cellular events as, e.g., DNA damage and repair).

The last theme deals with practical developments in clinical informatics, and more precisely with the elaboration of new medical information systems. As it is known, MIS is defined as a set of formal arrangements by which facts concerning the health and health care of individual patients are stored and processed in computers. The project DILEMMA will provide an integrated technology to support decision-making and information management in all phases of cancer care, including support for distant care (by general physicians) and home care. Also, the project HELIOS (Hospital Object Software Tools) is devoted to the creation of fully integrated medical software required for building critical parts of a Ward Information System.

Coordinator of the Research Program:
Prof. Petre Tautu

Divisions and their heads:

Medical and Biological Informatics:
Prof. Dr. Claus O. Köhler

Molecular Biophysics I:
Priv.-Doz. Dr. Sandor Suhai

Mathematical Models:
Prof. Petre Tautu

9

9.1 The Transparent Patient – On the Clinical Relevance of Raytracing

by Kirsten Meetz
and Hans-Peter Meinzer

Diagnostics and therapy control are two steps in therapy that rely heavily on decisions made by the physician on the basis of visual impressions. As a supporting tool for the clinician, the Heidelberg Raytracing Model for the visualization of medical objects has been developed at the Deutsches Krebsforschungszentrum.

Many diseases and pathological abnormalities can be diagnosed by simply looking at the patient or at the region of the body in question. New imaging techniques based on non-invasive methods supply an increasing amount of visual information. Tomographic imaging, for example, allows the physician "to take a look" into the patient by supplying a series of cross-sectional images of the body. Ideally, the distance between the sections is 1 mm; however, normally it is between 2 mm and 5 mm.

If the physician wants to interpret this image series, he has to mentally reconstruct a three-dimensional image from the sequence of individual sections. This method of reconstruction, however, is very inaccurate and subjective. Its quality depends very much on the physician's experience and on his knowledge about the imaged region. Thus, misinterpretations may occur.

Images that describe an extremely complex situation in particular tend to make excessive demands on the physician's imaginative capabilities, e.g., images in which the situation changes very much between neighboring slices. Only someone well-trained in the interpretation of sectional image series, e.g., a radiologist, is capable of gaining a more or less clear picture of the scene.

Three-dimensional visualization attempts to project the information contained in tomographic images from a three-dimensional onto a two-dimensional structure. This is done with an illumination model, which simulates the projection of the illuminated scene onto the eye of an observer. This model, which is presently under development, is based on physical regularities that describe the interaction of the light with the illuminated objects. The result of the modeling can be compared to a photograph, which displays a three-dimensional scene on a two-dimensional medium.

Heidelberg Raytracing Model

The Heidelberg Raytracing Model is based on a general raytracing approach developed by Kajiya. The goal is to model the interactions of the light with the illuminated objects. For this purpose, each light ray is traced from its source, which in this case is the light source, to its sink, which is the eye of the observer. All the changes the light ray is submitted to on its way are recorded. Since the Heidelberg raytracing approach is an achromatic model, all changes refer to a reduction in intensity. The results are black-and-white images, in which both the color of the objects and the color of the light are ignored.

Data of the Model

The Heidelberg Raytracing Model is used for the visualization of series of medical sectional images. These images are the only objective information about the three-dimensional scene that is to be illuminated. Since the output images are intended to be as faithful in the reproduction of details and as informative as possible, the Heidelberg Model is based on the original description of the scene without any changes. For this reason, the gray values of the digitized image series are taken as input data for the model. They form a three-dimensional data structure that indirectly contains information on the shape and on the arrangement of the objects to be visualized. Each element of this data structure describes the density of one point in space. Within the model, the gray values of the images, after having been mapped onto a range of values between zero and one, are interpreted as densities.

Since the Heidelberg Model is achromatic, the information on the color of the objects can be discarded. The arrangement of the objects is uniquely described by the density of each point in space. This is the basis for the modeling of the various interactions of the light with the objects.

The data structure presented here only reproduces the geometry of the illuminated arrangement and describes the objects with regard to their density. In addition to the image series, the model needs data on the properties of

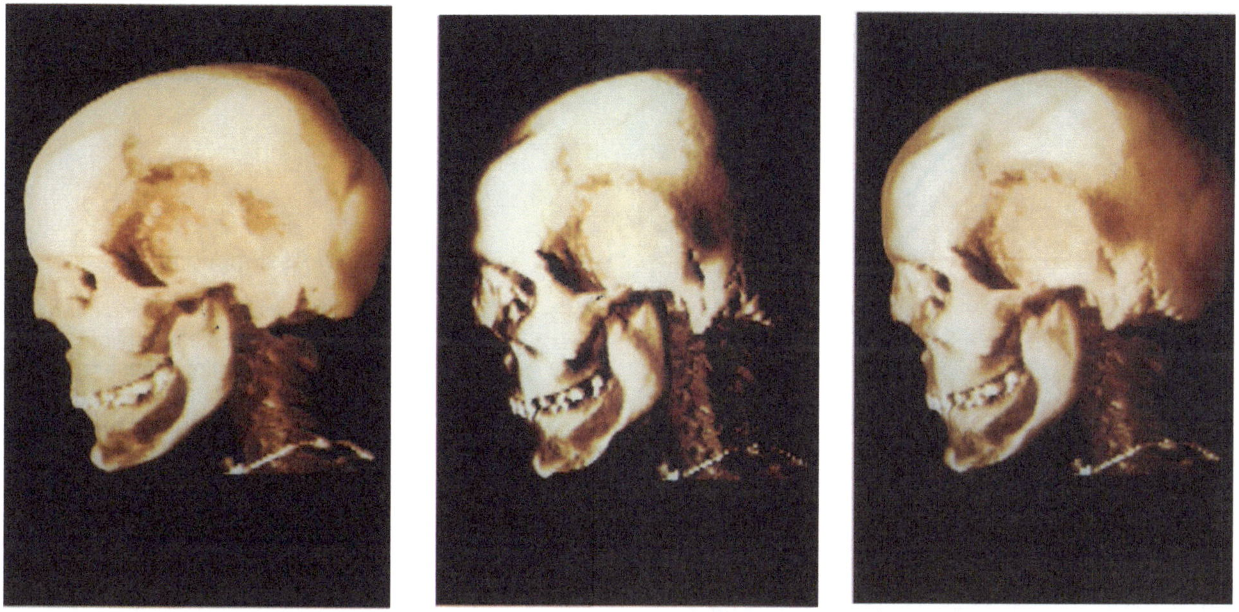

Figs. 123–125
The Heidelberg Raytracing Model serves to reconstruct three- dimensional images from the slice image series acquired using computed tomography. In the first processing step, the gray value images are transformed into density value images. Then, the illumination is modeled and the individual components of the interaction between the object and the light are calculated. The result is individual images, such as the image of diffuse reflection (Fig. 123) and the image of specular reflection (Fig. 124). The total image (Fig. 125) is produced by superimposing the component images.

the objects. These data are input in the form of a parameter list; they determine the nature of the interaction between the objects and the light. Thus, it is possible to take into consideration the objects' microscopic surface structure, which determines their reflectivity.

The result of the illumination is described with a two-dimensional data structure, which contains the image as seen by the observer. Each picture element (pixel) contains information on how much light from this point reaches the observer and contributes to the final image formed in his eyes.

Components of the Model

The components of the Heidelberg Raytracing Model can be subdivided into three groups: an image preprocessing component, a component for the modeling of the illumination, and a component for the final processing of the illumination results.

The modules of the second group simulate the three main interactions of light with objects in space: reflection, transmission, and scattering. Each of these interactions is described independently of the others in a separate model.

The physical reality of the illumination is thus reduced to the following basic components:

1) Transmission of the light: This component calculates which percentage of the originally emitted light intensity reaches each point in space and, finally, the observer.

2) Scattering: This gives the proportion of the incident light that is scattered towards the observer.

3) Reflection: In analogy to the scattering, it calculates the proportion of the light which is reflected toward the observer.

4) Superposition: This component summarizes the intensities of the light rays emitted towards the observer and which superimpose on his eyes.

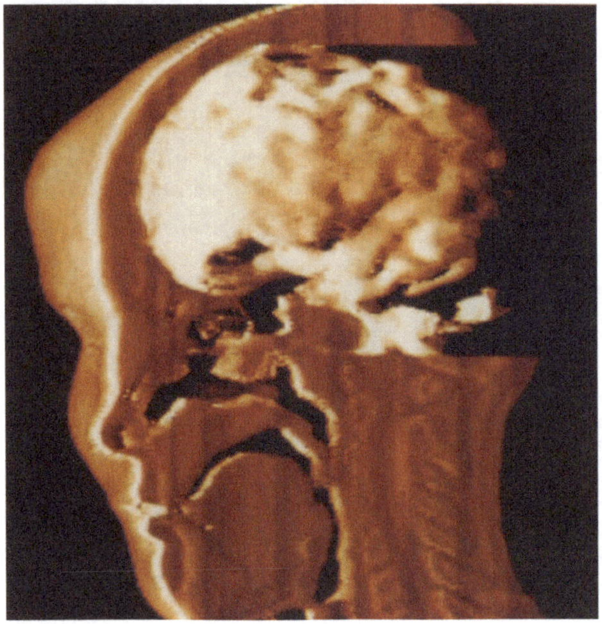

Fig. 126
The computer reconstructs a three-dimensional representation of the head from more than 100 slice images acquired with computed tomography.

The modeling of the transmission 1) is the first step in the illumination model. Here, the percentage of the emitted light arriving in each point of space is calculated. Scattering 2) and reflection 3) are combined under the term emission, and as such are the second modelling step. Finally, the image as seen by the observer is reconstructed with the aid of the superposition principle 4).

Before the modeling of the illumination, the data of the image series have to be converted into a suitable format. This is done by the modules of the image preprocessing group. Of special importance here is the transformation of the gray value images into density images, which is done by the component Raynorm. We plan to introduce further data preprocessing capabilities; however, these are not mandatory for the modeling of the illumination. Among these are, for example, the rotation of the scene to be illuminated, the segmentation of individual objects, and the enhancement of the gray values of certain image regions.

After the illumination has been modeled, the processed data have to be finished, i.e., converted into a format that is suitable for display. The final image is composed from several partial images that are the results of the various illumination components, such as reflection or scattering. Therefore, the total image is a composite of an image produced only by reflection, and of another image produced only by scattering.

Model Assumptions

In order to limit the modeling efforts, several simplifying assumptions have been made. One important assumption is that the various interactions of the light with the objects are independent of each other. When calculating the transmission, for example, only the portion of the light absorbed by the pixel is taken into consideration, whereas the reflected and scattered portions are neglected. The decoupling of the various components leads to a significant reduction of the modeling expenditure. Furthermore, it makes it possible to describe the various effects independently of each other and to construct the general model from small, independent partial models. Thus, the illumination model becomes more transparent and easier to understand.

One prerequisite for the separate modeling of the individual interactions is the assumption of the Low Albedo Case. It describes an illumination in which the intensity of the reflected and scattered light is so weak that it can be neglected as an additional light source. Thus, for the modeling of the light-matter-interaction only the rays emitted directly by the light source have to be traced and taken into account as incident irradiation.

In order to simplify the tracing of the light rays and the search for the points of interaction in space, it is assumed that all light rays propagate straight and parallel. The same is assumed for the viewing beams, which describe the path of the light from the objects into the observer's eye. These assumptions are equivalent to the light sources and the observer being infinitely far away from the illuminated scene.

In general, an illumination can be modeled with an infinite number of light sources. However, in order to reduce the modeling expenditure, the Heidelberg Raytracing Model uses only two light sources. Also, the positions of the light sources and of the observer are, in general, arbitrary. In the Heidelberg Model, however, they are defined in such a way that the modeling expenditure for the tracing of the light rays and the viewing beams can be minimized.

A further simplification makes it possible to apply the illumination model to each individual two-dimensional image of the series. Thus, time-consuming calculations in three dimensions can be avoided. The total image then is a composite of the partial images.

Modeling of the Components

For the purpose of clarity and transparency, the global model is subdivided into components, which will be described in more detail.

Raynorm

Module Raynorm preprocesses the series of sectional images serving as input data to the illumination model. It maps the image series, which contains the description of the scene to be illuminated, onto the range of values required by the model. This is done by two data transformations.

In analogy to the global model, the input data of module Raynorm consist of a description of the objects in space plus information on the range of gray values to be considered in the calculations.

The output data of module Raynorm also describe the three-dimensional arrangement. However, since these data range from zero to one, they are no longer gray values but densities. They are the basis for the modeling of the illumination.

Two subsequent transformations are the core of module Raynorm: a linear and an exponential transformation. The former only serves to map the input data onto the range of values required by the model. The exponential transformation serves to further manipulate the data. Thus, for example, it is possible to enhance objects with a specific range of density or gray values.

The data thus manipulated serve as input data for the illumination model; they range from zero to one.

Lightpath

This component actually traces the light rays on their way through the three-dimensional space. In this model, the optical path is the straight connection between the light source and each point in space, and from there to the observer.

Traveling from its source to the observer, the light loses intensity by absorption in each point in space. This attenuation is proportional to the density of the pixel considered.

For each point in space an energy balance establishes which proportion of the incident light is absorbed and how much is transmitted through the pixel. With the aid of transmission, the distribution of the light in space can be calculated. Note that reflection and scattering are not considered in the raytracing component.

Raytracing automatically introduces shadows. Shadows emerge when an object attenuates the light in such a way that another object situated behind the first one is illuminated more faintly or not at all. This effect is simulated by tracing the attenuation along the optical path. As a result, no objects are shown that lie behind another (opaque) object and therefore cannot be seen by the observer. The raytracing model automatically detects hidden objects and visualizes them as required.

Scatter

The component Scatter models the scattering of the light by particles; all other interactions between light and matter are neglected. It is assumed that the scattering towards the observer is directly proportional to the density of the scattering object. Neither the orientation of the rays, nor that of the normals to the surface of the object, nor the position of the observer are considered in the calculation of the scattering. This fact is based on the assumption that the scattering by a surface pixel only depends on its density and that it is completely independent of the surface's orientation in this point. In addition, it is assumed that the light is scattered uniformly in all directions. The position of the observer, therefore, does not need to be considered.

Phongshading

Module Phongshading models the reflection of the light. Just as in the case of scattering, only the portion of the light that is reflected towards the observer is considered. In contrast to scattering, however, light is reflected only off the surfaces of objects. The reflectivity of a pixel therefore depends on its location within an object's surface. Basis for this model is Phong's empirical equation of reflection. It serves for the modeling of diffuse and of specular reflections.

In the following, we will describe the principles of these two types of reflections.

Among the parameters are the normal to the surface N and the orientation of the incident light L. The position of the observer does not need to be considered, since here – as in scattering – the light is uniformly reflected in all directions.

The modelling of the specular reflection requires more parameters than that of the diffuse reflection. In addition to the incident light L, the orientation of the reflected light R, and the normal to the surface N, the position of the observer O also has to be known, since, according to the law of reflection, the light is reflected exactly in one direction. The calculation of the specularly reflected proportion of the incident light is based on Phong's equation.

Sampling

The component Sampling models the superposition of the light rays that, though emitted by different pixels, propagate along the same viewing beam. As input data it needs the results of the modules Scatter and Phongshading, as well as that of the component Lightpath.

In order to take into account the light conditions, the results of the modules Scatter and Phongshading are weighted in each point of space with the intensity of the light there. The result of the component Lightpath separately determines, for each point in space and for each light source separately, the intensity of the light there and its impression on the observer.

The superposition of the light intensities along one viewing beam is simulated by successive addition. This operation reduces the structure of the input data by one dimension. The result is two-dimensional images that differ by the types of interaction they describe.

The result of this component is, at the same time, the result of the illumination. In the final processing step they are composed to form the resulting image. In this last step, the results of the various components (of the specular and diffuse reflections and of the scattering) are used.

Image Composition and Normalization

This component "assembles" the modeling results for the various interactions and maps them onto a range of values suitable for display. The input data of this module are the images that are seen by the observer on the basis of the various types of light-matterinteractions. Among these are the results of the diffuse and specular reflections, and of scattering.

The total image, which in fact is the result of the Heidelberg Raytracing Model, is calculated on the basis of these results. Figures 123 through 125 show that the structure of the illuminated object becomes apparent only as a combination of all interactions.

The main component of this module is the linear combination of the reflection and scattering images which constitute the total image. The weights of the individual images are defined by parameters given by the user. These parameters can be considered as a specification of the objects' properties. If, for example, the user chooses a large weighting factor for the specular reflection "SPOT", the object in question will have a polished and therefore highly reflective surface. If, on the other hand, the parameter "DUST" is chosen to be large, the illuminated object will appear fuzzy. It then behaves like a non-compact, cloud-like object. If, by the choice of fixed parameters, the properties of the objects are to be independent of the illuminated scene, it is necessary to map the various component results onto a unique range of values before linearly combining them. Only then is the portion of the light being reflected calculated.

Results

A comparison between the Heidelberg Raytracing Model and other illumination models being used for the visualization of medical objects shows that the modeling expenditure of the Heidelberg model is relatively high; the result, however, is images of high quality.

On the one hand, this is due to the volume-oriented representation of the objects, which allows the use of the original data in the algorithm for the calculation of the illumination without segmentation. Thus, no information is lost and no errors can be introduced by segmentation.

On the other hand, the high-quality images of the Heidelberg raytracing algorithm are based on the comprehensive modeling of the interactions between light and objects. In this model, all volume elements of the illuminated scene are used for the calculation of the interactions. No selection or segmentation of pixels participating in the interaction is done.

All reactions of the light along the optical path and the viewing beam are considered in the model. By computing both the emission of the light (i.e., reflection and scattering) as well as absorption and transmission for all volume elements, the model produces realistic shadows. These are mandatory prerequisites for a correct interpretation of the image.

Furthermore, the modeling of the light-matterinteraction in each volume element and the subsequent superposition of the emitted light intensity along the viewing beams allows the representation of objects within their context. As an example, it is possible to show a brain tumor inside the head. For this, the skull and the tissue surrounding the tumor are represented semi-transparently. This method of representation supplies valuable information to the physician. On the basis of this information, for example, the physician can plan a surgical intervention or a radiotherapeutic treatment.

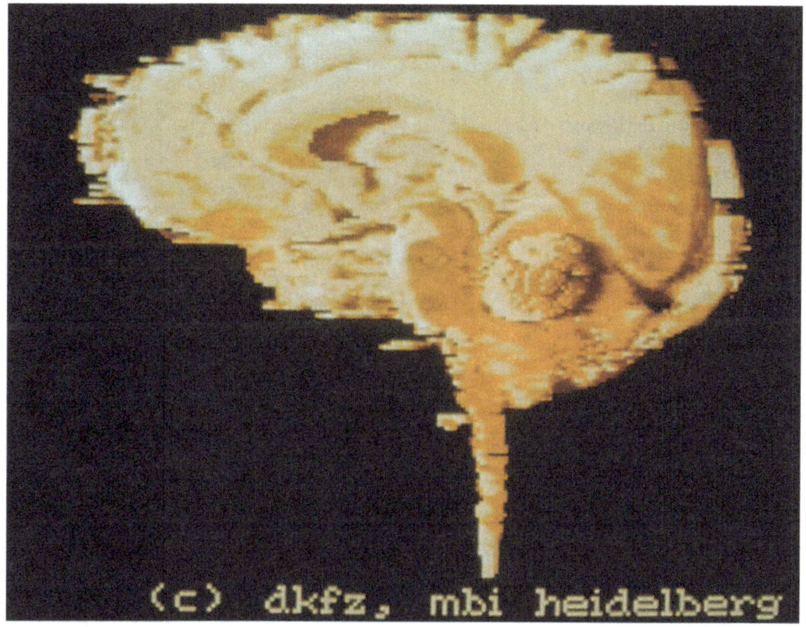

Fig. 127
Three-dimensional representations of soft parts are calculated on the basis of images acquired with magnetic resonance imaging. MR-images contrast the soft parts better than CT images.

Our experience with the Heidelberg raytracing algorithm shows that it is easier for the observer to interpret the scene if the images are moving, since only for moving objects do the spatial relationships become obvious. Therefore, rather than calculating a single view of the illuminated scene, we use the Heidelberg raytracing algorithm to calculate a movie sequence in which the illuminated object revolves about a coordinate axis.

The Heidelberg raytracing algorithm is an important tool for diagnostics and therapy. In collaboration with physicians, it is being further developed for use in the clinical routine. The focus of our work lies in an optimization of the computational speed and on the development of an easy-to-handle user interface.

Dipl.-Inform. Med. Kirsten Meetz
Priv.-Doz. Dr. Hans-Peter Meinzer
Division of Medical
and Biological Informatics

Participating staff

Hans Jürgen Baur
Judith Dilo
Dr. Uwe Engelmann
Irmhild Kocks
Ulrich Kreutzer
Konrad Preiser
Manuela Schäfer
Dr. Dinu Scheppelmann
Oliver Werner
Thomas Wolf

In collaboration with

Prof. Dr. Siegfried Hagl
Division of Heart Surgery,
Surgical University Clinic Heidelberg

Dr. Dr. Siegfried Jänicke
Cranio-facial Surgery Clinic,
Technical University Aachen

Prof. Patrice Degoulet
Hopital Broussais, SIM,
Paris, Frankreich

Prof. Nicholas A. Wright
Department of Histopathology,
Royal Postgraduate Medical School,
Hammersmith Hospital,
University of London,
England

Selected publications

Kreidel, K.: Ein Vergleich mehrer Verfahren zur dreidimensionalen Rekonstruktion von Objekten auf Rastersichtgeräten. Diplomarbeit. Universität Heidelberg, Fakultät für theoretische Medizin (1987)

Heyers, V.: Raytracing im Grauwertvoxelraum zur Visualisierung Medizinischer Schichtserien. Diplomarbeit. Universität Heidelberg, Fakultät für Physik (1988)

Sauerbier, F.: Automatische Segmentierung aus CT- und MR-Bildern mit Hilfe der topologischen Karte. Diplomarbeit. Universität Heidelberg, Fakultät für theoretische Medizin (1989)

Bertsch, H.: Die selbstlernende Merkmalskarte zur Bildsegmentierung und Klassifikation. Dissertation. Universität Heidelberg, Fakultät für theoretische Medizin (1990)

Engelmann, U.: Integrierte Wissensbasierte Bildanalyse. Dissertation. Universität Heidelberg, Fakultät für theoretische Medizin (1990)

Meetz, K.: Farbe in der 3D-Visualisierung medizinischer Schichtbildserien. Diplomarbeit. Universität Heidelberg, Fakultät für theoretische Medizin (1991)

Scheppelmann, D.: Analyse von Texturen in digitalen Bildern. Dissertation. Universität Heidelberg, Fakultät für theoretische Medizin (1991)

9.2 Genome Informatics – The Dowsing Rod Leading to Science under a Data Desert?

by Sándor Suhai and Martina Kieninger

Several large scale research projects have been initiated worldwide in the past years with the aim to uncover the genetic information stored in the genomes of higher organisms, including humans. Since it also became clear that cancer is intimately connected to alterations in the human genome, it is evident that the Deutsches Krebsforschungszentrum is very much interested and involved in several aspects of human genome research. There is, on the other hand, a justifiable fear in the biomedical science community that, while the results of this research might fundamentally contribute to our understanding of basic biological phenomena including cancer, the data production and accumulation at various levels of genome projects will so far exceed its assimilation that the volume of data itself might eventually prove an encumbrance for basic science and medicine. It is not surprising, therefore, that genome informatics, a new interdisciplinary research field on the borderline between genetics and computer science constitutes an integral part of all major genome projects. The present article is an attempt to explain why many scientists in the genome field sincerely hope that a close cooperation between two so different disciplines might help to overcome this difficult problem.

Fig. 128
Computer model of a synthetic DNA molecule, to which a cancer drug, cytostatic distamicine, is attached.

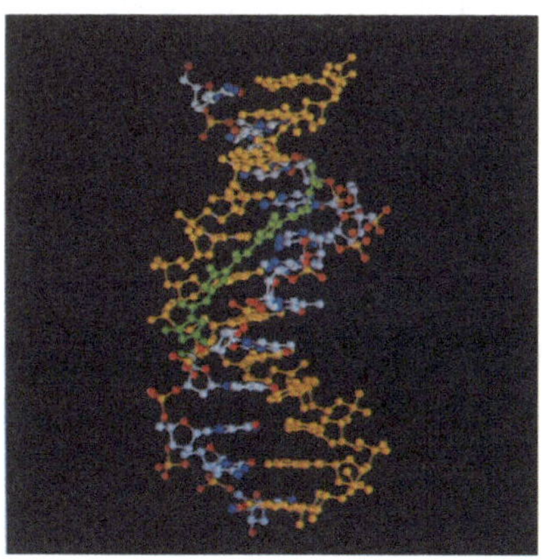

The Goals of Human Genome Research

The DNA sequence of every person's genome is the blueprint for his or her development from a single cell into a complex organism that is composed of more than 10^{13} (10 million million) cells. Encoded in the DNA sequence are not only our fundamental biological and mental capacities as human beings, but also the mutations and variations that cause or increase our susceptibility to many diseases, including cancer. Unprecedented advances in life sciences (molecular and cellular biology, biochemistry, genetics, structural biology, etc.) now provide these unique event in human history: For the first time, we can envision obtaining access to the complete sequence of the three billion nucleotides in human DNA, and to decipher much of the information contained therein. Since the human genome is remarkably stable, we shall be provided with a permanent base of knowledge concerning the genetic basis of all human beings. Although even the complete sequence of DNA in the human genome will not by itself explain human biology, it will serve as a great resource, an essential data bank that will facilitate future research in mammalian biology and medicine.

It can be anticipated that, to be able to solve such an enormous problem, the science community has to coordinate contributions from several countries and unify them by utilizing the synergetic effects provided by a supranational effort. In fact, besides several national human genome projects started in the past 2 years (e.g., in the United States, United Kingdom, France, Japan, and Italy), also the Commission of the European Communities (CEC) has initiated a Human Genome Ana-

Fig. 129
Computer model of a synthetic DNA molecule.

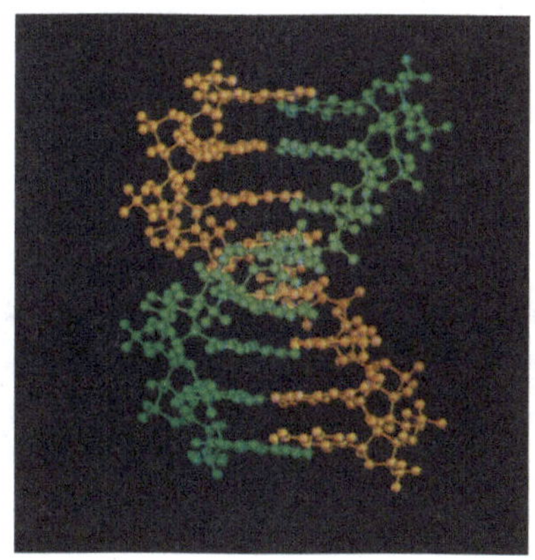

lysis (HGA) program with the participation of all the EC member countries. This program will complement the various national initiatives in Europe, and it seems clear from the input of funds and the rapidity with which genomic data are collected on both sides of the Atlantic that the science community is presently embarked on an international exercise in biology and human genetics on a scale that has never before been contemplated.

The HGA program, approved by the EC Council decision of June 29, 1990, has six major objectives (which will be explained in a bit more detail below):

1) improvement of the human genetic map,

2) physical mapping and construction of ordered clone libraries,

3) genome databases and informatics,

4) improvement of genetic technologies,

5) training and fellowships, and

6) ethical, social, and legal aspects of human genome research.

In connection with this research program, the EC is also implementing three major resource centers to coordinate and support genetic mapping, physical mapping, and genomic computing, respectively. This latter facility, the European Data Resource for Human Genome Research, will be established at the Deutsches Krebsforschungszentrum in Heidelberg (the other centers will be located at the Centre d'Etude de Polymorphisme Humain, Paris, and at the Human Gene Mapping Project, London).

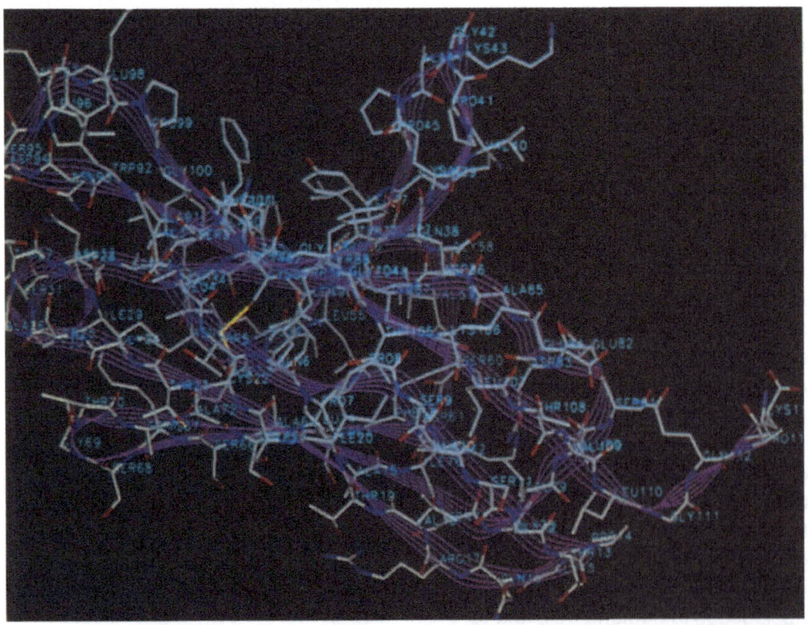

Fig. 130
Three-dimensional representation of the enzyme lysozyme.

Different Levels of Genome Data

Humans, like all living organisms, are composed largely of proteins. For humans these are roughly estimated to be of 100 000 different kinds. In general, each gene codes for the production of a single protein, and a gene and its protein can be related to each other by means of the genetic code. Therefore, scientists will be able to turn to the DNA sequence of the human genome and obtain detailed information on both the structure and function of any gene or protein of interest. In addition, all genes and proteins will be classified into large family groups that provide valuable clues to their functions. In this way, many previously unknown human genes and proteins will become available for biochemical, physiological, and medical studies. Though a number of specific regions of human DNA have already been analyzed, providing information about the structure of genes and their encoded proteins, both in normal and abnormal individuals, and about sequences that regulate gene expression, still only about 0.2% of the human genome is known at the nucleotide sequence level (including about 0.5% of our genes).

On the other hand, it is important to keep in mind that, though the knowledge of our genome at the level of its DNA sequence is an important future goal, it must not overshadow several short-term, intermediate goals of human genome research. One of the most urgent steps would be, for instance, to determine the order and spacing of all the genes that make up the genome. Such information is said to constitute a gene or genome map. One type of very useful genome map is the messenger RNA (mRNA) or exon map. Cellular enzymes transcribe or copy all of an organism's genes into mRNAs so that the functions of the genes can be expressed. Complementary DNA (cDNA) of all the mRNAs present in an organism can be synthesized enzymatically with reverse transcriptase. These cDNAs can then be cloned and used to locate the corresponding genes on a chromosome map. In this way, the genes can be mapped in the absence of knowledge of their function.

Another type of genome map would consist of an ordered set of the overlapping DNA clones (contigs) that constitute an entire chromosome. These DNA fragments are usually kept in bacteriophage or in yeast artificial chromosomes (YACs). Both the exon map and the ordered set of DNA clones are usually referred to as physical maps. Alternatively, the position of a gene can be mapped by following the effect of the expression of the gene on the cells containing it. Here, a map is constructed on the basis of the frequencies of coinheritance of two or more genetic markers. This type of genome maps is referred to as a genetic linkage map.

Maps of the human genome can be made at many different scales, or levels of resolution. Low-resolution physical maps have been derived from the distinctive patterns of bands that are observed along each chromosome by light microscopy. The physical association of genes with particular bands permits them to be mapped only approximatively, since a given gene might be assigned to a region of about 10 million nucleotides containing several hundred genes. On the other hand, such a bird's-eye view of the human genome provides a very useful first impression of its general organization and allows the systematic ordering of information coming from higher resolution techniques.

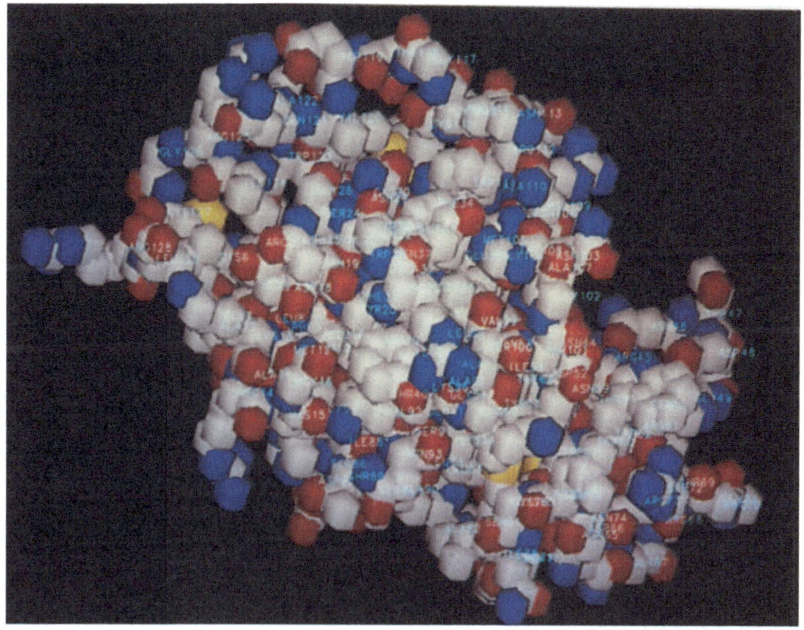

Fig. 131
Three-dimensional structure of an immunoglobulin.

Maps of higher resolution can be based, for instance, on sites in the DNA cut by special proteins called restriction enzymes. Each of these enzymes recognizes a specific short sequence of four to eight nucleotides (a restriction site) and cuts the genome at all occurrences of its sequence pattern. Since these patterns (sites) occur quite frequently, a high resolution map can be constructed by precisely determining the relative location of different restriction sites. Of particular value in human gene mapping are restriction sites that are highly variable (polymorphic) in the population. DNA lacking a specific restriction site yields a larger fragment when cut by the enzyme than does DNA containing the site; hence, the designation "restriction fragment length polymorphism" (RFLP). Hundreds of polymorphic restriction sites have so far been identified and mapped in the human genome and a number of diseaserelated genes have already been localized by determining the frequency of coinheritance of RFLPs and genetic diseases. Identifying a much larger number of useful polymorphic restriction sites should make it possible to map disease-related genes precisely enough to greatly facilitate the isolation of any human gene.

The ultimate physical map of the human genome will be its complete nucleotide sequence (of the length of three billion base pairs). Efficient strategies and technologies to perform this task are, however, not yet available and many pilot studies are focused on the sequencing of genes rather than non-coding DNA. Since only about 4–5% of the human genome encodes proteins, this is certainly a good strategy to begin with. It is not only the presently very high cost of sequencing ($2–$5 per base pair) that prevents full-scale genome sequencing in these days. An equally difficult problem is that DNA sequencing produces gene sequences much faster than the techniques of molecular biology can be applied to deduce their function. Obviously, the DNA sequence of an unknown gene (which is embedded in between long stretches of non-coding sequence regions, which are very difficult to localize) will be only a stepping stone in the process of ascertaining its function. The process of reverse genetics may be applied to produce probes and antibodies to identify the product, its cellular location, its time of appearance, etc. Sometimes the new sequence may be found (by computer comparison with databases) to be similar to that of a protein with a well-established function. Although at the moment such databases contain only a fraction of the sequences and functions of the genes of a cell, the list of the motifs that characterize specific functions and/or structures is growing almost daily and it becomes an increasingly important tool to identify the sequence in question.

Genome Research and Cancer

Humankind is afflicted by more than 3000 known, different, inherited disorders. Although their overall impact on human health is enormous, until recently, we have identified the responsible gene in fewer than 3% of all known inherited disorders. We have also learned in the past decade, largely through the application of molecular genetic tools, that deregulation of cell growth leading to cancer is caused by specific genetic abnormalities, i.e., mutations in growth-related genes that are either inherited or acquired during life. Inherited defects generally confer increased susceptibility to a particular form of cancer like malignant melanoma, cancer of the colon, certain kidney tumors, retinoblastoma, etc. The susceptibility gene for retinoblastoma has been identified, which now makes it possible to identify, by testing an individuals's DNA, those who need special surveillance for precancerous or early cancerous changes so that appropriate treatment can be applied at an early stage of disease. It will also be possible to counter the effects of inherited susceptibility more directly once the physiological effects of the various genes involved will be understood.

During one's lifetime, the copies of the genome contained in somatic cells undergo several mutations, either spontaneously, or as induced by environmental effects (various forms of radiation, substances interacting chemically with DNA, etc.). These mutations sometimes involve changes occurring in genes that regulate cell growth. Several dozen genes are today known that, when mutated in specific ways or overexpressed, deregulate cell proliferation. Some of these abnormal genes (called oncogenes) have been found in human cancer cells and seem to contribute to their tumorigenic properties. In several instances the proteins encoded by oncogenes have been shown to be altered forms of cell-growth simulators or the cellular receptors for growth stimulators. Other oncogenes encode proteins that are involved in the intercellular response of cells to growth stimulators. As a result of these findings, primary questions regarding cell growth and human cancer have come into sharp focus: What normal human proteins are involved in cell-growth, and how do they act? How do changes in one or more of these proteins cause cells to grow into tumors and to spread to distant organs? What genetic mechanisms underlie these changes? What is the spectrum of oncogenes or metastatis genes present in human tumors?

The availability of a map and DNA sequence of the human genome will help answer these questions. It will facilitate the isolation of genes that are homologous to known growth-related genes and the identification of previously undiscovered genes that play a role in cell growth and development. The characterization of the genes and proteins that regulate cell growth and are responsible for neoplasia and metastasis of tumor cells is likely to leed to more sensitive diagnostic and prognostic tests and to new approaches to the control of cancer.

To appreciate fully the functional significance of the biological information embedded in the human genome, detailed information about the genomes of other well-studied organisms must also be available for comparison. As evolution frequently conserves the critical structural or functional sequences of proteins and nucleic acids, knowledge of the structure of the genome of simpler organisms often facilitates functional understanding of the more complex human genome. Consequently, limited DNA sequence obtained for an unknown gene in one study often exhibits a structural homology with a known gene or protein during a computer search of corresponding databases established for other organisms. Such homologous relationships frequently permit biological and functional insights to be gained regarding the mechanism of action of an unknown gene, thus guiding further experimentation.

Genome Research and Informatics

The major products of human genome projects will be a series of linked data sets containing the genetic and physical location of all genes on each chromosome, plus the complete nucleotide sequence of the genome for humans and several model organisms. The primary focus of the informatics efforts associated with these projects is aimed first at the development of suitable database representations of the genetic and physical maps and their linkage to the DNA sequences, and the bibliographic databases representing the primary scientific and medical literature. The user community of these databases is widely dispersed and includes a broad range of scientific and medical disciplines ranging from molecular biology and medical genetics through computer science and mathematics.

One of the most important databases for human genome research is the Genome Database (GDB) located at Johns Hopkins University (Baltimore, Maryland, USA). This database provides complete location, ordering and distance information on human genetic markers, RFLPs, probes, and contigs linked to known human genetic diseases, as defined by the Human Gene Mapping Workshops 10.5, in Oxford, England, September 1990. Although there is currently no database (outside individual laboratories) to collect and organize the results of physical mapping studies, the GDB is in the process of incorporating such data in its structure. Managed together with GDB is the On-Line Mendelian Inheritance in Man (OMIM) database of Victor McKusick (School of Medicine, Johns Hopkins University), a text-based catalog of inherited human traits and diseases linked to GDB. Data on RFLPs, chromosomal assignments, and probes from the laboratory mouse are maintained in two mouse databases (DRHPL, maintained by the American Type Cell Culture Collection, ATCC, Rockville, Maryland, and GBase, maintained at the Jackson Laboratory, Bar Harbor, Main). As the linkage maps of mice and humans show a high degree of correspondence, it is likely that biological insights regarding the functional properties of the genomes of these two organisms will be derived from the linkage relationships first established in the genes of the other, thus reflecting our common evolution.

All of the above-mentioned databases have been developed and implemented in the United States (GDB is the only exception that has also been implemented in the UK). Though, in principle, they should be accessible also for European scientists through computer networks, it turned out in practice that such overseas connections are not yet stable, and are very expensive. Therefore, one of the first activities of the previously mentioned European Data Resource for Human Genome Research at the Deutsches Krebsforschungszentrum will be to maintain a copy of those databases in Heidelberg, and to provide access and service to them for continental Europe.

Several databases contain important data sets based on the molecular sequence of biopolymers. First among these are the nucleic acid databases: GenBank (collected by Intelligenetics, Inc., Moutain View, California, and Los Alamos National Laboratory through a contract from the National Institute of General Medical Sciences, NIH, Bethesda, Maryland), the EMBL Nucleotide Sequence Data Library (European Molecular Biology Laboratory, Heidelberg), and the DNA Database of Japan, DDBJ. These three agencies maintain an international collaboration which makes available a timely and accurate collection of all known DNA and RNA sequences from any organism. The output of the three databases is now functionally equivalent and comprises over 50 million base pairs of sequences from more than 2500 different organisms. A new nucleotide sequence database, GenInfo, based on journal scanning, with connections to the patent literature and to several genome projects, is scheduled to be available in 1991 by the National Center for Biotechnology Information (Bethesda, Maryland). The information in these databases contains many features required for intelligent and efficient use of the data. Annotated features of both RNA and DNA sequences (e.g., regulatory signals, coding sequences, mRNA splice sites, ribosome binding sites) are attached to each sequence in the GenBank/EMBL/DDBJ collection, when such information is known. Although at present more than 95% of the new protein sequences are derived from the determination of the nucleotide sequences of genes or messenger RNAs, the protein databases are currently separate from GenBank/EMBL/DDBJ.

The Protein Identification Resource (PIR) is the major protein sequence database with international connections to Germany (Martinsried Institute of Protein Sequences) and to Japan (Kyoto University). PIR's data set (complete protein amino acid sequences) is the result of additional analysis of published protein and DNA sequences intended to eliminate errors and oversights in the reported literature. Two further protein sequence databases, Swissprot and GenPept, are very useful to molecular biologists as they contain, in addition to the protein sequences of PIR, the translated open reading frames of experimentally determined unknown sequences. As for nucleic acid sequences, information on many features of protein structure (e.g., motifs, secondary structures) are also contained in the sequence annotation. These features are sometimes catalogued separately or can be inferred by the use of appropriate software.

The ultimate source of protein structural information, the crystallographic coordinates, are collected in the Protein Data Base (PDB) in Brookhaven, New York. Structural information based on nuclear magnetic resonance data is also available in the BioMagRes, BMR, database. An extensive collection of structural data on complex carbohydrates, CarbBank, exists, but there is no counterpart for lipids.

There are some very important catalog databases that make available knowledge of organisms and strains to the scientific public. Foremost among them is the American Type Culture Collection (ATCC, Rockville, Maryland), which makes available a vast array of strains and cell lines from different organisms. Also in this category are the various stock centers (e.g., the Escherichia coli Genetic Stock Center at Yale University), which maintain and provide to the research community an extensive collection of mutant strains. Some of these collections are now being organized in relational databases which will allow on-line access and user queries. As the information on particular topics is frequently found in different databases, there is a trend to set up comprehensive, organism-specific databases. Besides the ones mentioned above for humans and mice (GDB and GBase), respectively, efforts are under way to establish an E. coli database which will contain all genetic, DNA, and protein sequences and, possibly, biochemical information on the genes and gene products from this best-studied organism. Other useful small databases are HIVSSA, a collection of all HIV sequence data (Los Alamos National Laboratory), and the Restriction Enzyme Database, RED (Cold Spring Harbor Laboratory, New York), which lists the properties of all known restriction endonucleases.

Finally, there are large bibliographic databases that contain the relevant information on all articles published in scientific journals. MEDLINE, assembled by the National Library of Medicine (Bethesda, Maryland), attempts comprehensive coverage of the biomedical literature. CAS ONLINE furnishes abstracts of the scientific literature entries found in Chemical Abstracts, whereas BIOSIS reports research in the entire life sciences area.

Much of the data collected in the databases described above needs to be manipulated by sophisticated mathematical and computational tools to be of maximum use. Efforts by molecular biologists, computer scientists, and mathematicians during the past decade resulted in the development of several new algorithms and software packages for nucleic acid and protein sequence homology searches (designed primarily to reveal functional similarities in proteins and common structural motifs in either proteins or nucleic acids), for the support of the planning and performing of largescale mapping and sequencing experiments, and for the identification of protein coding regions of genomic DNA, etc.

Access of Genome Databases through Computer Networks

The establishment of global computer networks has completely changed the way scientists gather and disseminate information and conduct collaborative research. On-line access via modem over computer networks allows remote users to manipulate data in many distant databases and to download either raw data itself or the computed results of these searches. With the advent of high-speed national networks, distribution of the databases and their updates is increasingly easily via File Transfer Protocol (FTP) procedures that gradually replace the mailing of tapes or CD-ROMs. Electronic mail is also becoming more widely used, both for the depositing in and accessing of the databases, as well as initiating collaborations.

In mid-1990, with the support of the Federal Ministry for Research and Technology, the Deutsches Krebsforschungszentrum installed a dedicated computer for the German biomedical community to serve as a center for biocomputing and networking. This facility, called GENIUSnet (Genetic Interactive Unix System network), provides access to all important sequence databases together with the analysis software environment HUSAR (Heidelberg Unix Sequence Analysis Resources) for about 300 scientists in Germany who make use mostly of the national scientific computer network WIN (Wissenschaftsnetz). GENIUSnet also serves as the German node in EMBnet (European Molecular Biology network), a collaboration of about a dozen national biocomputing centers, including EMBL, to coordinate data and software exchange and communication within Europe.

Genome databases are still being distributed as "flat files" without any structure, each institution is developing its own (in most cases incompatible) software to structure and analyze them. An important task in the next years will be the establishment of standardization and compatibility, not only in the various transaction protocols for communication (different networks use different standards), but also to ensure the compatibility of data formats and to allow connectivity of the various databases. The ultimate aim here must be a user interface that requires minimum computer or database knowledge and allows access to data in a variety of databases. For instance, the investigation of a single problem in molecular biology may require that the user extract information from different databases dealing with evolution, physical and genetic maps, clone libraries, sequence, structure, etc.

In somewhat longer terms, the basic philosophy of data entry and maintainance has to be changed. Scientists in the lab, who understand the full meaning of the new data, should be enabled (through appropriate software and computer network) to place it into the proper context within the database and to establish its relation with existing knowledge. Beyond software supporting basic annotation, automatic error-checking and consistency proofs, they will have to possess more advanced analytic tools, for instance, to be able to optimize homologies to related sequences during submission (which should then become part of the database), to define pointers for highly informative sites (e.g., protein binding sites, structural motifs, regulatory sequence patterns), etc. Such information should also form the basis to cross-link different databanks (sequence, structure, enzyme, vector, etc.). Parallel to our proceeding with major genome projects, we will have to make the transition from centralized to distributed database management systems that handle data distributed among a number of interconnected machines that may be physically remote from each other. Major data generation centers should serve as local nodes to this network that update the primary data collection only at regular intervals.

Future Challenges for Genome Informatics

The present day organization of genomic databases reflects the fact that genome research has been aimed, up until now, at decoding the structure and function of single genes or small groups of genes. Our existing databanks are nothing more than an additive collection of information about a few thousand of nearly independent genes. If molecular genetics will attempt to search for the overall logical structure of larger genomes and ask questions about how, during development or function, different parts of these genomes interact with each other, we will need far more sophisticated database structures and retrieval tools than are in use now. Principally, the organization and investigation of such highly branched structures will be possible only by using completely new software tools like artificial intelligence programming techniques, object oriented databases, etc.

To be able to build comprehensive pictures of complicated genomes, databases should also support the need to view the data in different contexts at the same time, i.e., from a physical point of view (mapping, taxonomy) or from a functional one (encoded gene products, their structure and interactions, etc.).

To provide such a flexibility, the databases will have to be richly structured and profoundly linked so that one will be able to take data stored primarily under one organizational scheme and reorganize them according to the structure of some other data set to which they are to be linked. In addition, there is an important missing link between high-level (low-resolution) and low-level (high-resolution) genetic databases and an urgent need for physical map database(s) of the human genome. Supplementary information on organization and coordination (who is doing what?) will also become increasingly important as genome research is imaginable only as a collaborative international effort.

One of the most serious factors limiting the more rapid integration of the new methods and practical tools provided by genome informatics to the biomedical science community is the ignorance or reluctance of the potential users (or both). Thus, to reap the full value of the analysis and subsequent application of the biological information embedded in the databases, a serious educational effort in computer science and genome informatics is needed in the biomedical sciences. In fact, a successful genome informatics requires the strong interaction of computer-literate biologists with mathematicians, software engineers, and programmers who are, in turn, at ease with the life sciences. For this purpose, a deliberate effort seems to be indispensable to teach courses, establish new postdoctoral training programs, and possibly develop undergraduate curricula to provide suitably trained experts to populate this new field.

Another urgent task is to provide flexible, cheap, functional connectivity to all biomedical scientists – one with a transparent infrastructure. This requires the development of standards for text and graphical representation of genetic map data, database application interfaces, and syntax languages, all in a hardware-independent fashion, if possible. Although the use of electronic means for accessing and sharing biological information is increasing steadily, only a small part of the total scientific community actually participates in and enjoys the advantages of today's technology in their research programs. Perhaps the Human Genome Analysis program offers a visible international example of the power of distributed, shared small science projects linked via international networks, now with the power to tackle in a concerted fashion a unified big science objective.

Dr. Sándor Suhai
Dipl.-Chem. Martina Kieninger
Division of Molecular Biophysics I

Participating scientists

Dr. Bernd Drescher
Dipl.-Math. Karl-Heinz Glatting
Dipl.-Biol. Matthias Hage
Dr. Eckhard Krauss
Dr. Otto Ritter

In collaboration with

Dr. Kurt Böhm
Central Data Processing,
Deutsches Krebsforschungszentrum

Dr. Martin J. Bishop
Universität Cambridge,
Computer Laboratory,
Cambridge, England

Dr. Marc Lathrop
Centre d'Études du Polymorphisme Humain,
Paris, Frankreich

Dr. Hans Lehrach
Imperial Cancer Research Fund,
London, England

Prof. Victor McKusick
Johns Hopkins University,
School of Medicine,
Baltimore, Maryland, USA

Dr. Jean Thierry-Mieg
Centre National de la Recherche Scientifique,
Montpellier, Frankreich

Prof. Peter Pearson
Johns Hopkins University,
Medical School,
Welsh Medical Library,
Baltimore, Maryland, USA

Dr. John Sulston
MRC – Molecular Biology Laboratory,
Cambridge, England

Selected publications

Suhai, S.: Computational Methods in Cancer Research – The Hierarchy of Genomic Information. Interdisc. Science Rev. 14, 225–232 (1989)

Suhai, S.: Computer-Aided Analysis of Biomolecular Sequence and Structure in Genome Research. In: Genome Analysis in Domestic Animals, Eds. H. Geldermann and F. Ellendorff, Verlag Chemie, Weinheim, pp. 81–104 (1990)

Suhai, S.: Modelling of Protein Structures on the Basis of Sequence Data. In: Modern Methods in Protein- and Nucleic Acid Resach, Ed. H. Tschesche, W. de Gruyter, Berlin, pp. 395–422 (1990)

Suhai, S.: Bioinformatics Aspects of Genome Research – Current Methods and Emerging Trends. J. Clin. Chem. Clin. Biochem. 28, 373–374 (1990)

Suhai, S.: The Electronic Structure of Parallel ß-Pleated Sheets in Proteins. Int. J. Quant. Chem. 39, 122-140 (1991)

Suhai. S.: On the Structure Dependence of the Polarizability of Polyenes. Molecular Engineering 1, 115–129 (1991)

Central Facilities

Central Library

The Central Library collects, catalogs, and provides scientific literature for the Deutsches Krebsforschungszentrum. In addition, it looks after the eight libraries of the former Institutes that exist in the Center.

The library is not only accessible to the staff of the Center, but also to guests. Due to its location in the vicinity of the University of Heidelberg's natural sciences and medical institutes and to the University Clinic, it is also much used by University members, especially students and physicians. The Central Library also provides services for the Tumor Center Heidelberg/Mannheim and for the Cancer Information Service (KID).

In accordance with the Center's working program, the library focuses on literature on tumor biology, mechanisms of carcinogenesis, cancer risk factors, cancer prevention, and research on cancer diagnosis and therapy. The library contains about 63000 volumes and subscribes to 880 journals. The eight departmental libraries contain an additional 12000 monographs and 300 journals.

The classified arrangement of books makes it possible to find the literature without using the library's catalog. By open access shelving about 80% of the literature are freely accessible to employees of the Center and to guests. Only older literature is placed in the

Fig. 132
Reading room.

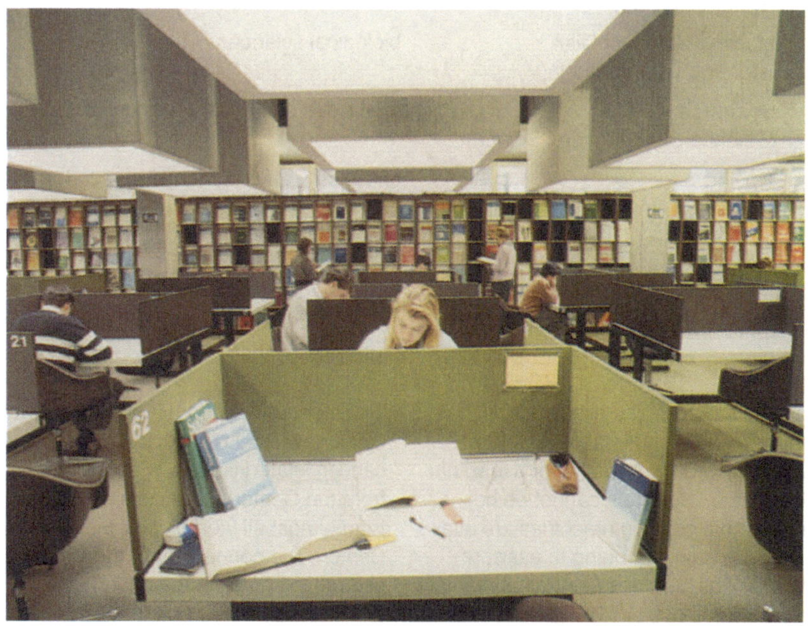

Selection of the data bases available in the information center

Data base	Specialty
BIOSIS (Biosciences Information Service)	entire biological sciences
CA Search (Chemical Abstracts Search)	chemistry, biochemistry
Cancerlit (Cancer Literature)	oncology
Cancer Compact Disk – for end-user searching	oncology
Embase (Excerpta Medica Data Base)	biological sciences, pharmacy
FSTA (Food Science and Technology Abstracts)	nutrition and food sciences
INIS (International Nuclear Information System)	nuclear medicine
Medline (Medical Literature Analysis and Retrieval System Online)	biological sciences
Medline Compact Disk – for end-user searching	biological sciences
Scisearch (Science Citation Index Search)	total exact sciences, multidisciplinary
Toxline (Toxicology Information Online)	toxicology, environmental research

closed storage. The reading room has more than 70 workplaces. Books can be borrowed for 2 weeks for use within the Center. Journals cannot be borrowed, but copying machines are available. Its main aim being to assist research, the Center's Central Library is a reference library.

The menu-guided, on-line monographs catalog, which is a special catalog on cancer-related issues, is accessible from the Center's terminals and thus from almost all workplaces within the Center. The connection of the Center's central computer to the postal data net (Datex-P) and to the German Research Net (DFN) allows out-of-house scientists to access the Center's data base.

The Information Center, which is part of the Central Library, supplements the in-house means for literature information by providing on-line access to several international biomedical and scientific data banks such as Medline and Scisearch. About 60 data banks, including factual data banks that give direct information without recourse to the literature, are presently being used. The on-line connections comprise the data base supplier Data-Star in Bern, the Dialog Information Service in Palo Alto (U.S.A.), the DIMDI (German Institute for Medical Documentation and Information) in Cologne, and the STN (Scientific and Technical Information Network) in Karlsruhe.

Head:
Wiss. Bibl. Rolf-Peter Kraft (provisional)

Central Animal Laboratory

Progress in biomedical research is the cornerstone to improvement in human and animal health, quality of life, and life expectancy. Animal experiments, despite the fact that alternatives are being developed, are still indispensable for classical disciplines. The use of animals for research, though, has been reduced to an absolute minimum. Animal experiments have made a major contribution to our knowledge of biomedical interactions, especially to the understanding of the extremely complex nature of cancer. However, especially in the field of fundamental research, animal experiments still appear indispensable. They are largely concerned with the development of methods for improved diagnosis and treatment of tumors, as well as with obtaining information on the possibilities of cancer prevention.

The Central Animal Laboratory consists of five barrier units, an isolator station divided into four subwards, and a conventional (open) animal sector which, however, is losing its importance. The main task of this central facility is to ensure that all types of animals used in research (mice, rats, (to a certain extent) rabbits, guinea pigs, chickens, etc.) are housed, fed, taken care of, and medically looked after in accordance with today's requirements (animal protection laws, theories of animal behavior). The laboratory is authorized to issue instructions to all users on aspects of hygiene and the keeping of laboratory animals. The animal laboratory is run by professionals, including veterinarians specialized in microbiology and laboratory animal science, administrative personnel, diagnostic and laboratory animal technicians, the majority of whom have been trained in our center. The head of the laboratory and his deputy are, in accordance with the recommendations of the German Research Society (Deutsche Forschungsgemeinschaft), directly responsible to the Management Board of the Foundation and personally responsible for the observance and enforcement of all national and international laws, regulations, and orders concerning the keeping of laboratory animals. The same is true for internal regulations which govern the rights and duties of operators and users.

It is the staff's task to not only operate the animal laboratory and to supervise the general care of animals, but also to give advice on the characteristics of test animals and suitable animal models. The staff is also involved in the planning and implementation of animal experiments.

Furthermore, it is an important objective of the Central Animal Laboratory to pass on basic knowledge and skills associated with laboratory animals and animal experiments. Thus, since 1990 (and in the future, twice a year) we have held a "Basic course on animal experiments" for Diploma (Master's degree) and Ph.D. students in biology, the veterinary sciences, and medicine.

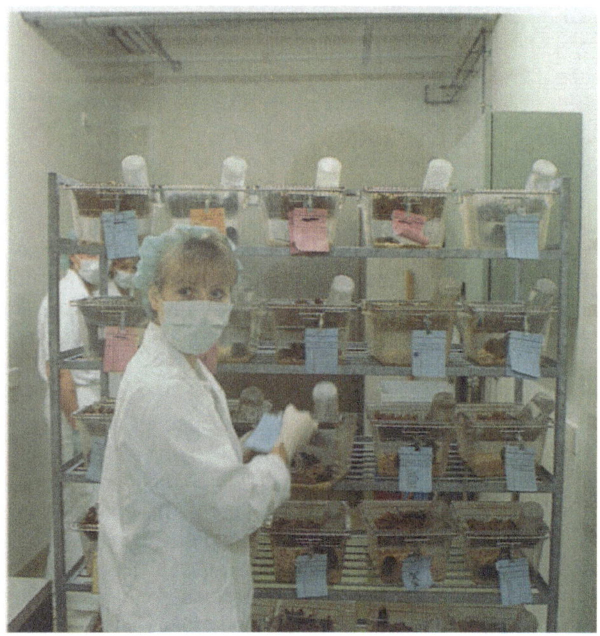

Fig. 133
A laboratory animal technician feeding rats in the animal laboratory.

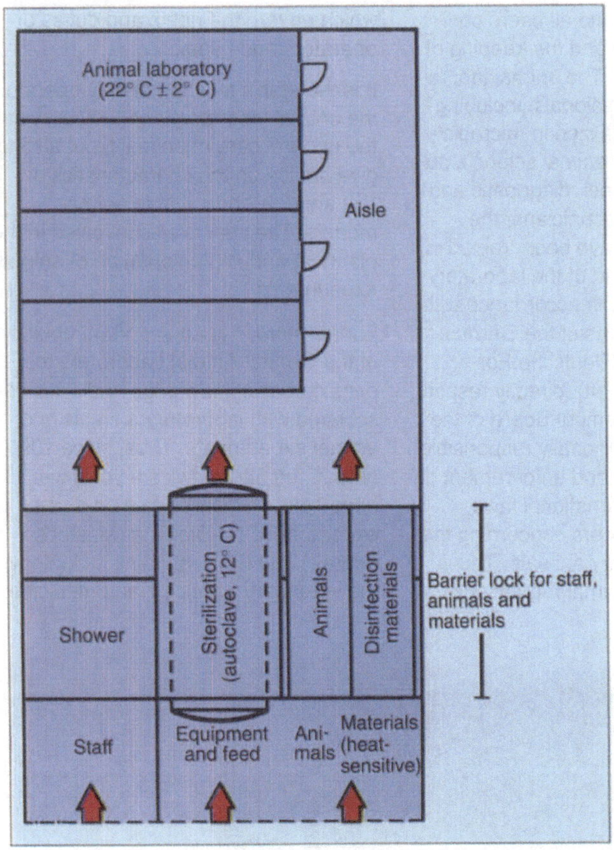

Fig. 134
Functional plan of a "closed system". Technicians, animals, and materials have to pass a barrier to enter the animal laboratory. The technicians take a shower and change their clothes; all materials are sterilized. These measures protect the infection-free animals from diseases.

Successful completion of this course is a prerequisite for admission to, and work in, the animal laboratory.

Even before the new law on Animal Protection became fully effective in 1987, questions dealing with the protection of animals (to be more precise, applications for permission to carry out animal experiments) were discussed in, and decided by, the internal animal protection commission (ITSK), established in 1985. It is the task of this commission to weigh the need for animal experiments (project by project) against the benefit that might be gained from the new knowledge. This commission, which was created on the initiative of the Deutsches Krebsforschungszentrum, is also responsible for assessing the objective and ethical justification for animal experiments. The central laboratory receives additional assistance from six animal welfare officers (biologists, veterinarians, medical surgeons), each responsible for one area. They are not bound by directives, but are independent and only responsible to their own conscience; they are involved in individual projects as advisers and supervisors from the application through completion.

In the planning of scientifically based animal experiments, the needs of biometry and statistics are now routinely considered at an early planning stage; thus, the necessity for a later repetition of experiments is greatly reduced. The statistical analysis of the experiments further reveals ways of controlling and reducing systematic errors in the results.

Many chemico-physical or meteorological environmental factors may influence the biology and physiology, i.e., the reactions and measurement data of our animals. It is of enormous importance for the standardization of the "measuring device," (which in this case is the test animal) that the scattering of the results and deviations from the norm should be minimized. Elaborate technical equipment in and outside of the animal laboratories ensure that a standard climate (temperature: 20 +/– 2°C, relative humidity: 55%) and lighting conditions are maintained at all times. Thus, endogenously regulated daily and seasonal biorhythms can be maintained and accounted for. By providing a balanced nutrition appropriate to the species (standard diet), as well as personal care from qualified staff (experimental animal technicians) we come very close to the goal of a total standardization of the environment.

Part of this is, from the point of view of animal protection, the microbiological standardization of the experimental animals in our care. Constructional and organizational precautions (standards of the barrier or isolator principles) can, together with specific hygienic measures, ensure with sufficient certainty that infective agents (in the case of small rodents, more than 60 different viruses, bacteria, and parasites) are prevented from being introduced into the stocks, which would result in erroneous experimental results. The microbiological-diagnostic laboratory of the Central Animal Laboratory has a graded program for permanent infection surveillance (for both animals arriving and those in care), and the most modern diagnostic methods for the direct and indirect detection of infective agents (serology: IFA, ELISA, HI, CF). The microbiological status of all laboratory animals is known at any time and can thus be considered in the evaluation of the experiments, or used as the basis for improving the animal stock's health status.

The conversion of animal laboratories from open to closed (standardized) units (the barrier system for SPF (specified pathogen-free) animals was introduced in 1988 (Fig. 134) was carried out to reduce the physiological and pathophysiological variables as far as possible and, thus, to raise the value of the experimental results. In this way the total number of animals required has been reduced by two-thirds. The cost of keeping such SPF animals is considerable, but absolutely essential for scientific, ethical, and legal reasons.

Head:
Dr. med. vet. Uwe Zillmann

Deputy:
Dr. med. vet. Werner Nicklas

Central Spectroscopy

The Central Spectroscopy Department provides spectroscopic services for all divisions of the Deutsches Krebsforschungszentrum. These services range from routine analytical tasks and quality control to structure determination of synthetic and natural products, as well as intensive cooperation in long-term research projects requiring sophisticated techniques such as in vivo NMR spectroscopy.

Fig. 135
Two-dimensional spectroscopic images of an oligopeptide fragment (46 amino acids) of the beta-tubulin protein. The image was taken with a nuclear magnetic resonance imager. It is possible to resolve nuclear magnetic resonance signals from individual amino acid side chains.

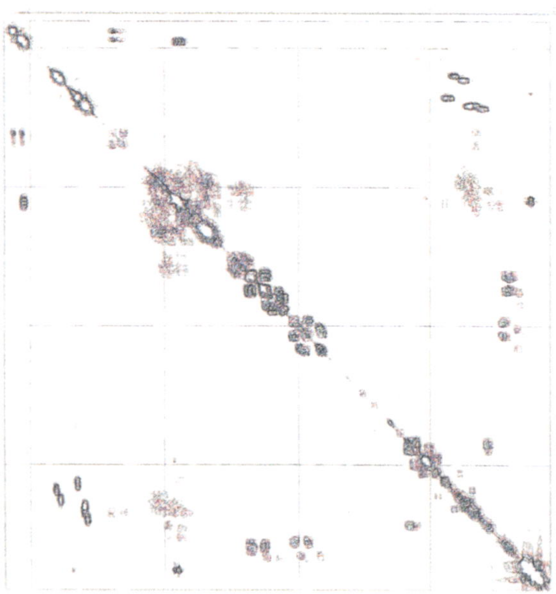

The techniques offered include:

a) high-resolution mass spectromety (MS) with electron impact (EI), chemical ionization (CI) and fast-atom bombardment (FAB) methods, and coupling with a gas chromatograph (GC/MS);
b) infrared and visible/UV spectroscopy;
c) circular dichroism (CD);
d) nuclear magnetic resonance (NMR) spectroscopy:
- routine $^{1}H^{13}C^{19}F^{31}P$ NMR with a 250 MHz (5.8 Tesla) instrument.
- state-of-the-art multinuclear NMR with a 500 MHz (11.7 Tesla) instrument offering high sensitivity and the most modern one- andc two-dimensional NMR techniques for in vitro solutions, cell suspensions, and tissue samples.
- a "super wide bore" 300 MHz (7.0 Tesla) system with a 15 cm vertical magnet for both in vitro spectroscopy with large samples and in vivo spectroscopy with large samples and in vivo spectroscopy and imaging with mouse and rat animal models.

The Spectroscopy is committed to acquirin and further developing the most modern spectroscopic techniques and methodology and applying them to biochemical and biological problems in cancer research. Some of the collaborative research projects being pursued are:

a) structure elucidation of natural products and derivatives that exhibit tumor promoting activity (GC, MS, NMR);
b) structure elucidation of substances involved in chemical carcinogenesis as well as compounds developed for chemotherapy (IR, MS, NMR);
c) structure elucidation of oligosaccharides and oligopeptides, fatty acids and their metabolites (GC/MS, FAB, NMR);
d) conformation of peptides and proteins in solution (^{1}H-NMR);
e) optimization of the synthesis and purification of ^{18}F-labelled substrates that are being used for positron emission tomography (PET): in vitro analysis of the metabolites of such substrates and in vivo monitoring of uptake and metabolism (^{1}H-, ^{19}F-NMR);
f) investigation of fluoropyrimidine metabolism (chemotherapy with 5-FU or 5-FdUrd) by the in vitro analysis of metabolites in plasma, urine, and tissue samples from patients and the in vivo study of metabolism in tumor-bearing mice (^{19}F-NMR);
g) investigation of polyamine metabolism and the possible use of fluorinated polyamine analogs for

monitoring tumor metabolism and therapy (^{19}F-NMR);

h) quantitation of phosphate metabolites and investigation of phospholipid metabolism in cultured tumor cells and solid tumors: monitoring the effects of various therapy modalities (^{31}P-NMR).

Particularly in the application of NMR techniques it is our goal to contribute to the more detailed biochemical understanding of tumor metabolism and therapy and provide information which can guide the use of NMR and PET in clinical practice and assist in the interpretation of the result obtained and in the development of improved therapy regimens.

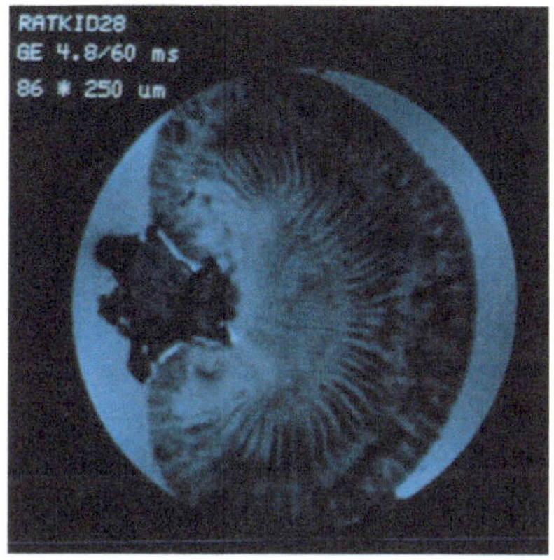

Fig. 136
Nuclear magnetic resonance microscopy of a rat's kidney.

In addition to the collection of spectroscopic data, the Central-Spectroscopy is actively involved in developing efficient techniques for the archiving, documentation and analysis of spectra by means of a computer-based information system called SPEKTREN. This data bank and search system has been reorganized in a relational form and includes MS, IR, and ^{13}C-NMR data as well as other physical data and a two-dimensional structural representation of each compound. Both our own measured spectra and data from the literature and other data banks have been incorporated. The program allows for the automated analysis of spectra and the correlation of spectroscopic and structural features (substructure and similarity search). Current developments involve the coding of three-dimensional structures (stereochemistry), incorporation of the Cambridge Crystallographic Data Files and the inclusion of pharmacological and toxicological data.

Finally, the Central Spectroscopy is acquiring and developing a powerful collection of software tools for computer-assisted molecular modeling. Routines for generating, manipulation and comparing structures interactively, for minimizing static conformational energy, and for simulating the dynamics of molecular motion are bein made available as a service for groups interested in structure-activity relationships, drug design and protein engineering. This software will augment and facilitate the use of our spectroscopic data bank and protein sequence and crystal structure data banks and will complement the rapidly growing techniques of molecular biology and their applications in cancer research.

Head:
Dr. William E. Hull

Deputy:
Priv.-Doz. Dr. Wolf-Dieter Lehmann

Central Service of Radiation Protection and Dosimetry

The function of the Central Service of Radiation Protection and Dosimetry is to ensure adequate protection of the staff, the working area and the surroundings against the hazard of ionizing radiation and radionuclides used in the Deutsches Krebsforschungszentrum. All divisions and project groups, the research reactor, the cyclotron, and the large-scale diagnostic and therapeutic equipment are to be monitored.

In nearly all divisions and in all project groups radioactive labelled compounds with mainly beta-emitting radionuclides are used in in vitro and in vivo experiments; in three divisions radiopharmaceuticals and ionizing radiation are also used in diagnosis and therapy, as well as in animal studies.

The following amounts of radionuclides are purchased per year: beta-emitting radionuclides amounting to a total activity of about 120 gigabecquerel (GBq), beta-gamma emitters amounting to approximately 350 GBq, and, solely for use in nuclear medicine, the generator-produced radionuclide molybdenum-99 with an overall activity of about 1000 GBq. Because of their short half-life, pure positron emitters totalling between 2000 and 3000 GBq are produced immediately on the spot in the cyclotron.

Fig. 137
Control measurement of possible contamination by radioactive substances with a hand-body-clothes monitor.

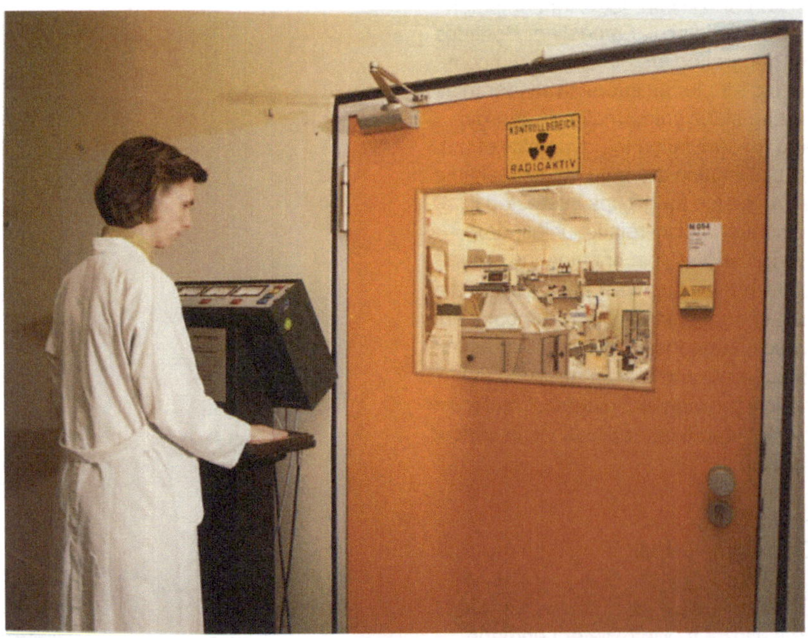

The following examples illustrate the variety of work of the Central Service of Radiation Protection and Dosimetry: monitoring the exposure of staff and monitoring contamination in laboratories; monitoring and dosimetric measurement of the experimental large-scale equipment; monitoring and documentation of the purchase and production of radioactive materials; central registration, selection and storage of radioactive waste; separation into radioactive and non-radioactive waste; delivery to the officially licensed depots or companies.

In addition to the radiation protection duties concerning the staff and their working areas, as well as the fulfillment of requirements imposed by the authorities, the Service also carries out radiation protection tasks for patients within research studies, such as dosimetric measurements and calculations for positron emission tomography (PET). These tasks concern the radiation exposure of patients and of technical and medical staff. The effective dose for patients given the usual activity of 500 megabecquerel (MBq) was calculated via the individual organ doses at about 5 millisievert (mSv) for a PET examination with nitrogen-13 glutamate and at about 15 mSv for an examination with F-18-labeled 5-fluorouracil.

In cooperation with the Division of Biophysics and Medical Radiation Physics the possible radiation exposure of staff members working in positron emission tomography was investigated. This exposure can be measured by the ambient doses in the area surrounding the tomograph. The ambient doses were measured and calculated at various positions with a distance between 1.9 and 5.3 meters from the center of the tomograph. For 700 PET examinations per year the measured annual doses ranged between 3.80 mSV and 0.86 mSv. The calculated annual doses ranged between 4.21 mSv and 0.90 mSv. The background effect of 0.70 mSv is included in these values.

The good agreement of calculated and measured ambient doses shows that the calculation method applied is suitable for prospective dose estimates if the character and number of scheduled examinations are known and structural characteristics are taken into account through experimentally determined factors of geometry.

Furthermore, the Central Radiation Protection operates a whole-body counter, which serves for incorporation monitoring of specific staff groups within personnel dosimetry and for activity measurements on thorotrast patients within a EURATOM study carried out by the Division Oncological Diagnostics and Therapy.

In 1990, the old compact cyclotron was dismantled and disposed of via the special waste depot of the Land Baden-Württemberg. The parts of the plant had a total weight of about 27000 kg and a rather small activity: at the end of last year it amounted to not more than 20 GBq. The majority of the activity has a half-life of approximately one year; not more than 2 GBq of it has a half-life of about 5 years.

In 1991, a highly efficient new cyclotron was installed. Together with the inspector and the authority in charge, the Central Radiation Protection is currently working on the operating permit for the new plant and the regulations for the handling of the radioactive substances produced. This requires extensive measurements of ambient dose rates and exhaust air activities.

Head and Radiation Protection Officer:
Dipl.-Phys. Otto Krauss

Deputies:
Dipl.-Ing. (BA) Mechthild Kämmer
Dipl.-Phys. Dr. Wolfgang Kübler

Research Reactor TRIGA in Heidelberg

On August 26, 1966, the first research reactor, TRIGA Heidelberg I, was put into operation at the former location of the Deutsches Krebsforschungszentrum on Berliner Strasse.

From 1972 to 1978 the research reactor TRIGA Heidelberg II was built in the new building of the Deutsches Krebsforschungszentrum with newly designed reactor safety systems and peripheral devices. The fuel elements were transferred from TRIGA Heidelberg I and are still being used. TRIGA Heidelberg II was put into operation on February 28, 1978 in the new building of the Deutsches Krebsforschungszentrum in the Neuenheimer Feld. TRIGA Heidelberg I was shut down and disposed of.

TRIGA reactors are very reliable irradiation devices and have a very low susceptibility to disturbances. The Center's reactor is operated and maintained by a team of three staff technicians. Repairs are carried out in the reactor cyclotron machine shop. Regular inspections according to the German Nuclear Power Law are conducted in collaboration with the Technical Control Board South- West. Since 1978, seven malfunctions were reported, but only the repair of the rotary irradiation system required a significant interruption of the reactor operation. All other malfunctions could be eliminated by exchanging electronic devices.

The reactor is mainly used for neutron activation, both in medical and biological research, as well as for material testing. In general, only neutron activation can detect small traces of metals in samples. In contrast to atomic absorption, neutron activation makes it possible to detect several elements simultaneously. In general, neutron activation analysis requires irradiation times of 50 hours and more.

The in-core irradiation positions are primarily used for operations that require a high neutron flux, such as the production of radionuclides for examinations in nuclear medicine. Since August 1966, about 11 700 experiments have been conducted with TRIGA Heidelberg II. TRIGA Heidelberg I and II have produced 2310 MW and 4890 MW in thermal energy, respectively, making a total of 7200 MW. Since 1978, about 30 000 samples have been irradiated in TRIGA Heidelberg II. During the past 10 years, the daily radiation time has increased continuously from about 5 to about 11 hours per working day. On average, the reactor has been operated 180 days per year; 30 days are required for reliability checks and tests, and 20 days for maintenance and repair.

The general trend has shifted to longer irradiation times and more irradiation samples per experiment. TRIGA Heidelberg II may also be used by scientists of the University of Heidelberg, the Nuclear Sciences Research Center in Karlsruhe, and the University of Karlsruhe. In special cases, experiments have also been conducted for universities outside the region and for several industrial companies.

In September 1990, the 11th European TRIGA User's Conference took place in the Deutsches Krebsforschungszentrum. 50 scientists from 11 European countries, the USA, Japan, and northern African countries attended the meeting. The TRIGA User's Conference takes place at regular intervals and serves to exchange experiences among the TRIGA users and is thus a useful international platform for exchanging and discussing all related matters.

General manager:
Prof. Dr. Walter Lorenz

Operational manager:
Dr. Wolfgang Maier-Borst

Deputy operational manager:
Dipl.-Phys. Otto Krauss

Cyclotron

A New Cyclotron for Cancer Diagnosis

How fast and to what extent does a kidney resume functioning after transplantation? Is the myocardium threatened by infarctation and, if so, to what extent? Which part of the lung is blocked by a carcinoma, and how aggressive is the tumor growth? Will chemotherapy succeed? Does a tumor respond to a specific therapy? All these questions can be addressed directly and without delay with the help of radioactively marked ("radiolabeled") substances.

Nuclear-medical function diagnosis, i.e., the in vivo detection of radiolabeled biomolecules and their metabolism, makes it possible to quantify physiological processes non-invasively and highly specifically and sensitively. Images of the distribution of radioactivity within the organism (scintigrams) show the temporal process of tracer accumulation and diffusion in the examined region. These scintigrams are the basis for the physician's assessment of the organ's functioning and of the kind and extent of pathological alterations.

A radioactive nuclide with specific physical and chemical properties serves as the "label" of its host molecule, the "chemical spy". Upon decaying, the nuclide must emit an energy quantum which is within the sensitivity range of the available detection devices (80 to 500 keV), the chemical process of integrating the nuclide into the host molecule must be fast, and the nuclide must not change the typical metabolic behavior of the host molecule. In addition, it must decay rapidly, i.e., its half-life must not be long compared to the duration of the examination. This makes sure that the patient's exposure to radiation remains small and that several examinations can be carried out in short intervals.

Some of these short-lived radionuclides with half-lives of minutes or a few hours decay so fast that they have to be produced at the site of their use. The most effective production technique is the transformation of stable isotopes by irradiation with charged particles, in most cases with protons and deuterons, which are the nuclei of the light and the heavy hydrogen. In order to be able to overcome the repulsive forces of the target nucleus, these subatomic projectiles have to be accelerated to high energies. Only then are they able to penetrate the target nucleus and to alter its structure in such a way that it becomes unstable (radioactive). Later, the radioactive nucleus spontaneously decays into a stable state, a process which is accompanied by the emission of positive or negative electrons and hard electromagnetic radiation (gamma rays). These rays can be detected outside the body.

The atomic projectiles are produced in small electromagnetic circular accelerators, so-called compact cyclotrons. The first cyclotron was built in 1930 in Berkeley, California, by the

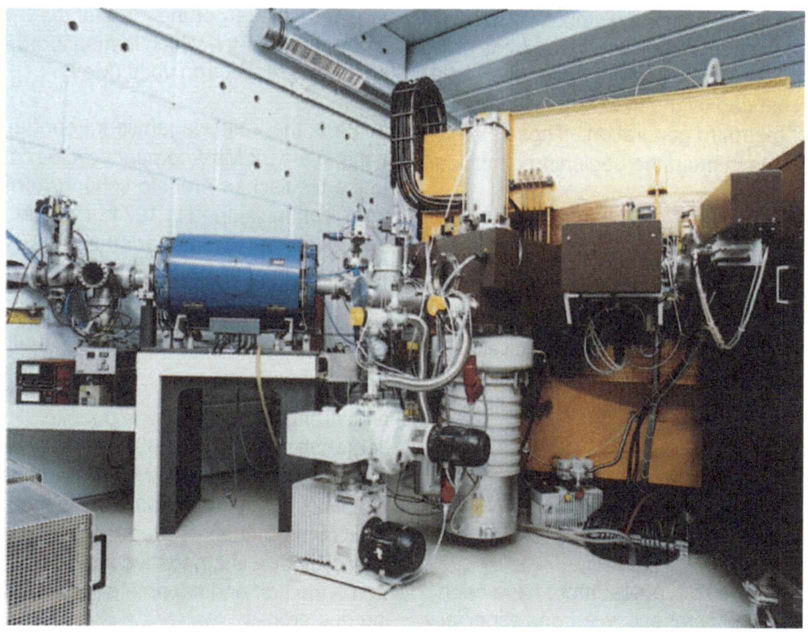

Fig. 138
The new cyclotron of the Deutsches Krebsforschungszentrum. It produces radioactive nuclides, which are used, for example, to study the metabolisms of tumors and their change after therapy.

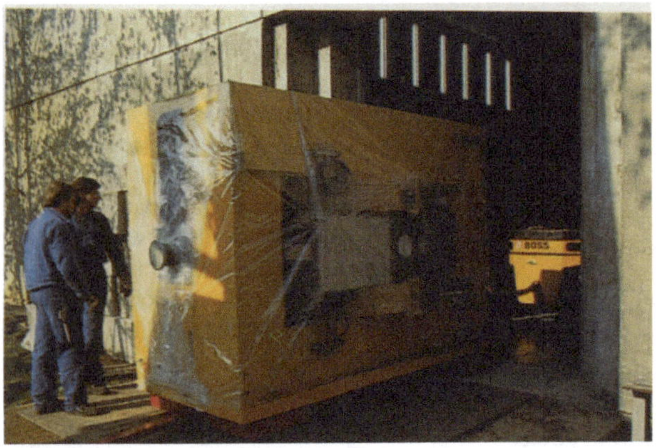

Fig. 139
Delivery of prefabricated components for the new cyclotron from Sweden.

American physicist Ernest Lawrence. Five years later, his brother, the physician John Lawrence, and his colleague, Joe Hamilton, conducted self-experiments to study the distribution of the vital element potassium in the body using radioactive potassium-38 that had been produced by the then largest cyclotron of the "third generation". These experiments marked the beginning of nuclear medicine.

The advantage of nuclear transformation with charged particles is the fact that the product of the reaction is an isotope of another chemical element, which can be separated chemically from the irradiated original substance, the target. It is then available with a high grade of purity, i.e. with high specific activity. It is thus possible to effectively radiolabel extremely small, non-toxic amounts of specific pharmacons.

Since the late 1960s, there have been available compact cyclotrons especially designed for the production of radionuclides. Inside a cyclotron a strong magnetic field forces hydrogen or helium nuclei to move on helical paths; several times per cycle the particles are accelerated by a strong radiofrequency. The highest energy of the projectiles is mainly given by the diameter of the magnet – the larger the magnet the higher the energy, which is measured in millions of electron volts (MeV).

In 1968, the Volkswagenwerk Foundation gave a 22 MeV compact cyclotron to the Deutsches Krebsforschungszentrum; commissioned in 1971, it was in use for almost 20 years for the production of radionuclides as well as for the dosimetry and radiobiology of fast neutrons and charged particles.

After 28 months of construction, a new and stronger cyclotron was put into operation on April 25, 1991. It produces 32 MeV protons and 15 MeV deuterons (nuclei of heavy hydrogen) with higher ionic currents than its predecessor. The new cyclotron is a negative ion cyclotron – the first one capable of accelerating deuterons.

The new cyclotron will be mainly used for producing known radionuclides that are suited for investigating the metabolism of tumors and their behavior after therapy on the basis of an innovative diagnostic technique, the positron emission tomography (PET). Among the radionuclides produced are the "physiological" radioisotopes, which, due to their specific nature or their chemical bond, do not change the metabolic behavior of the radiolabeled substrates: carbon-11, nitrogen-13, oxygen-15 and, above all, fluorine-18. The higher energies provided by the new cyclotron will result in a significantly higher yield and a longer life of the target system, in particular, in the case of the most important positron emitter, fluorine-18. Higher initial activities are of long-term importance, since the process of radiolabeling highly specialized biomolecules is becoming ever more complicated and thus slower, and since the degree of chemical purity needed today requires complex purifying processes. The loss of radioactivity during these processes has to be compensated for by higher initial activities.

In addition, higher energies and beam currents make it possible to develop long-lived radionuclides for the detection and tracing of slow biological processes (for example, with radiolabeled antibodies) for research purposes and, eventually, for application in medicine.

The charged particles, as well as the fast neutrons produced with their help, also serve as tools for radiobiologic investigations. The activation analysis with ions or neutrons offers numerous new possibilities in applied research, which might be of interest for scientists within and outside of the Deutsches Krebsforschungszentrum.

As a brief summary, it can be said that higher particle energies and currents lead to higher yields of the traditional radionuclides for development of new radiolabelling methods of higher specificity and purity. They also have a higher operational reliability and offer a broader potential for further research areas.

Guest scientists are invited to make use of the existing technologies. Thanks to this new cyclotron we are able to supply clinical partners in our region with short-lived radionuclides for development of their own diagnostic techniques, such as in positron emission tomography.

Head:
Prof. Dr. Walter Lorenz

Operating Manager:
Dr. Gerd Wolber

Central Data Processing

Almost all divisions of the Deutsches Krebsforschungszentrum use programs and the computing capacity of central computers which are accessible directly via terminals, personal computers or work stations. The spectrum of applications comprises the following focal points:

- Recording of laboratory data, e.g., by digitalization and storage in a form appropriate for data processing.
- Running of data banks, e.g., for DNA sequences, for spectra, experimental animals, and literature.
- Statistical analysis, e.g., of laboratory and animals trials.
- Image processing, e.g., for cell and organ sections.
- Simulations and calculations, e.g., for models of cell division and interactions between molecules.
- Presentation of the results by text processing, graphs, and diagrams.

The Department of Central Data Processing (ZDV) supports users in their data-processing applications by the adaptation of instrument interfaces for recording of laboratory data with microcomputers, by transport of data to the appropriate evaluation computer or terminal via a local area network (LAN), by the operation of centrally available computers, and by provision of programs for user groups. Additionally, the tasks include training and counselling in the use of data processing, programming, and result presentation. Users who wish to employ personal computers in order to carry out individual data-processing independently are supported by the ZDV in the selection, configuration, and operation of their computer.

The central data-processing is carried out with IBM 3090 and 4341 and two Convex 210 computers with the operating systems VM/CMS and Unix, in two operator shifts. 30 decentralized computers and about 230 terminals and personal computers in the Deutsches Krebsforschungszentrum are connected via a local computer network.

External, directly connected users are institutes and clinics of the University of Heidelberg via the data networks of the Federal Post Office (Datex-L, Datex-P). Access to the computers of the Deutsches Krebsforschungszentrum is also available to other authorized users.

In addition, by the connection of a computer to the EARN computer network and to the science networks WIN, BeLWü and Internet a worldwide exchange of data and information is possible for all users, especially with other research facilities and universities. There are high-speed computer connections to the University Computer Center and to the Center of Molecular Biology in Heidelberg.

The program languages available on the computers of the ZDV are Cobol, Pascal, C, APL, PL/1, and Fortran. The following generally recognized software packages are implemented: for statistics: SAS; for data banks: SQL; for graphics: Tellagraph, SAS/Graph; for word processing: Script, TEX. The own developments of the Deutsches Krebsforschungszentrum are frequently applied, e.g. for DNA sequence analysis: Husar.

The Central Data Processing gives support to all scientific research activities and service facilities in the Deutsches Krebsforschungszentrum in the use of the computer as a tool of modern research and is therefore organized as a central facility.

Head:
Dr. Kurt Böhm

Safety

The Safety Division is directly assigned to the Scientific Board of the Deutsches Krebsforschungszentrum. It advises the heads of divisions and all staff on matters related to safety provisions and waste disposal. In addition, it is in charge of environmental protection. The division has three safety engineers as well as a laboratory and clerical staff.

The diversity and quantity of the scientific research carried out at the Center and the infrastructure involved require adherence to a wide range of laws, regulations, guidelines, and standards. The spectrum covers, for example, the Waste Disposal Law, the Genetic Engineering Law, and instructions on how to deal with cytostatic agents.

Cancer research is not conceivable without the use of dangerous substances, especially carcinogenic and mutating agents. However, repercussions for the environment are prevented by advising the researchers and by establishing the necessary safety measures. The same applies for genetic engineering. Advisory work, the inspection of safety facilities and disinfection procedures, and the compilation of internal operating instructions are of utmost importance for optimization of biological safety.

Regular inspections, reports of defeciencies, the identification of possible sources of danger, the monitoring of workplaces for possible contamination, as well as the training for and the testing of safety precautions also play a key role in the work of the safety division.

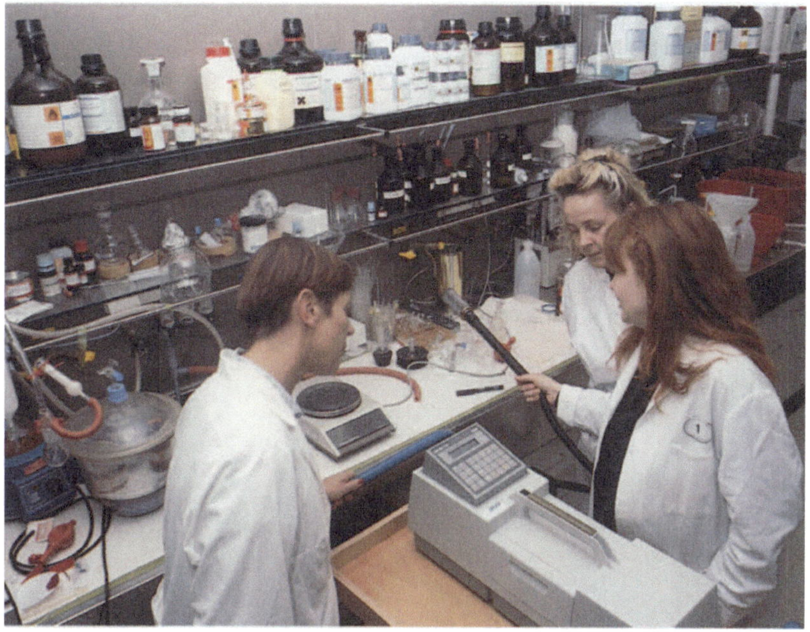

Fig. 140
Technicians of the Safety Division conducting routine measurements in a laboratory.

The Safety Division's laboratory is equipped with modern, mobile instruments for monitoring the air. Close cooperation has been established with the Center's Divisions of Environmental Carcinogens and Central Spectroscopy, as well as with the section responsible for waste disposal. The main areas of collaboration are in chemical conversions, in the determining of important factors, and in the classification and declaration of problem waste. The safety engineer, who also serves as the waste disposal officer, is responsible for advising staff and carrying out inspections.

Of course, in all matters relating to safety at work, the Safety Division closely cooperates with the medical officer and the staff council. The comparatively low number of incidents recorded at the Deutsches Krebsforschungszentrum has only been achieved as a result of this joint effort.

The committee for safety at work consists of the safety officers, who are usually scientifically trained, and of specialists for technical matters and radiation protection. It regularly discusses safety problems and recommends new measures. The chairperson is the head safety engineer.

10

Great importance is attached to the work of external boards and committees, such as the Mutual Industrial Accident Insurances (Berufsgenossenschaften), the Association of German Safety Engineers (VDSI), or the Association of Major Science Research Institutions (AGF).

Head:
Edgar Heuss (safety engineer)

Deputies: Annekathrin Kollenda (safety engineer)
Matthias Beyer (safety technician)

Appendix

Evaluation of Results

In 1989, the third round of the evaluation of the institutes and project groups of the Deutsches Krebsforschungszentrum began. Since 1983, internal presentations of the scientific work and external evaluations of the divisions have alternated in regular intervals. The internal presentations of the activities are supervised by the Scientific Council, the coordinators of the Research Programs, and the Management Board. Each division's scientists give a lecture on their work and their results and present plans and prospects for future activities.

The final assessment of the research work takes place after discussion with the heads of the divisions and projects. Each division has to present its work every 2 or 3 years. Consequences of the evaluations may be new scientific priorities, a redistribution of resources, the exchange of personnel, an increase or reduction in office or laboratory space and investments.

These internal evaluations supplement the external assessments which take place every 5 years. These external assessments are supervised by the Scientific Committee of the Board of Trustees. The results are discussed by the Scientific Council and implemented in agreement with the Board of Trustees and the Management Board. In 1989, external committees evaluated the scientific work of the Institute of Experimental Pathology and of the Institute of Cell and Tumor Biology. The work of the Institute of Virus Research, of the Project Group Applied Tumor Virology, which is the nucleus of a Research Program having the same name, and of the Institute of Biochemistry was evaluated in 1990. In 1991, the Institute of Immunology and Genetics, the Division of Applied Immunology, the Project Group Tolerance and Immune Response, the Division of Cell Biology, and the Project Group Cytogenetics were subject to external evaluation.

The appointment of two new Division heads extended and partially re-oriented the Center's research program. In the Institute of Biochemistry, the Division of Developmental Genetics was established by appointing Prof. Dr. Bernhard Mechler as its head. The research work done in the Division of Molecular Biology of the Cell II in the Institute of Cell and Tumor Biology was re-oriented by appointing Prof. Dr. Ingrid Grummt as its head. In addition, the Project Group Molecular Biophysics, headed by lecturer Dr. Sándor Suhai, was established as a new division.

Three new project groups were established: "Molecular Biology of Aging", headed by Dr. Heinz D. Osiewacz, "Tumor Promotion in the Liver", headed by Priv.-Doz. Dr. Michael Schwarz, and "Biochemical Cell Physiology", headed by Priv.-Doz. Dr. Walter Pyerin. These projects are to last for a period of 5 years. Meanwhile, Dr. Osiewacz was appointed head of a division.

The large number of projects financially supported by national and international organizations for the promotion of scientific research indicates the multitude and breadth of the Center's research activities. In 1989, a total of 204 research projects were financially supported by external organizations. This figure rose to 241 in 1990.

The publication of the results of the scientific work in national and international scientific journals is another factor in the evaluation of the Center's performance.

New divisions and project groups

Three divisions and the same number of project groups were established in the Deutsches Krebsforschungszentrum in 1989 and 1990.

In 1989, the delicate fruit fly (Drosophila melanogaster) was brought into the Division of Developmental Genetics, headed by Prof. Dr. Bernard Mechler. The tiny insect serves as a model organism for investigating the role of tumor suppressor genes in the genesis of tumors. These genes normally help to control the division and differentiation of cells. However, if they are lost or changed, the cell loses a decisive control mechanism. It degenerates and a tumor develops. Meanwhile, it was possible to isolate such a gene in Drosophila. Presently, the division's scientists are trying to find out the exact role and functioning of this gene. On the basis of their experience with Drosophila, they investigate whether such tumor suppressor genes also exist in humans.

In 1990, Prof. Dr. Ingrid Grummt took over as head of the Division of Molecular Biology of the Cell II. Her research work aims at understanding the molecular mechanisms that link the cells' growth and the activity of the genes involved. Cancer cells are characterized, for example, by the fact that they proliferate uncontrolled and that they do not differentiate. The higher the growth rate of a cell symplasm, the more proteins that are synthesized, and the higher the need in ribosomes which transcribe the genetic information into proteins.

The investigations focus on the following "switches": How does the activity of genes in mammalian cells depend on the rate of cell proliferation, and how are the involved genes turned on and off? So far, the scientists have succeeded in understanding the regulatory mechanism that allows the cells to react to a multitude of growth stimulating and inhibiting substances which determine the state of the cell from outside.

The Project Group Molecular Biophysics, headed by Priv.-Doz. Dr. Sándor Suhai, was upgraded to a division in mid-1990. The scientists examine the structural properties of

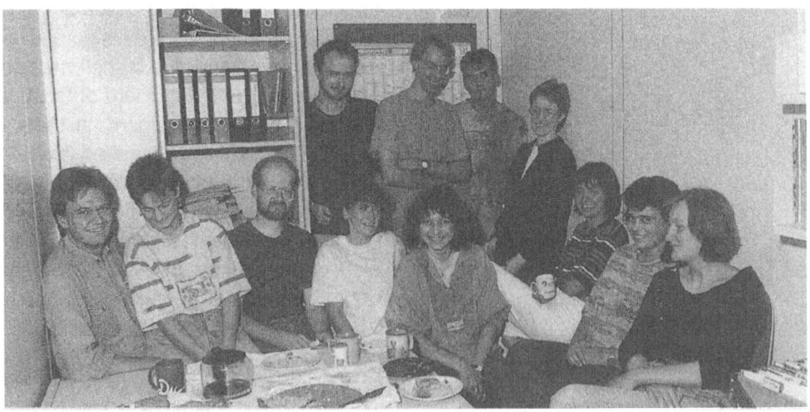

Fig. 141
Collaborators of the Division of Molecular Biology of the Cell II with their department head Prof. Dr. Ingrid Grummt (third to right).

nucleic acids and proteins, which are the functional units of all cells. They employ advanced methods of mathematics, physics, and computer science. As an aid to molecular-biological cancer research, biophysicists are developing powerful computer programs. These help to analyze the connection between molecular structure and biological function. In addition, such programs facilitate the communication with international gene and molecular-biological data bases.

By installing new project groups, the Deutsches Krebsforschungszentrum promotes young scientists who contribute to cancer research with particularly promising and innovative concepts. For the same purpose, the new Statutes and Articles of the Deutsches Krebsforschungszentrum, in effect since August 1991, make it possible to install divisions for a limited time of 6 years.

Since 1989, the Deutsches Krebsforschungszentrum has installed three new project groups: "Molecular Biology of Aging," "Tumor Promotion in the Liver," and "Biochemical Cell Physiology," raising the total number of project groups to 10.

Why does the incidence of cancer increase with age? The Division of Molecular Biology of Aging, headed by Dr. Heinz D. Osiewacz since 1990, uses the ascomycete Podospora anserina as a model system for the investigation of aging processes. Using these relatively simple organisms, the researchers investigate the basic processes that cause the cell to age and, eventually, to die. They observe the effects of artificially produced genetic defects on aging processes, and plan to eventually validate their results on human connective tissue cells in vitro.

Since 1990, the Project Group Tumor Promotion in the Liver has been headed by Priv.-Doz. Dr. Michael Schwarz. The group investigates a particular class of substances that stimulate the growth of a tumor cell without causing cancer themselves. As a con-

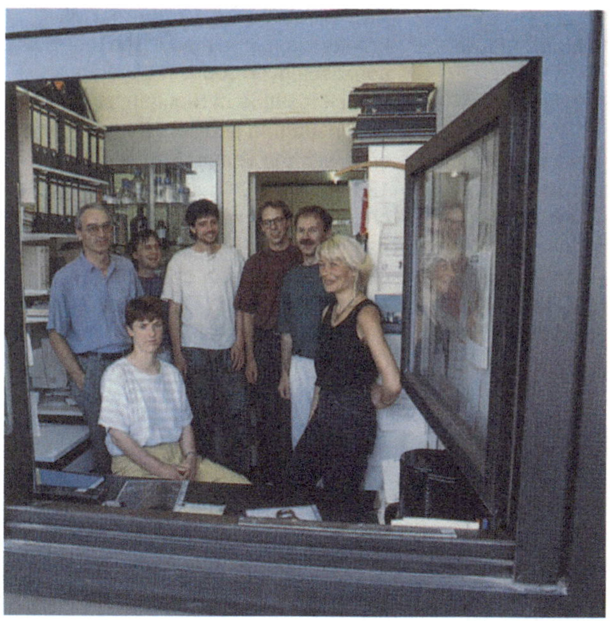

Fig. 142
Project Group Tumor Promotion in the Liver with the head of the group, Priv.-Doz. Dr. Michael Schwarz (left).

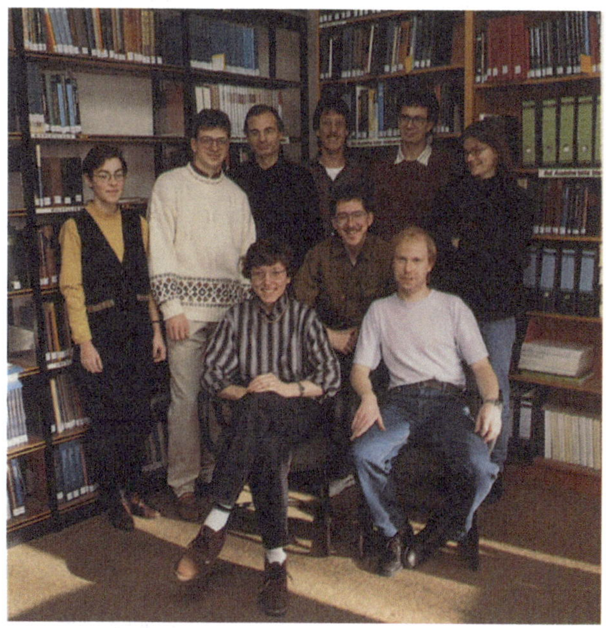

Fig. 143
Project Group Biochemical Cell Physiology with the group's head, Priv.-Doz. Dr. Walter Pyerin (third to left).

tribution to cancer prevention, it is one of the project group's goals to determine the activity of tumor stimulating substances in concentrations that are low but nonetheless relevant for the human organism. Also, the project group is investigating these substances' mechanisms of action.

The Project Group Biochemical Cell Physiology, headed by Priv.-Doz. Dr. Walter Pyerin, was established in mid-1990. The scientists' work focuses on a complex enzyme system, whose center is cytochrome P450. It is the keystone of the metabolism of the cell and controls the transformation of substances that may influence the genesis and growth of tumors. The key enzymes are in turn regulated by so-called protein kinases, which influence the regulation of cell growth in multiple ways. These protein kinases are the second subject of investigations of the new project group's research.

Awards and appointments

Again in 1989 and 1990, scientists of the Deutsches Krebsforschungszentrum were granted numerous awards and honors.
Heinz Maier Leibnitz Award 1988 (Dr. Bernd Arnold)
Varian Award 1988 of the Germen Society of Medical Physics (Dr. Karl-Heinz Höver, Bernd Michael Hesse, and Prof. Dr. Walter Lorenz)
Walter J. Johnson Award 1988 (Dr. Georg Krohne)
von Recklinghausen Award 1989 of the German Society of Endocrinology (Dr. Thomas Klenner and Dr. Franz Wingen)
Paul Martini Award 1989 (Prof. Dr. Stefan C. Meuer)
Award of the Eureopean Society for Medical Oncology (Dr. Lothar Schweigerer)
Gerhard Domagk Award 1989 (Prof. Dr. W. Jens Zeller, Guan Chen, Dr. Eva Frei, and Priv.-Doz. Dr. Manfred Kaufmann)
Ludolf Krehl Award 1989 (Dr. Bruno Bethsch)
Farmitalia Carlo Erba Award 1989 and Dr. Joszef Obrath Award 1989 (Prof. Dr. Manfred Volm, Dr. Michael Bak, and Dr. Jürgen Mattern)
Walther and Christine Richtzenhain Award 1989 (Dr. Uwe Stähle)
Gottfried Wilhelm Leibnitz Award of the German Research Society 1989 (Prof. Dr. Ingrid Grummt)
Claudius Galenus Award 1990 for "Drug Research at a University" (Prof. Dr. W. Jens Zeller)
San Marino Award of Medicine 1990 (Prof. Dr. Stefan C. Meuer)
Otto Westphal Award 1989/90 (Dr. Ulrich Pessara)
Walther and Christine Richtzenhain Award 1990 (Dr. Thomas Bortfeld, Dr. Wolfgang Pfau, and Dr. Falk Weih)
Falcon Award 1991 (Dr. Petra Boukamp and Dr. Rudolf Leube)
Award for Natural Sciences of the Fritz Winter Foundation (Prof. Dr. Ingrid Grummt)
Kind Philipp Award 1991 for Oncological Research in Pediatrics (Prof. Dr. Peter Krammer)
Karl Freudenberg Award 1991 (Dr. Peter Lichter)
INSTAD Award of the Institute for Standardization and Documentation and Ernst Krokowski Award 1991 (Priv.-Doz. Dr. Dr. Ulrich Abel, scientist at the Tumor Center Heidelberg/Mannheim).
Prof. Dr. Rolf Flügel was awarded a fellowship by the Foundation for the Promotion of Cancer Research, Tokyo.
In 1989, Prof. Dr. Walter Lorenz was granted the honorary badge Alma Mater Lipsiensis of the University of Leipzig.
Also in 1989, Prof. Dr. Werner W. Franke was appointed to the international scientific council of the Max Planck Institute of Biochemistry in Martinsried. In addition, he was honored with the Robert Feulgen Lecture 1989 by the Austrian Society for Histochemistry and with the Tinsley R. Harrison Lecture 1989/90 by the University of Alabama School of Medicine.
Also in 1989, Prof. Dr. Gerhard van Kaick was elected First Chairman of the German Society of Ultrasound in Medicine.
In the same year, Prof. Dr. Günter Hämmerling was elected Secretary General of the European Network of Immunology Institutes.
Also in 1989, Prof. Dr. Erich Hecker was elected member of the German Academy of Natural Scientists Leopoldina.

In the same year, Priv.-Doz. D. Sc. Ethel-Michele de Villiers was appointed honorary member of the Polish Dermatological Society.
Also in 1989, Prof. Dr. Jürgen Wahrendorf was appointed to the Scientific Advisory Council of the Research Center for Environment and Health of the Society for Radiation Research (GSF).
In the same year, Prof. Dr. Dietrich Schmähl (†) was again appointed to the scientific advisory council of the project "European Research Center for Measures of Air Pollution Abatement".
Beginning in July of 1989, Prof. Dr. Harald zur Hausen began his 2-year term as the Chairman of the Society of Major Research Institutions (AGF). In addition, he was admitted as a honorary member of the Polish Dermatological Society. In 1990, he was admitted as a member of the Academia Europea and as an honorary member to the Japanese Cancer Society. In 1991, Prof. zur Hausen was elected external member of the Polish Academy of Sciences.
In 1990, Priv.-Doz. Dr. Bernd Kimmig was honored with the Hermann Holthusen Ring of the German Roentgen Society.
In the same year, Prof. Dr. Erich Hekker was appointed to the Golden Anniversary Committee of the McArdle Laboratory for Cancer Research in Madison, Wisconsin, USA.
Also in 1990, Prof. Dr. Klaus Munk was appointed honorary member of the Japanese Cancer Society.
In the same year, Prof. Dr. Stefan C. Meuer was appointed to the founding committee of the "Center of Molecular Medicine" in Berlin-Buch and to the advisory council "Oncology" of the German Land Baden-Württemberg.

Awards granted by the Deutsches Krebsforschungszentrum

Three awards for extraordinary achievements in cancer research and the early detection of cancer are granted in cooperation with the Deutsches Krebsforschungszentrum.

For more than 10 years the Wilhelm and Maria Meyenburg Foundation has granted awards for extraordinary accomplishments in cancer research. The award includes a donation of 30000 Deutsche Marks. The Management Board of the foundation also supports research projects of scientists of the Deutsches Krebsforschungszentrum and their cooperation partners.

In 1989, the Meyenburg Award was bestowed on to Prof. Dr. Peter Herrlich, Director of the Institute of Genetics and Toxicology of the Nuclear Research Center in Karlsruhe, Germany, and of the Institute of Genetics of the University of Karlsruhe. In particular, the award was granted for the molecular-biological research that has led to a better understanding of the effect of cancer-stimulating environmental factors on the cells of the body.

In 1990, the Meyenburg Award was presented to Prof. Dr. Rainer Storb, head of the program "Transplantation Biology" of the Fred Hutchinson Cancer Research Center in Seattle, Washington, USA. The award was granted for his pioneering research that has contributed to establishing bone marrow grafts as a therapy for acute leukaemia and serious anemia.

The Meyenburg Award in 1991 was given for the research done by Dr. Hans-Georg Rammensee, head of the working group Immunobiology of the Max Planck Institute for Biology in Tübingen. His work has led to a better understanding of how killer cells recognize exogenous and altered endogenous proteins.

Fig. 144
Prof. Dr. Harald zur Hausen with the winners of the 1990 Walter and Christine Richtzenhain Award: Dr. Thomas Bortfeld (left), Dr. Wolfgang Pfau (second to left), and Dr. Falk Weih (second to right).

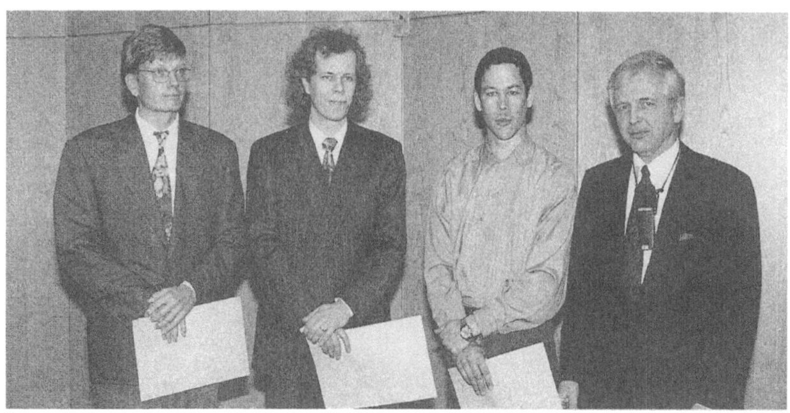

The Walther and Christine Richtzenhain Award is given by the Deutsches Krebsforschungszentrum on an alternating annual basis to doctoral students from Heidelberg or to German scientists for research in the field of experimental cancer research. It includes a grant of up to 15000 Deutsche Marks from the estate of Walther and Christine Richtzenhain.

In 1989, Dr. Uwe Stähle received the award for his dissertation on the structural and functional characterization of elements of the genetic material that plays a role in the effect of a specific group of hormones.

The following year, the Walther and Christine Richtzenhain Award was awarded equally to three persons: Dr. Thomas Bortfeld, who worked on new planning methods for cancer radiotherapy, Dr. Wolfgang Pfau, who investigated the mode of action of certain carcinogenic plant components, and Dr. Falk Weih, who used a model system to examine a common mechanism of gene regulation.

As a stimulus and as an award for outstanding activities in the field of early detection of cancer, the Deutsches Krebsforschungszentrum granted the Ernst von Leyden Award for the first time in 1990. The award, which was donated by the Röhm Pharma GmbH, includes an award of 20000 Deutsche Marks. The prize is supervised by the Department of Press and Public Relations of the Deutsches Krebsforschungszentrum.

The award was presented to both Prof. Dr. Eckhard W. Breitbart, deputy director of the University Dermatological Clinics Hamburg-Eppendorf, and to Dr. Jochen Aumiller, editor-in-chief of the Münchener Medizinische Wochenschrift. Prof. Dr. Breitbart, a dermatologist, founded the "Commission for the Early Detection of Skin Cancer" of the German Dermatological Society and, in 1989, initiated a successful nationwide campaign for the early detection of skin cancer. During more than a decade, Dr. Aumiller, who is a journalist, has devoted his extensive journalistic work to the early detection of cancer, which he di-

Fig. 146
Prof. Dr. Eckhard W. Breitbart (center) of the University Dermatological Clinics Hamburg-Eppendorf and science journalist Dr. Jochen Aumiller (right), editor-in-chief of the Münchner Medizinische Wochenschrift, receive the 1990 Ernst von Leyden Award from Prof. Dr. Harald zur Hausen (left).

Fig. 145
Presentation of the 1990 Meyenburg Award to Prof. Dr. Rainer Storb, Seattle (second to left), by the managing board of the Meyenburg Foundation, Dr. Marion Meyenburg (second to right), Prof. Dr. Klaus Munk (right), and Dr. Wolfgang Henkel (left).

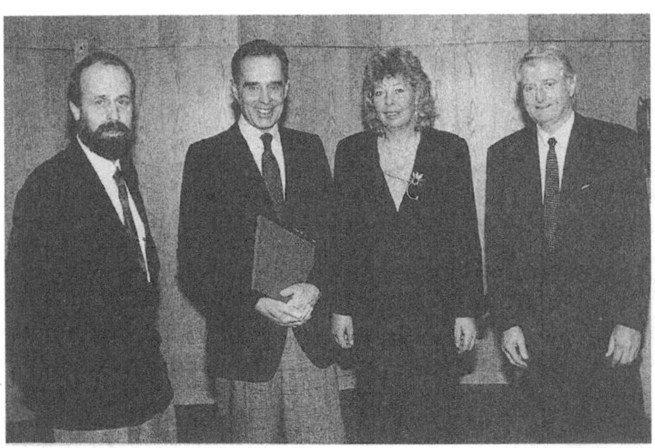

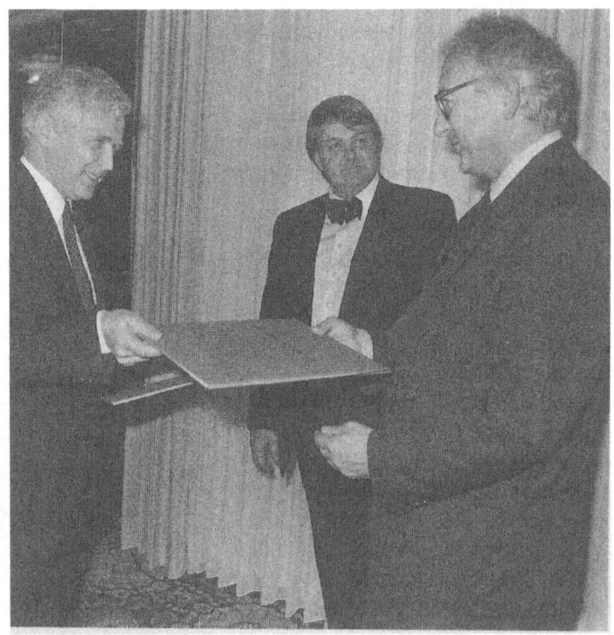

rected both to the general public and to practicing physicians.

Under difficult circumstances and with the greatest personal effort the two pathologists have achieved that the number of women undergoing cytological screening in Mecklenburg-Vorpommern has raised up from 1,5% in 1965 to 53% in 1989.

For many years, the physician Ernst von Leyden (1832–1910) was chairman of the German Central Committee for Cancer Research and director of the 1st Clinic for Internal Medicine at the Charité in Berlin. He is known as a pioneer in cancer research in Germany.

Publications

The results of the scientific work of the Deutsches Krebsforschungszentrum are published on a regular basis in the listing "Veröffentlichungen aus dem Deutschen Krebsforschungszentrum". By the end of 1989, the year of its 25th anniversary, the Center's scientists had published a total of 8897 scientific articles. Out of these, 5514 were published in scientific journals, 741 were diploma theses, dissertations and habilitations, and 347 were books and articles in handbooks that appeared in 1988 and 1989.

These publications are supplemented by thousands of lectures held at scientific congresses and for the interested general public.

The listing is published every year and can be ordered by any interested party.

It is the task of the Center's Department of Press and Public Relations to make the results of the research known to the general public and to explain its significance in the prevention, the early detection, and the therapy of cancer. The Department maintains permanent contacts with all media and with interested citizens (see the article on Press and Public Relations).

12

International and National Collaboration

The integration of the research activities of the Deutsches Krebsforschungszentrum into international research concepts is documented by the high percentage (approx. 50%) of joint publications with scientists from other research institutes in Germany and abroad. The research program of the Deutsches Krebsforschungszentrum comprises cooperation with researchers from a total of 29 countries. On the national level there is cooperation with more than 30 universities and 70 other research institutes. The cooperation with the University of Heidelberg is centered around the joint clinical-experimental projects within the Heidelberg/Mannheim Tumor Center. By 1992, this cooperation could look back on 12 years of history. Of special interest in the field of fundamental research is the collaboration within the special research programs of the Deutsche Forschungsgemeinschaft, namely, the special research program Nr. 229 "Molecular mechanisms of gene expression and differentiation" and Nr. 123 "Stochastic mathematical models".

In 1990/91 the management of the Deutsches Krebsforschungszentrum committed itself to supporting and securing the research potential of the scientific centers at Berlin-Buch, East Berlin. The Deutsches Krebsforschungszentrum participated in the international expert assessment of the Zentralinstitut für Krebsforschung (Central Cancer Research Institute) at Berlin-Buch and supported the evaluation of the biomedical research institutes of the former GDR by delegating a staff member to the Scientific Council. There is an intensive contact and scientific exchange between researchers from East Berlin and their colleagues from the Deutsches Krebsforschungszentrum. The establishment of another scientific center which focuses on cancer research and is coupled with a research clinic is considered by the Deutsches Krebsforschungszentrum as a promising chance to intensify clinical cancer research in Germany.

Collaboration on the basis of bilateral agreements with other countries has been continued and intensified. The cooperation with the United States is based on the "Memorandum of Understanding" with the American National Cancer Institute (NCI) in Bethesda, Maryland. The agreement concluded with the National Council of Research and Development (NCRD) in Israel has secured twelve years of highly successful scientific cooperation with scientists in various Israeli research institutions, including the Ben Gurion University, Tel Aviv University, the Hebrew University of Jerusalem, the Weizmann Institute of Science, the Technicon in Haifa and the Hadassah University Medical Hospital in Jerusalem. Close contacts have also been established in the field of administration, in particular with the Weizmann Institute, which has lead to the dispatch of delegations from Israel and from Germany, as well as to an intensive exchange of administrative solutions.

For the 15th time the "Directory of On-Going Research in Cancer Epidemiology" has been published in collaboration with the International Agency for Research on Cancer (IARC) in Lyon, France. This guide presents information on all current research projects in the field of cancer epidemiology all over the world. The printed version is supplemented by a diskette so that all data are also available on computer.

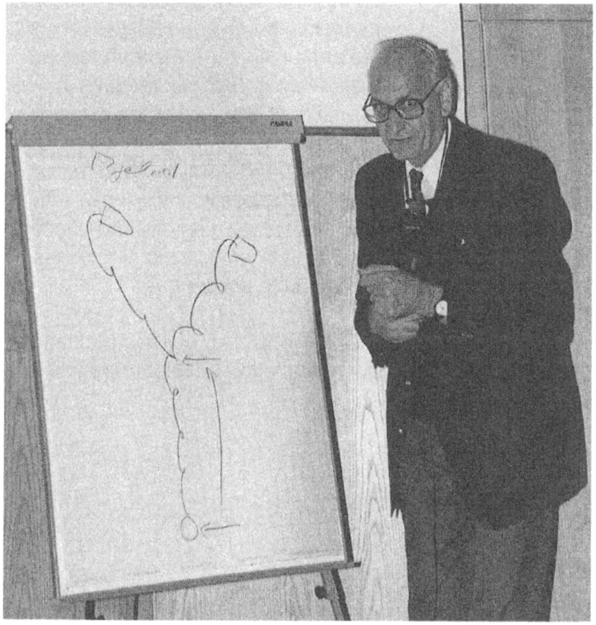

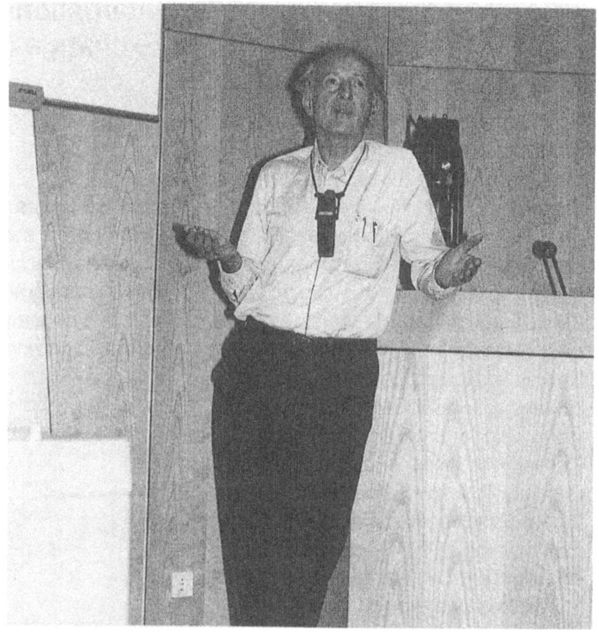

Figs. 147, 148
On the 25th anniversary of the Deutsches Krebsforschungszentrum in October 1989, a symposium on new concepts in oncology was held. The photos show Prof. Dr. Leo Sachs (Fig. 147) of the Weizmann Institute, Rehovot, Israel, and Prof. Dr. George Klein (Fig. 148) of the Karolinska Institute, Stockholm, Sweden, delivering their lectures.

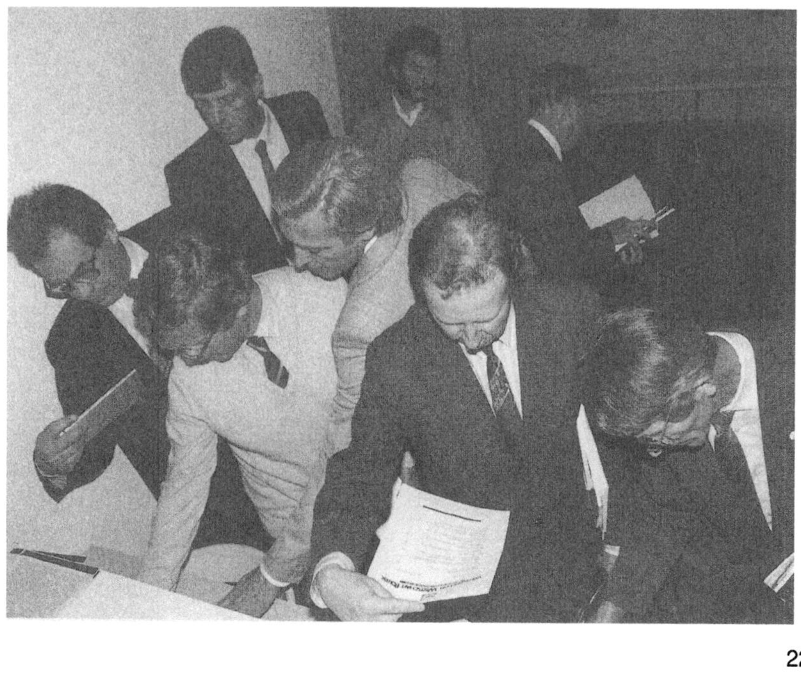

Fig. 149
After the opening of the Iron Curtain, the Deutsches Krebsforschungszentrum invited Czechoslovakian scientists for an exchange of information, especially on research structures and means for the advancement of research. The exchange, which is continued on a regular basis, helps to reconstruct the research system of the former CSFR.

The collaboration with the Academy of Medical Sciences of the former USSR has been continued on the basis of guest scientist stays. The research program agreed upon with the Tanzania Tumour Centre in Dar es Salam comprises projects in molecular biology, epidemiology, and clinical research. On the organizational, technical, and humanitarian levels this cooperation is being supported by the society "Tanzania Tumor Support" whose members are scientists from the Deutsches Krebsforschungszentrum and other citizens of Heidelberg. The society provides help for the Tanzania Tumour Centre in the form of regular donations of scientific and medical instruments, by providing technical equipment and staff training at the Deutsches Krebsforschungszentrum, as well as by collecting clothes and money.

Direct contacts between scientists from different nations continue to be a characteristic feature of the research work. Official agreements are particularly supportive when there is a question of the use of special funds.

International Scientific Exchange

Science needs the exchange of ideas and it profits substantially from the discussion with guest scientists. This is true particularly for cancer research which is concerned with nearly all fields of medicine and most fields of natural science.

On the one hand, the research stays for a limited time give the guests an insight into certain lines of research and enables them to learn techniques in which scientists of the Deutsches Krebsforschungszentrum are preeminent. On the other hand, they serve to recruit scientists with specific know-how, with which they can rationally complement the scientific work at the Deutsches Krebsforschungszentrum.

A further objective of international collaboration is the development and im-

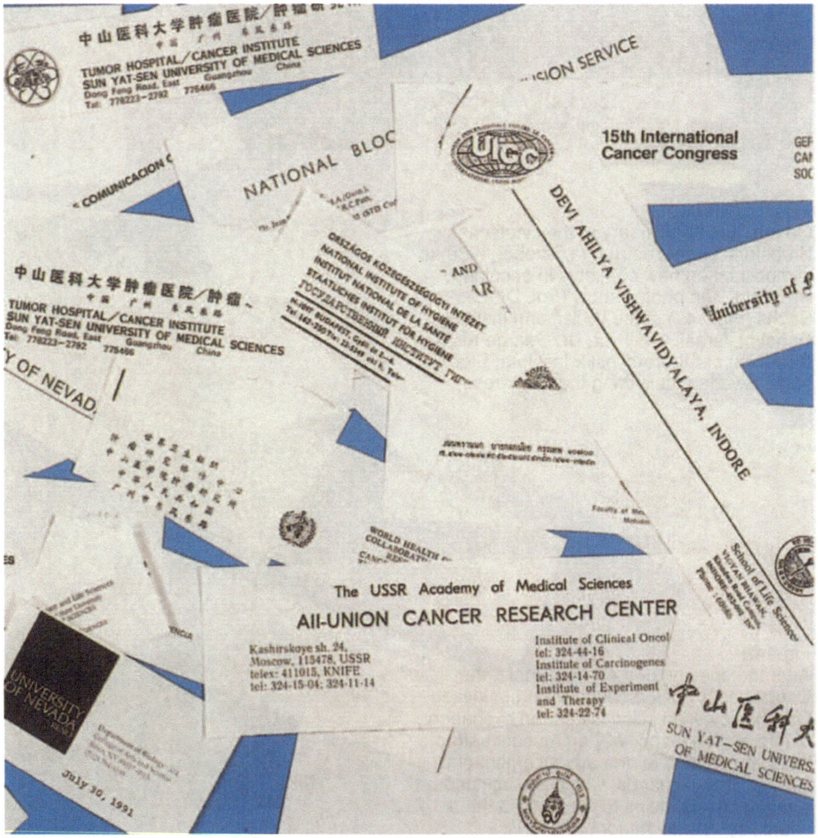

Fig. 150
Scientists from all over the world exchange information.

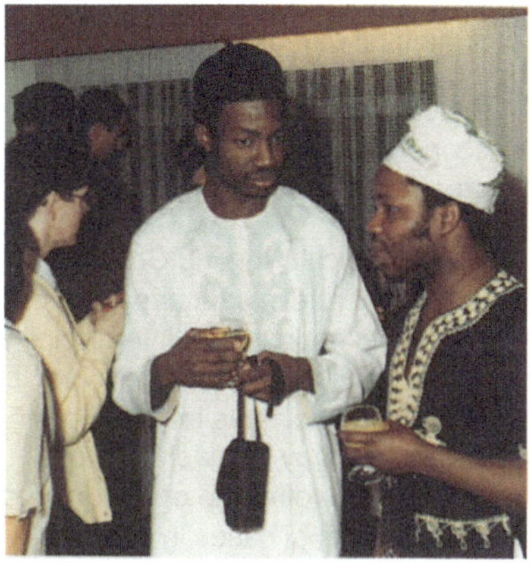

Fig. 151
Spring reception for guest scientists in one of the guest houses of the Deutsches Krebsforschungszentrum.

Fig. 152
In the framework of joint projects, or to study new methods that are of interest for cancer research in Germany, scientists of the Deutsches Krebsforschungszentrum are offered the possibility to work in foreign research institutions. In 1991, Dr. Hartmut Richter was given a one-year sabbatical to work at the Laboratory of Molecular Carcinogenesis of the National Institute of Environmental Health Services in North Carolina, USA.

plementation of joint projects and programs in the field of cancer research.

The figures of recent years impressively show the intensity of international and national collaboration in the Deutsches Krebsforschungszentrum:

In 1988, 1989, and 1990, a total of 544 guest scientists from 38 countries worked at the Deutsches Krebsforschungszentrum.

In addition to internal grants and scholarship programs the guest scientists were supported by the following organizations:

German Academic Exchange Service (DAAD)

Humboldt Foundation

German Research Association (DFG)

Study Foundation of the German Nation

Meyenburg Foundation

European Molecular Biology Organization

NATO

Council of Europe

Catholic Academic Exchange Service

Konrad Adenauer Foundation.

Furthermore, there is an active international and national collaboration.

In the guest houses of the Center in Heidelberg, 41 completely fitted residential units (one-room to three-room apartments) are available for the guest scientists.

In view of the intensive international research contacts the guest houses are still completely used to capacity. Thus, they still cover their costs.

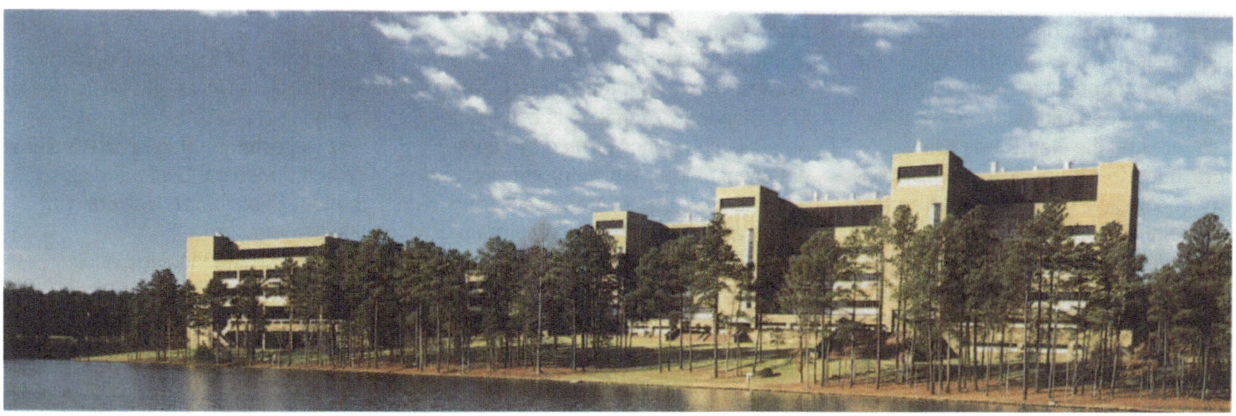

Tumor Center Heidelberg/Mannheim

Twenty-five years ago, the Oncological Working Group Heidelberg and, 7 years later, the Oncological Working Group Mannheim were founded. The fight against cancer in Heidelberg had started much earlier, however: the First International Cancer Congress was held in Heidelberg; in 1906, the first interdisciplinary cancer research institute in Europe was established in Heidelberg, and – following this tradition – in 1964 the Deutsches Krebsforschungszentrum was founded by K. H. Bauer, at that time the director of the Surgical University Clinic in Heidelberg.

On January 1, 1979, the Tumor Center Heidelberg/Mannheim was established. As designated, it links the University Clinics in Heidelberg and Mannheim and Thorax Clinic in Heidelberg-Rohrbach (which is supported by the Social Insurance Institution of Baden) to the Deutsches Krebsforschungszentrum. It is the goal of this collaboration to practically assure the best possible care for cancer patients in the area and to develop new impetuses for diagnosis and therapy of malignant diseases by cooperative research programs between clinics, theoretical institutes, and the Deutsches Krebsforschungszentrum. This interdisciplinary oncological unit has gained a clear profile and has proven its value; it is now a fast track between research on, and the fight against cancer. Its goal is the rapid translation of the latest research results into clinical practice. Results of basic research can be applied directly to patient care, and the experiences gained in patient care point the way to further research in the field of oncology.

The Tumor Center Heidelberg/Mannheim, as the organizational framework for this close collaboration between research and clinical practice, also has a broad variety of administrative and coordinating duties, such as organizing collaboration in basic research, organizing advanced and vocational training programs, and editing "guidelines for a standardized diagnosis, therapy, and follow up care." The goal is to help improve patient care by passing on verified research results and intensifying the exchange of experiences, not only in the Tumor Center's institutions, but in the whole region. This is supported by a close collaboration with other tumor centers and oncological research programs.

The wide range of the Tumor Center's institutions necessitates an effective coordinating, interdisciplinary body. This is the Tumor Center's Steering Committee, consisting of 14 members who are the representatives of the contracting parties, the local practitioners, and the chairmen of the Oncological Working Groups Heidelberg and Mannheim. The Steering Committee defines the foci of research, and coordinates the work of the Tumor Center. The Steering Committee is assisted by an advisory council formed by representatives of the medical profession and the sciences, and of individuals from industry and public life. The chairman of the Steering Committee is Prof. Dr. Christian Herfarth, who also heads the coordinating and the administrative office; this allows the smooth coordination of activities between the various partners.

The work of the Tumor Center concentrates on the following topics:

- the care of cancer patients,
- cooperative cancer research, and
- organizational-editorial work.

The Oncological Working Groups play an important role in cancer patient care. They help to improve the interdisciplinary collaboration in clinical oncology by establishing guidelines for the diagnosis and therapy for each kind of tumor. They also offer the opportunity to discuss individual cases in an interdisciplinary colloquium, which meets on a weekly basis. This forum develops plans for the diagnosis and therapy of individual patients and presents them as written recommendations following consideration of the latest scientifically proven methods. This forum also answers inquiries from private practicioners of the region and from all over Germany.

The clinical institutions participating in the Tumor Center have established specialized oncological units which make it possible to both give the patients qualified care, and to work scientifically. These oncological units are

- the section of Surgical Oncology of the Surgical University Clinic Heidelberg,
- the Department of Internal Medicine V of the Medical Clinic and Outpatient Clinic of the University of Heidelberg,
- the section of Oncology and Hematology of the Pediatric University Clinic Heidelberg,
- the section of Orthopedic Oncology of the Foundation Orthopedic University Clinic Heidelberg,

- the Oncological Center at the Clinics of Mannheim of the section Specialized Oncology of the III. Medical Clinic, and
- the Oncological Department of the Thorax Clinic Heidelberg- Rohrbach of the Social Insurance Institution of Baden.

In addition, all clinics of the University treat tumor patients. The psychosocial follow-up plays an essential role in the rehabilitation of tumor patients. In 1979, a psychosocial rehabilitation institution was established within the Tumor Center as an integrated oncological department. This institution offers advanced teaching programs for physicians, psychologists, nursing staff, social workers, and all professionals who work in the treatment, care, and follow-up care of tumor patients (head: Priv.-Doz. Dr. Reinhold Schwarz).

The goal of advanced oncological training in medical care is to improve tumor patient care under special nursing and psychosocial aspects. Since 1988, advanced clinical professional courses for nursing in oncology have been organized at the Tumor Center Heidelberg/Mannheim. These courses consist of theoretical classes, hospital visits, and practical education.

One of the Tumor Center's main tasks is organizing the collaboration between the Deutsches Krebsforschungszentrum and the clinics. In the past, this cooperative cancer research has worked mostly on large-scale projects which were selected after invitation and evaluation by an international committee of experts.

These projects are mostly directed at specific organ tumors, but also encompass very broad research concepts in molecular biology, immunology, pathology, and morphology in connection with clinical therapy concepts using the latest imaging technologies. A large-scale project is composed of many individual sub-projects in clinical practice and basic research, which are each organized by coordinators. The Tumor Center supports the following large-scale projects:

A. Colon Carcinoma

(Coordinators: Prof. Dr. Peter Schlag, Surgical University Clinic Heidelberg, and Prof. Dr. Volker Schirrmacher, Institute of Immunology and Genetics of the Deutsches Krebsforschungszentrum)

Subprojects:

1. Cellular surface structures in the colorectal carcinoma relevant for prognosis.
(Project heads: Dr. Axel von Herbay, Dr. Karin Koretz, and Prof. Dr. Peter Möller, Pathological Institute of the University of Heidelberg)

2. Adhesion and glycosylation of colorectal tumor cells isolated from human biopsies.
(Project heads: Dr. Wolfgang Kemmner, Prof. Dr. Reinhard Brossmer, Institute of Biochemistry of the University of Heidelberg)

3. Investigation of the spontaneous expression of natural T- cell ligands in colon carcinoma and its inductability by IFN or/and TNF.
(Project heads: Prof. Dr. Peter Möller, Dr. Karin Koretz, Pathological Institute of the University of Heidelberg)

4. Application of a vaccine isolated from modified and autologous tumor cells: increasing the vaccine activity and establishing an immunological monitoring for therapy control.
(Project head: Prof. Dr. Peter Schlag, Surgical University Clinic Heidelberg)

5. Characterization of the cellular immune response of patients with colon carcinoma under adjuvant ASI treatment.
(head of the project: Prof. Dr. Volker Schirrmacher, Institute of Immunology and Genetics of the Deutsches Krebsforschungszentrum)

6. Study on immune therapy using human effector cells in nude SCID mice.
(Project head: Prof. Dr. Volker Schirrmacher, Institute of Immunology and Genetics of the Deutsches Krebsforschungszentrum)

7. Isolation, identification, and characterization of antigens isolated from patient serum after active specific immunization.
(Project head: Prof. Dr. Peter Michael Kloetzel, Institute of Molecular Genetics of the University of Heidelberg)

8. Development and application of intense-field NMR spectroscopy and NMR imaging for the characterization and therapy of tumors in patients and animal models.
(Project head: Dr. Dr. William Hull, Central Spectroscopy of the Deutsches Krebsforschungszentrum)

B. Bronchial carcinoma

(Coordinator: Prof. Dr. Peter Drings, Thorax Clinic Heidelberg-Rohrbach)

Subprojects:

1. Inhibition of the cytokine-dependent activity of immunocompetent cells by

growth factors of bronchial carcinoma cells with autocrine activity.
(Project heads: Dr. Jürgen Fischer, Thorax Clinic Heidelberg- Rohrbach, and Prof. Dr. Peter Krammer, Institute of Immunology and Genetics of the Deutsches Krebsforschungszentrum)

2. Molecular basis of tumor-induced or tumor-associated immune deficiency in patients with small-cell bronchial carcinoma.
(Project heads: Prof. Dr. Stephan Meuer, Institute of Radiology and Pathophysiology of the Deutsches Krebsforschungszentrum, and Priv.-Doz. Dr. Hans-Georg Mahnke, Thorax Clinic Heidelberg-Rohrbach)

C. Malignant lymphomas and leukemias

(Coordinator: Priv.-Doz. Dr. Bernd Dörken, Medical University Clinic and Outpatient Clinic Heidelberg)

Subprojects:

1. Differentiation antigens on neoplastic B-cells – monoclonal antibodies for diagnosis and therapy of B-cell neoplasias.
(Project head: Priv.-Doz. Dr. Bernd Dörken, Medical University Clinic and Outpatient Clinic Heidelberg)

2. Therapy of B-cell leukemias and malignant lymphomas with anti-idiotypic monoclonal antibodies and testing new therapeutic strategies on the SCID and HID mouse model.
(Project heads: Dr. Gerhard Moldenhauer, Dr. Peter van Endert, Prof. Dr. Günther Hämmerling, Institute of Immunology and Genetics of the Deutsches Krebsforschungszentrum, and Dr. Bernhard Heilig, Medical University Clinic and Outpatient Clinic Heidelberg)

3. Enzymes of the purine metabolism in malignant lymphatic cells – starting points for a specific therapy with enzyme inhibition.
(Project head: Dr. Daniela Männel, Institute of Immunology and Genetics of the Deutsches Krebsforschungszentrum)

4. Structural and functional characterization of surface expressed and secreted antigens of cells of lymphatic leukemias and malignant lymphomas of the B-cell type.
(Project head: Dr. Reinhard Schwartz-Albiez, Institute of Immunology and Genetics of the Deutsches Krebsforschungszentrum)

5. Lymphokine receptors on leukemia and lymphoma cells.
(Project heads: Dr. Klaus-Michael Debatin, Pediatric University Clinic Heidelberg, and Prof. Dr. Peter Krammer, Institute of Immunology and Genetics of the Deutsches Krebsforschungszentrum)

6. Function of differentiation antigens for regulating the proliferation of normal and neoplastic B-cells.
(Project head: Dr. Antonio Pezzutto, Medical University Clinic and Outpatient Clinic Heidelberg)

7. B-cell system and B-cell lymphomas associated with epithelium under special consideration of the primary mediastinal (thymic) B-cell lymphoma and of the primary gastrointestinal lymphoma.
(Project head: Prof. Dr. Peter Möller, Pathological Institute of the University Heidelberg)

8. Investigation of recombinant hematopoietic growth factors for application in patients under large-dose chemotherapy and autologous bone marrow and blood stem cell transplantation.
(Project head: Dr. Reiner Haas, Medical University Clinic and Outpatient Clinic Heidelberg)

9.1. Labelling of antibodies with heavy metal nuclides: new ligands.
(Project head: Dr. Jochen Schuhmacher, Institute of Radiology and Pathophysiology of the Deutsches Krebsforschungszentrum)

9.2. Tumor localization using bi-specific antibodies.
(Project heads: Dr. Siegfried Matzku, Dr. Margot Zöller, Institute of Radiology and Pathophysiology of the Deutsches Krebsforschungszentrum)

9.3. Radioimmunotherapy of malignant melanomas and B-cell lymphomas.
(Project heads: Dr. Heiner Bihl, Radiological University Clinic Heidelberg, and Dr. Siegfried Matzku, Institute of Radiology and Pathophysiology of the Deutsches Krebsforschungszentrum)

10. T-cell function and clonal analysis of “graft versus leukemia” effects in patients after autologous bone marrow transplantation.
(Project heads: Priv.-Doz. Dr. Bernd Dörken, Medical University Clinic and Outpatient Clinic Heidelberg, and Prof. Dr. Stephan Meuer, Institute of Radiology and Pathophysiology of the Deutsches Krebsforschungszentrum)

11. Induction of a “graft versus host” disease after autologous stem cell transplantation.
(Project head: Dr. Reiner Haas, Medical University Clinic and Outpatient Clinic Heidelberg)

D. Neurooncology

(Coordinators: Dr. Gabriele Schackert, Neurosurgical University Clinic Heidelberg, and Prof. Dr. Dr. Michael Wannenmacher, Radiological University Clinic Heidelberg)

Subprojects:

1. Stereotactic convergent beam irradiation.
(Project heads: Priv.-Doz. Dr. Dr. Bernd Kimmig, Radiological University Clinic Heidelberg, Dr. Karl-Heinz Höver, Institute of Radiology and Pathophysiology of the Deutsches Krebsforschungszentrum, and Dr. Bernd Wowra, Neurosurgical University Clinic Heidelberg)

2. Stereotactic conformation therapy of brain tumors.
(Project heads: Prof. Dr. Dr. Michael Wannenmacher, Radiological University Clinic Heidelberg, Prof. Dr. Wolfgang Schlegel, Institute of Radiology and Pathophysiology of the Deutsches Krebsforschungszentrum, and Dr. Bernd Wowra, Neurosurgical University Clinic Heidelberg)

3. Biological and molecular biological investigations of gliomas and their recurrences and of brain metastases/ Immunotherapy on brain tumors: activation of monocytes/macrophages.
(Project heads: Dr. Gabriele Schackert and Dr. Friedrich Albert, Neurosurgical University Clinic Heidelberg)

4. Localized carrier-mediated chemotherapy.
(Project heads: Dr. Bernd Wowra, Neurosurgical University Clinic Heidelberg, and Prof. Dr. Jens Zeller, Institute of Toxicology and Chemotherapy of the Deutsches Krebsforschungszentrum)

5. Oncogenes in pediatric and neuronal tumors/Identification and characterization of NMYC-induced angiogenetic activity.
(Project heads: Prof. Dr. Manfred Schwab, Institute of Chemotherapy of the Deutsches Krebsforschungszentrum, and Dr. Lothar Schweigerer, Pediatric University Clinic Heidelberg)

E. Mammary carcinoma

(Coordinators: Prof. Dr. Manfred Kaufmann, Gynecological University Clinic Heidelberg, and Prof. Dr. Peter Möller, Pathological Institute of the University of Heidelberg)

Subprojects:

1. Biochemical and immunological monitoring of epithelium-specific proteins (keratins) in homogenates and supernatants of primary tumors and metastases (lymph nodes, bone marrow, other metastases): correlation of histological and immunocytological results for the monitoring of malignancy and prognostic criteria.
(Project head: Prof. Dr. Manfred Kaufmann, Gynecological University Clinic Heidelberg)

2. Monoclonal antibodies against mammary carcinoma. Further development of own specific monoclonal antibodies against TAG 12 to applicability in the human system and clinical phase-O-study.
(Project heads: Prof. Dr. Gunther Bastert, Gynecological University Clinic Heidelberg, Dr. Heiner Bihl, Radiological University Clinic Heidelberg, and Dr. Siegfried Matzku, Institute of Radiology and Pathophysiology of the Deutsches Krebsforschungszentrum)

3. Expression of aromatase and tumor growth in the mammary carcinoma.
(Project head: Priv.-Doz. Dr. Walter Pyerin, Institute of Experimental Pathology of the Deutsches Krebsforschungszentrum)

4. Preparation of peptide and antibodies specific to the mammary carcinoma by means of endogenous human retroviruses.
(Project head: Prof. Dr. Rüdiger Hehlmann, Gynecological Clinic of the Clinics of the City of Mannheim)

F. Malignant melanoma

(Coordinators: Priv.-Doz. Dr. Wolfgang Tilgen, Dermatological University Clinic Heidelberg)

Subprojects:

1. Active immunization with human monoclonal anti-idiotypic antibodies: establishing a therapy model.
(Project heads: Priv.-Doz. Dr. Margot Zöller, Institute of Radiology and Pathophysiology of the Deutsches Krebsforschungszentrum, and Priv.-Doz. Dr. Wolfgang Tilgen, Dermatological University Clinic Heidelberg)

2. Preclinical testing of the ability of Napavin, a new laser- activated Vinca alkaloid, to overcome resistance against cytostatics in melanoma in an experimental system.
(Project heads: Prof. Dr. Herwig Ponstingl, Institute of Cell and Tumor Biology of the Deutsches Krebsforschungszentrum, Priv.-Doz. Dr. Wolfgang Tilgen, Dermatological University Clinic Heidelberg, and Dr. Siegfried Matzku, Institute of Radiology and Pathophysiology of the Deutsches Krebsforschungszentrum)

3. Adoptive immunotherapy.
(Project head: Dr. Ulrich Keilholz, Medical University Clinic and Outpatient Clinic Heidelberg)

G. Thyroid carcinomas

(Coordinators: Prof. Dr. Michael Trede, Surgical Clinic of the Clinics of the City of Mannheim, and Prof. Dr. Klaus-Henning Usadel, Department of Internal Medicine II of the Clinics of the City of Mannheim)

Subprojects:

1. Epidemiology of thyroid carcinomas in the North of Baden- Württemberg and the northern Palatinate.
(Project heads: Dr. Johannes Winter, Surgical Clinic of the Clinics of the City of Mannheim, Dr. Reiner Frenzel-Beyme, Institute of Epidemiology and Biometry of the Deutsches Krebsforschungszentrum, and Prof. Dr. Heinz Buhr, Surgical University Clinic Heidelberg)

2. Case-control study on the ethiology of thyroid tumors.
(Project head: Dr. Reiner Frenzel-Beyme, Institute of Epidemiology and Biometry of the Deutsches Krebsforschungszentrum)

H. Differentiation labels of the cytoskeleton

Epidermal cytoskeleton differentiation markers for the improvement of the diagnosis of tumors of the skin and other organs.
(Project heads: Prof. Dr. Werner Franke, Institute of Cell and Tumor Biology of the Deutsches Krebsforschungszentrum, and Prof. Dr. Ernst G. Jung, Dermatological Clinic of the Clinics of the City of Mannheim)

I. Research on radiotherapy

(Coordinators: Prof. Dr. Dr. Michael Wannenmacher, Radiological University Clinic Heidelberg, and Prof. Dr. Walter Lorenz, Institute of Radiology and Pathophysiology of the Deutsches Krebsforschungszentrum)

Subprojects:

1. Combined neutron-photon therapy.
(Project heads: Priv.-Doz. Dr. Dr. Bernd Kimmig, Radiological University Clinic Heidelberg, and Dr. Karl-Heinz Höver, Institute of Radiology and Pathophysiology of the Deutsches Krebsforschungszentrum)

2. Brachytherapy.
(Project head: Dr. Peter Fritz, Radiological University Clinic Heidelberg)

J. Epithelial tumors of liver and kidney

Microbiochemical and molecular-biological analysis of early stages and precursors of epithelial tumors of liver and kidney.
(Project heads: Prof. Dr. Peter Bannasch, Institute of Experimental Pathology of the Deutsches Krebsforschungszentrum, and Priv.-Doz. Dr. Gerd Otto, Surgical University Clinic Heidelberg)

K. Human Papilloma viruses

Detection of E6 and E7 proteins of the human Papilloma viruses type 16 and 18 with monoclonal antibodies in the cervical carcinomas.
(Project heads: Prof. Dr. Gunther Bastert, Gynecological University Clinic Heidelberg, and Prof. Dr. Lutz Gissmann, Institute of Virus Research of the Deutsches Krebsforschungszentrum)

L. Tumors of the aero-digestive tract

Carcinomas of the squamous epithelium of the upper aero-digestive tract.
(Project head: Prof. Dr. Hagen Weidauer, ENT University Clinic Heidelberg)

Research thrives on the evolution of concepts and on renewed questions and accents. In the past 2 years, the Tumor Center Heidelberg/Mannheim has developed a new concept which better correlates new focuses of work to methodological research; this was supported by the experts who reviewed the listed projects in the summer of 1989. New research topics have thus been planned for the 1990s that will devote more attention to methodological problems. The following research programs are planned to start in 1992:

Research program I: Immunological and molecular-biological approaches for tumor diagnosis.
Coordinators: Prof. Dr. Peter Möller, Pathological Institute of the University of Heidelberg, and Dr. Gerhard Moldenhauer, Institute of Immunology and Genetics of the Deutsches Krebsforschungszentrum

Research program II: Biological response modifiers and molecular therapy concepts.
Coordinators: Prof. Dr. Stephan Meuer, Institute of Radiology and Pathophysiology of the Deutsches Krebsforschungszentrum, and Priv.-Doz. Dr. Bernd Dörken, Medical University Clinic and Outpatient Clinic Heidelberg

Research program III: Locoregional tumor therapy – research in radiotherapy including diagnostics.

Coordinators: Prof. Dr. Gerhard van Kaick, Institute of Radiology and Pathophysiology of the Deutsches Krebsforschungszentrum, and Dr. Günther Gademann, Radiological University Clinic Heidelberg

Research program IV: Heterogeneity of tumor cells, metastatic spread, and resistance.
Coordinators: Prof. Dr. Peter Schlag, Surgical University Clinic Heidelberg, and Prof. Dr. Werner W. Franke, Institute of Cell and Tumor Biology of the Deutsches Krebsforschungszentrum

These research activities were supplemented by collaboration with other tumor centers and organizations, such as the European Organization for Research on Treatment of Cancer (EORTC), with the Swiss Working Group for Clinical Cancer Research (SAKK), and with the oncological working groups of the German Cancer Society.

In the past, the Tumor Center has developed a large variety of organizational and editorial activities.

The activity of the clinical institutions of the Tumor Center makes it possible to apply in practice the results of the theoretical-clinical research on a great number of cancer patients. The high professional standard of the clinics and research institutions of the Tumor Center assures the scientific-clinical as well as the technical collaboration with other national and international centers. Not only the national and international collaboration with other tumor centers play an important role for the Tumor Center Heidelberg/Mannheim, but also the collaboration with large institutions of clinical cancer research (the National Cancer Institute of the USA, the Swiss Working Group for Clinical Cancer Research; the European Organization for Research on Treatment of Cancer, EORTC, and associations of various disciplines in the German Cancer Society).

Documentation and biological statistics are an essential part of the assignment to research and patient care. The documentation of standardized data about cancer patients in the form of a standardized clinical documentation is an essential prerequisite for progress in diagnostics, therapy, and the follow-up care of cancer patients. Such a tumor documentation is intended to monitor the individual course of the disease of every cancer patient until healing or death. The tumor documentation at the Tumor Center Heidelberg/Mannheim consists of a clinical cancer register of all affiliated clinics.

The Tumor Center regularly conducts advanced training programs which are sponsored by the Oncological Working Groups Heidelberg and Mannheim in collaboration with the Academy for Medical Advanced Training of the Physician's District Chamber of North Baden. These training programs take place at a spring symposium in Heidelberg and at an autumn symposium in Mannheim. They present research topics and new therapeutic approaches of the participating clinics. Most presentations are interdisciplinary, in accordance with the cooperative character of cancer research and cancer treatment.

The advanced training programs underline the Tumor Center's aim to act as a link between clinic and practice in diagnostics, therapy, and follow-up care, and to pass on results of cancer research already being applied in the clinics of the Tumor Center Heidelberg/Mannheim to private practicioners and clinicians. At the same, the center aim to stimulate an intense exchange of information and a sensitive coordination of interdisciplinary action. The advanced training symposiums since 1988 have covered the following topics:

- "The Malignant Melanoma – Treatment Concepts and New Diagnostical Methods" (February 6, 1988)
- "Oncology for Practitioners – Prevention, Care and Follow-up" (December 3, 1988, and December 1, 1990)
- "Combination Therapy Modalities in Oncology" (January 28, 1989)
- "Diagnosis and Therapy of Cancer-related Pain" (February 3, 1990)
- "The Unknown Primary Tumor" (February 2, 1991)
- "The Geriatric Tumor Patient" (October 5, 1991)

One important medium for spreading up-to-date and verified knowledge of tumor treatment is a series of publications jointly edited by the Oncological Working Groups Heidelberg and Mannheim under the title "Guidelines on Diagnosis, Therapy, and Follow-up Care". These publications, known as the "Green Series", are constantly actualized and supplemented and cover topical oncological matters. The recommendations are binding for the members of the Oncological Working Groups Heidelberg and Mannheim; the individual application, however, lies in the responsibility of the treating physician. So far, the following brochures have been published, partially as revised editions:

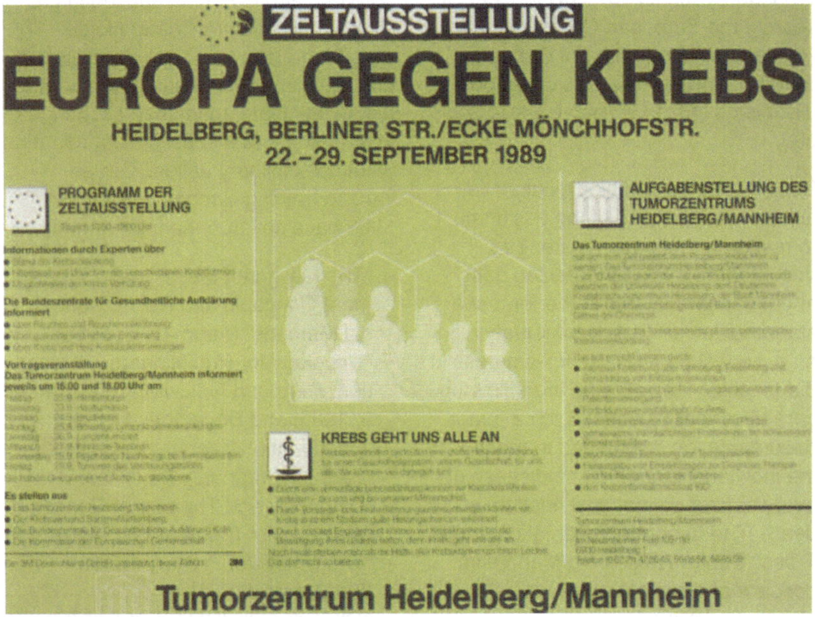

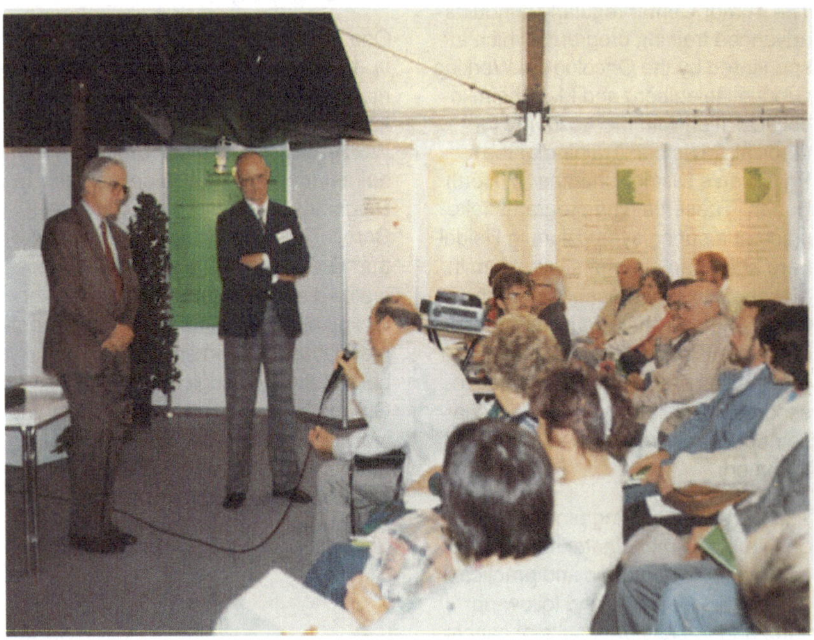

Fig. 153/154
In a tent exhibition that was organized on the occasion of the Cancer Information Year, the Tumor Center Heidelberg/Mannheim addressed itself to the citizens of Heidelberg and informed them of cancer diagnosis, therapy, and prevention.

1. "The Bronchial Carcinoma" – 1st edition July 1979, Vol. 8
2. "Gastrointestinal Tumors" – 1st edition January 1981, Vol. 9, 12, 15, 17
3. "The Malignant Melanoma" – 3rd revised edition February 1987
4. "Soft Tissue Sarcomas in Adults – 3rd unrevised edition July 1985
5. "Morbus Hodgkin" – 2nd unrevised edition July 1985
6. "The Mammary Carcinoma" – 3rd unrevised edition November 1984
7. "Non-Hodgkin Lymphomas" – 2nd unrevised edition July 1985
8. "Malignant Tumors of Lung, Pleura, and Thymus" – 1st edition November 1985, re-edition of the brochure "The Bronchial Carcinoma"
9. "The pancreatic carcinoma" – 1st edition January 1986
10. "The Renal Cell Carcinoma" – 1st edition January 1986
11. "The Thyroid Carcinoma" – 1st edition May 1986
12. "The Colorectal Carcinoma" – 1st edition January 1987
13. "Social Legislation in the Medical and Social Rehabilitation of Cancer Patients" – 1st edition September 1989
14. "Diagnosis and Therapy of Cancer-related Pain" – 1st edition January 1990
15. "The Stomach Carcinoma" – 1st edition January 1990

16. "Malignant Tumors of the Efferent Urinary Tract" – 1st edition December 1990
17. "The Esophagus Carcinoma" – 1st edition January 1991

In 1991, the following publications were added to the series:

- "Malignant Tumors of the Male Genitals" – 1st edition
- "The Renal Cell Carcinoma" – 2nd revised edition
- "The Malignant Melanoma" – 3rd revised edition
- "The Malignant Tumors of Lung, Pleura, and Thymus" – re-edition.

These brochures are offered free of charge to cooperating and interested physicians as a diagnostic and therapeutic aid. One copy of each of these brochures may be ordered free of charge from the coordinative and administrative office of the Tumor Center Heidelberg/Mannheim, Im Neuenheimer Feld 105/110, D- 6900 Heidelberg, Germany, phone +6221/472645.

In 1989, the Tumor Center Heidelberg/Mannheim took advantage of its 10th anniversary as an opportunity to inform the general public about cancer and the Center's various activities in fighting cancer. In collaboration with the Cancer Association of Baden-Württemberg, the European Commission, and the Federal Center for Health Education, and as a part of the "European Cancer Information Year," an information tent was set up from September 22 to 29, 1989, in which the public was introduced to the diagnosis and treatment of malignant diseases. During 1 week, about 8000 visitors from all over the region visited the exhibit.

Coordinating Committee for Cancer Research of the Association of Major Research Institutions (Arbeitsgemeinschaft der Großforschungs-einrichtungen)

The Deutsches Krebsforschungszentrum is one of the 13 institutions that have joined to form the Association of Major Research Institutions (Arbeitsgemeinschaft der Großforschungseinrichtungen, AGF), which has a total of 20000 employees. The AGF has assumed, among others, the responsibility of rationally and purposefully coordinating the research of its member institutions. In 1983, the Coordinating Committee for Cancer Research was constituted. It is made up of representatives of the Deutsches Krebsforschungszentrum (DKFZ), the Society of Radiation and Environmental Research in München-Neuherberg (GSF), the Society of Biotechnological Research in Braunschweig-Stöckheim (GBF), the Nuclear Research Facility in Karlsruhe-Leopoldshafen (KfK), and the Nuclear Research Facility in Jülich (KFA). Of these, the Deutsches Krebsforschungszentrum is the only one that has devoted all of its activities to cancer research. Notwithstanding that, the other institutions provide important contributions to cancer research.

Presently, the members of the committee are:

Prof. Dr. Peter Bannasch, DKFZ, chairman,
Prof. Dr. John Collins, GBF,
Prof. Dr. Ludwig E. Feinendegen, KFA,
Prof. Dr. Dres. h. c. Harald zur Hausen, DKFZ,
Prof. Dr. Peter Herrlich, KfK,
Prof. Dr. Heinz Höfler, GSF,
Prof. Dr. Stephan Meuer, DKFZ, and
Prof. Dr. Wolfgang Wilmanns, GSF.

Dr. Horst Metzler of the Deutsches Krebsforschungszentrum is responsible for the organization of the committee.

The committee gives advice on research work done by the member institutions in the field of cancer research. It also helps to avoid overlaps by installing joint research projects. It prepares and publishes a list of the member institutions' research activities in the field of cancer research on a regular basis. This list is available upon request.

The activities of the committee have resulted in organizing three symposia (all in Heidelberg), which were attended by internationally renowned scientists. The first symposium, held in 1986, dealt with "Cancer Risks: Strategies for Elimination". The second symposium was held in 1988 on "Cancer Therapy: New Trends"; and the third one, organized in 1991, dealt with "Cancer Diagnosis: Early Detection". Invited speakers, moderators, journalists and scientists from Belgium, Denmark, Germany, France, Great Britain, India, Japan, Canada, Austria, Sweden, Switzerland and the USA attended. The proceedings of all three symposia have been published by Springer Verlag Berlin, Heidelberg, New York, and Tokyo and they were praised in numerous internationally scientific journal reviews. An indication of the relevance of these publications might be the fact that the first two editions have nearly sold out.

The proceedings of the symposium "Cancer Diagnosis: Early Detection" have just been published by Springer Verlag. Aside from the proceedings, the symposia were mentioned in numerous news magazines.

In addition, the Coordinating Committee for Cancer Research of the AGF has assumed the role as mediator for the coordination of the German-Indian cooperation in cancer research. The large number of projects planned and the published results of fruitful joint projects have encouraged the committee to plan a German-Indian symposium on recent results in cooperative cancer research in Heidelberg in October 1992. The cooperation with cancer researchers from India also conveys comprehensive information on the status of cancer diseases in the societies of underdeveloped and developing countries, the age structures of which differ significantly from that in Europe, as a consequence of which only some types of cancer occur more commonly. The cooperation between Germany and India in the field of cancer research is part of AGF's endeavor to promote research in and for the developing countries.

Organs of the Foundation

As provided by § 7 of its Statutes and Articles, the Foundation has the following organs:

- the Board of Trustees with the Scientific Committee,
- the Management Board, and
- the Scientific Council.

The Board of Trustees

As provided by § 8 of the Statutes and Articles of the Foundation, the Board of Trustees supervises the legality, expediency, and economy of the conduct of the Foundation's transactions. It decides on the aims of research and important research policy and financial affairs of the Foundation. In addition, it determines the principles of management and those governing efficiency control, and it sets up long-term financial plans including programs for development and investment. Normally, the Board of Trustees convenes twice a year.

In 1989/1990, the Board of Trustees mainly dealt with the following tasks:

- Assessment of the results of the external evaluations of the institutes of Toxicology and Chemotherapy, of

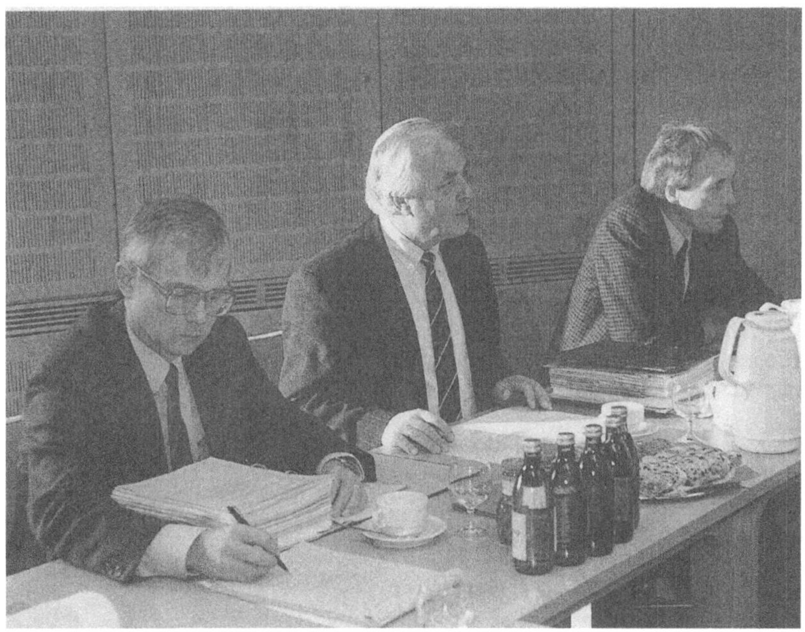

Fig. 155
Meeting of the Board of Trustees: The chairman, undersecretary Dr. Josef Rembser of the Federal Ministry for Research and Technology *(center)*, the vice-chairman, assistant secretary Dr. Heribert Knorr of the Ministry for Science and Research of the Land Baden-Württemberg *(right)*, and principal Dr. Konrad Buschbeck of the Federal Ministry for Research and Technology *(left)*.

Experimental Pathology, of Virus Research, and of Cell and Tumor Biology.
- Appointment of the Administrative Member of the Management Board, Dr. Reinhard Grunwald, for a second term of five years.
- Appointment of Prof. Dr. Ingrid Grummt as the head of the Division "Molecular Biology of the Cell II".
- Foundation of the Division "Molecular Biophysics".
- Foundation of the project "Molecular Biology of Aging" and appointment of Dr. Heinz D. Osiewacz as its head.
- Establishment of the project "Tumor Promotion in the Liver" and appointment of Priv.-Doz. Dr. habil. Michael Schwarz as its head.
- Establishment of the project "Biochemical Cell Physiology" and appointment of Priv.-Doz. Dr. Walter Pyerin as its head.
- Continuation of the project "Structural Gene Analysis and Transcriptor Organization" and re-appointment of Prof. Dr. Michael Trendelenburg as its head.
- Continuation of the project "Molecular Biology of Mitosis" and re-appointment of Prof. Dr. Herwig Ponstingl as its head.
- Approval for the foundation of clinical cooperation units with the Deutsches Krebsforschungszentrum and the University of Heidelberg.
- Considerations regarding the working structure of the Center.

As provided by § 10 of the Statutes and Articles of the Foundation, the Scientific Committee prepares the decisions of the Board of Trustees in all scientific matters. In particular, it is responsible for the continuous evaluation of the results of the research work by scientific expertise. Aside from elaborating the basis for decisions for the Board of Trustees, the Scientific Committee appoints consultative commissions, composed of leading international scientists, for external evaluations of the Deutsches Krebsforschungszentrum institutes.

The Management Board

As provided by § 14.1 of the Statutes and Articles, the Management Board directs the Foundation. It consists of at least one scientific and one administrative member (§ 15.1). The Board of Trustees appoints the members of the Management Board after consultation with the Scientific Council (§ 15.2).

Since May 1, 1983, Prof. Dr. med. Dres. h.c. Harald zur Hausen has directed the Management Board as its chairman and as its scientific member. In May 1988, he was re-appointed for a second five-year term. Since July 1, 1984, Dr. jur. Reinhard Grunwald has been the administrative member of the Management Board. In 1989, he was reappointed for a second five-year term.

In a multi-disciplinary, complex and necessarily decentralized research institution the traditional management functions of planning, decision making, and supervision, are less hierarchically structured. Scientific management is primarily based on encouraging and promoting ideas, coordinating processes, and balancing multiple interests.

Thus, when defining the scientific program of the Deutsches Krebsforschungszentrum, the Management Board focuses on considering how to initiate and to terminate Research Programs, how to distribute the Center's resources depending on performance, and how to further improve organizational processes. The collaboration with the Foundation's committees and its sponsors and the cooperation with scientific partners in Germany and abroad are important aspects of the work of the Management Board. The experiences and the results of the analyses of the work completed so far have been integrated into a restructuring plan which is to give the Center the flexibility that it needs for continued success. An important instrument is the internal evaluation of all scientific divisions. The Chairman and Scientific Member is supported in his task by the scientific consultants of the Management Board.

The work of the Management Board is considerably supported by advisory committees. In the past, the Management Board has delegated the following tasks to permanent commissions: selection of scientists for awards, bonuses, upgrading, and tenure, assessment of all applications for the use of laboratory animals in the Center according to the German Law on Animal Protection, and examination of all applications and supervision of all work and installations subject to the German Gene Technology Law.

Other tasks are delegated to ad hoc committees. The Management Board is supported in its work by staff departments and by the administration.

Biological Safety Commission

Most areas of molecular biology, which tries to elucidate fundamental biological problems with methods of genetic engineering, are now, after many years of being supervised by the Central Commission on Biological Safety, subject to the Law on the Regulation of Genetic Engineering (in short, Genetic Engineering Law).

The Genetic Engineering Law and the accompanying regulations, such as that on compulsory record-keeping on all work in genetic engineering in research and industry (Regulation on Record-Keeping in Genetic Engineering), the Regulation on Safety Stages and Safety Measures for Genetic Engineering in Genetic Engineering Installations (Genetic Engineering Safety Regulation), and the Regulation on Application and Registration Procedures according to the Genetic Engineering Law (Genetic Engineering Procedural Rules Regulation) have as a consequence that all experiments have to be prepared (and planned) with great precision, both scientifically and administratively. There are more than 50 pages of specimen forms to be completed, accompanied by 15 pages of instructions explaining how to fill these out. The Genetic Engineering Law and the Genetic Engineering Safety Regulation describe the tasks of, and the requirements for becoming a biological safety officer. The biological safety officer, who should be especially and thoroughly trained in the application of the Genetic Engineering Law and the accompanying regulations, supervises and checks all relevant work in research and industry.

The Deutsches Krebsforschungszentrum is too large an institution to be supervised by only one biological safety officer. As early as November 1990, the Management Board established a Biological Safety Commission and has, after a statutory hearing of the staff council, appointed its members. At present, the commission is formed by 12 scientists of the Center.

In numerous discussions among its members and with the administration of the State of Baden-Württemberg in Tübingen, which supervises the correct application of the Genetic Engineering Law, the commission has tried to realize the directives of the Genetic Engineering Law and its accompanying regulations (which, in part, are rather obstructive for basic research) in a way that takes account of the public interest in supervision, control, and a minimization of the risk of handling genetically altered organisms, as well as the interest of there searchers in advancing their sciences.

The Biological Safety Commission serves (as does the internal Animal Protection Commission) as a "clearing institution" between the supervising authority (the regional administrations of Karlsruhe and Tübingen) and the scientists. The work of both commissions is characterized by the high personal commitment of its members.

Chairman:
Prof. Dr. Claus Hobe Schröder

Internal Animal Protection Commission

The Animal Protection Law in its wording of the "Proclamation of August 18th, 1986" (Official Bulletin I p. 1319), amended by article 56 of the Law of August 20th, 1990 (Official Bulletin I, p. 1762) and article 3 of the Law of August 20th, 1990, strictly regulates the carrying out of animal experiments. In addition, the experimenter has to observe the regulation on reports on experimental animals and their marking of May 20th, 1988, and the regulation on the reporting of experimental animals of August 1st, 1988. The keeping of experimental animals is also regulated by a guideline of the European Communities.

Animal experiments are still necessary for experimental cancer research, the development of models for the disease, and the examination of new substances which might open new paths in therapy and diagnosis. Though new substances or methods can be pretested with cell cultures and pain-free systems such as explanted organs; they can still not completely substitute for animal experiments.

The number of animal experiments and the number of small rodents (mice and rats) used in the Center have been continuously reduced over the past years. This is partly due to the fact that all applications for approval of animal experiments and all notifications on the use of animals for the explantation of organs are thoroughly deliberated by the legal animal welfare officers and the internal animal protection commission. It was founded by the Board of Trustees in 1984. This commission, which is formed by several scientists from the

Center and one layman, mainly considers the scientific necessity of the animal experiments applied for, while the Animal Protection Law charges the animal welfare officers with the supervision of the management and execution of the animal experiments with respect to animal protection. The animal welfare officers and the commission also elaborate internal standards for the execution of animal experiments. Part of this work has gained significance outside the Deutsches Krebsforschungszentrum. For example, the internal instruction on the keeping of tumor bearing animals has become generally accepted by the legal authorities and is now obligatory for all animal experiments in Nordbaden. Presently, 200 applications for animal experiments have been approved in the Deutsches Krebsforschungszentrum; in addition, there is a large number of notifications.

Chairman:

Prof. Dr. Stefan Meuer

The Scientific Council

The Scientific Council advises the Board of Trustees and the Management Board in all significant matters of a scientific nature. In some matters of particular importance, the decisions of the Management Board have to be confirmed by the Scientific Council.

In particular, the Scientific Council deals with research projects and research programs, appointments, the use of research results, the control of the effectiveness, the advancement of

Member of the Scientific Council (January 1990–January 1992)

Dr. Dirk Breitkreutz
Institut für Biochemie

Prof. Dr. Werner Wilhelm Franke (Chairman)
Institut für Zell- und Tumorbiologie

Prof. Dr. Erich Hecker
Institut für Biochemie

Prof. Dr. Hans-C. Kaerner
Institut für Virusforschung

Dr. Jürgen Kartenbeck
Institut für Zell- und Tumorbiologie

Prof. Dr. Dymitr Komitowski
Institut für Experimentelle Pathologie

Prof. Dr. Peter Krammer
Institut für Immunologie und Genetik

Prof. Dr. Walter Lorenz
Institut für Radiologie und Pathophysiologie

Prof. Dr. Rudolf Preussmann
Institut für Toxikologie und Chemotherapie

Dr. Walter Pyerin
Institut für Experimentelle Pathologie

Dr. Wolfgang Schlegel
Institut für Radiologie und Pathophysiologie

Prof. Petre Tautu
Institut für Epidemiologie und Biometrie

Prof. Dr. Jürgen Wahrendorf
Institut für Epidemiologie und Biometrie

Dr. Klaus Wayss (Deputy Chairman)
Institut für Experimentelle Pathologie

Dr. Jens Zeller
Institut für Toxikologie und Chemotherapie

Dr. Hanswalter Zentgraf
Institut für Virusforschung

Members of the Scientific Council (as of February 1992)

Prof. Dr. Werner Wilhelm Franke (Chairman)
Dr. Jürgen Kartenbeck
Research Program Cell Differentiation and Carcinogenesis

Prof. Dr. Norbert Fusening
Prof. Dr. Friedrich Marks
Research Program Tumor Cell Regulation

Dr. Norbert Frank
Prof. Dr. Jürgen Wahrendorf
Research Program Cancer Risk Factors and Prevention

Prof. Dr. Stefan Meuer
Dr. Klaus Wayß (Deputy Chairman)
Research Program Diagnostics and Experimental Therapy

Prof. Dr. Walter Lorenz
Dr. Wolfgang Schlegel
Research Program Radiological Diagnostics and Therapy

Prof. Dr. Lutz Gissmann
Dr. Elisabeth Schwarz
Research Program Applied Tumor Virology

Prof. Dr. Peter Krammer
Dr. Gerhard Moldenhauer
Research Program Tumor Immunology

Dr. Sándor Suhai
Prof. Petre Tautu
Research Program Bioinformatics

scientific communication, the cooperation with universities and other research institutions, budget planning, and investment plans.

Since the new Statutes and Articles went into effect in 1991, the new structure of the Deutsches Krebsforschungszentrum, which integrates the divisions as the scientific units of research into Research Programs, has been reflected, among others, by a new composition of the Scientific Council. The Scientific Council now consists of the coordinators of the Research Programs and an equal number of elected representatives of the scientific staff.

Normally, the Scientific Council convenes once a month. In its work and in the preparation of its decisions, the Scientific Council is supported by a permanent secretary and several expert committees.

With the introduction of the new Statutes and Articles on August 10, 1991, the Scientific Council had to be reconstituted. Since the Deutsches Krebsforschungszentrum presently has eight Research Programs, the Scientific Council has 16 members.

Staff Council

by Brigitte Hobrecker, chairperson

The Staff Council exercises its rights and duties as provided by the Law on Staff Representation of the State of Baden-Württemberg. The fact that of the employees less than 50% have a permanent contract creates some obvious, but nonetheless serious problems: temporary contracts, a high turnover and a lack of continuity in the entire personnel hierarchy. As a result, the employees may lose a sense of responsibility for their work; insufficient care may make it difficult to observe the safety regulations for the workplace.

The structural changes that have been realized in the Deutsches Krebsforschungszentrum are based on the idea that only research projects that are limited in time and depend on temporary employment can yield excellent scientific results. However, this does not consider the fact that pressure and stress, and the fear of unemployment as a consequence of temporary employment all burden the employee and adversely affect his or her research work.

The advancement of young scientists is one of the main concerns of the Management Board. The Staff Council has long requested that the situation of doctoral students be improved. These employees, working on scientific projects, are excluded from the Federal Salary Scale (BAT). In recent years the Staff Council has made numerous efforts to negotiate a special collective wage agreement for doctoral students.

Presently, the collective bargaining is suspended; however, internal transitional regulations have been worked out that improve the financial situation of the doctoral students. In the period under review, the Staff Council engaged in the following projects:

- elaboration of rules for data privacy protection while filing and processing data related or relatable to an individual; and
- signed a working agreement on the reduction of hours of the work weak, and on the newly installed system HICOM.

Members of the Staff Council (as of August 1992)

Dieter Baumgartl, member of the board
Joachim Buchholz, member of the board
Grit Brettschneider
Hanspeter Götz
Siegfried Herz
Edgar Heuss
Brigitte Hobrecker, chair
Heinrich Lerchl
Heinrich Schmitt, deputy chairman
Rolf Schmitt, member of the board
Ruth Wittmann

15

Administration

Functions and Organisation

As a service facility, the administration of the Deutsches Krebsforschungszentrum assumes central administrative tasks and specific functions for the divisions and central facilities. It prepares and implements decisions taken by the organs of the foundation, notably by the Management Board. Its work is influenced by the various individual requirements of the scientists and numerous laws and regulations for public foundations.

In this "field of tension" the administration tries to rapidly, pragmatically, and unbureaucratically execute its tasks. The major part of administrative work is in the fields of personnel, financing, procurement, supervision of projects, and technical services.

In the period under review, the administration:

- supervised the construction of the buildings for the Research Program "Applied Tumor Virology" and the Communication Center;
- organized the establishment of divisions and project groups;
- organized the scientific restructuring of the Center;
- supervised the project "Reorganization of Administrative Data Processing", which is designed to integrate the data processing solutions developed by the specialized departments and to develop them into a modern communication system;
- drafted, in collaboration with the Staff Council and the Scientific Council, general principles on data protection on personal computers;
- drafted and put into effect concepts for asbestos clearance;
- supervised the installation of the Center's new telephone system (HICOM 380);
- drafted, in collaboration with the Staff Council, working agreements on the realization of the collective reduction of working hours and the introduction and application of the salary and wage accounting system LOGA;
- developed, together with the Scientific Council, models for an effective assignment of personnel and means, equipment management, development of a modern storage concept, and further development of procurement management;
- supervised the disposal of solid and liquid toxic wastes in accordance with new stricter regulations;
- drafted a model for improving the situation of the Center's doctoral students.

New divisions and project groups were established despite the government's job-cutting policy, because since 1982 all vacancies due to fluctuation have been filled only after strict examination by the Management Board and the Scientific Council.

The Deutsches Krebsforschungszentrum committed itself to promoting young scientists and has further intensified this activity with the aid of grants. By the end of 1990, 193 doctoral students, 62 diploma students, 23 post- doctoral students, and 5 scholars supported by the Center's special funds worked in the Center.

A further important task of the administration is the custody of bequests. In accordance with the wish of various benefactors, estates are used completely or in part as awards granted to scientists with eminent achievements in cancer research, or to exceptional doctoral dissertations in cancer research. Laboratories or research projects are dedicated to other benefactors.

Of special importance are the Meyenburg Award, granted annually by the Wilhelm and Maria Meyenburg Foundation, and the Walther and Christine Richtzenhain Award.
In the period under review, the winners of the Meyenburg Award (which was endowed with DM 25 000 until 1989, and DM 30 000 since 1990) were:

1989, Prof. Dr. med. Peter Herrlich, director of the Institute of Genetics and Toxicology at the Nuclear Research Center Karlsruhe, for his research work in molecular biology, in particular for the clarification of gene regulation by tumor promoters;

1990, Prof. Dr. med. Rainer Storb, head of the program "Transplantation Biology" of the Fred Hutchinson Cancer Research Center in Seattle, Washington, USA., for his pioneering work on bone marrow transplantation in cancer therapy;

1991, Dr. rer. nat. habil. Hans-Georg Rammensee, head of the Research Group Immunology of the Department of Immunogenetics at the Max Planck Institute of Biology in Tübingen, for his extraordinary studies on the identification of cell-associated antigen fragments and their detection by T-cell receptors as an important component of specific immune response.

The winners of the DM 15 000-Walther and Christine Richtzenhain Award, which (alternatingly) in one year is awarded for scientific work in Germany, and in the following year for dissertations in Heidelberg research institutions, were

1989, Dr. rer. nat. Uwe Stähle for his dissertation on "Structural and Functional Characterization of DNA Elements Mediating Steroid Induction of Gene Expression";

1990, Dr. rer. nat. Thomas Bortfeld for his dissertation on "New Methods for Solving the Inverse Problem in Radiotherapy Planning", Dr. rer. nat. Wolfgang Pfau for his dissertation on "DNA Adducts of Aristolochia Acids", and Dr. rer. nat. Falk Weih for his dissertation on the "Regulation of Gene Expression through cAMP Signal Transmission Chains".

General Administration

The Department of General Administration coordinates

- committees,
- project management,
- patents, licenses,
- graphics, printing, and
- photo documentation.

The group "Committees" prepares the bi-annual meetings of the Management Board and its committees.

By the end of 1991, the working group "Project Management" had handled a total of 216 research and associated projects (207 projects in 1990).

Financial means were allocated to

- thirty-eight projects of Federal Institutions (Federal Ministry of Research and Technology, Federal Ministry of Youth, Family, Women, and Health, Federal Ministry of the Environment, Natural Protection, and Reactor Safety, Federal Ministry of Food and Agriculture, Federal Health Agency, Federal Environment Agency);
- ninety-five projects of other institutions (Federal Agency for Labor Safety and Accident Research, various professional associations, European Community, German Cancer Association, Meyenburg Foundation, and industrial cooperations);
- fifty-eight projects of the German Research Association as parts of Special Research Project No. 229 "Molecular Mechanisms of Gene Expression and Differentiation";
- eleven projects of the Federal Government as parts of the German-Israeli Cooperation Program;
- nine projects, financed by the donations to the Deutsches Krebsfor-

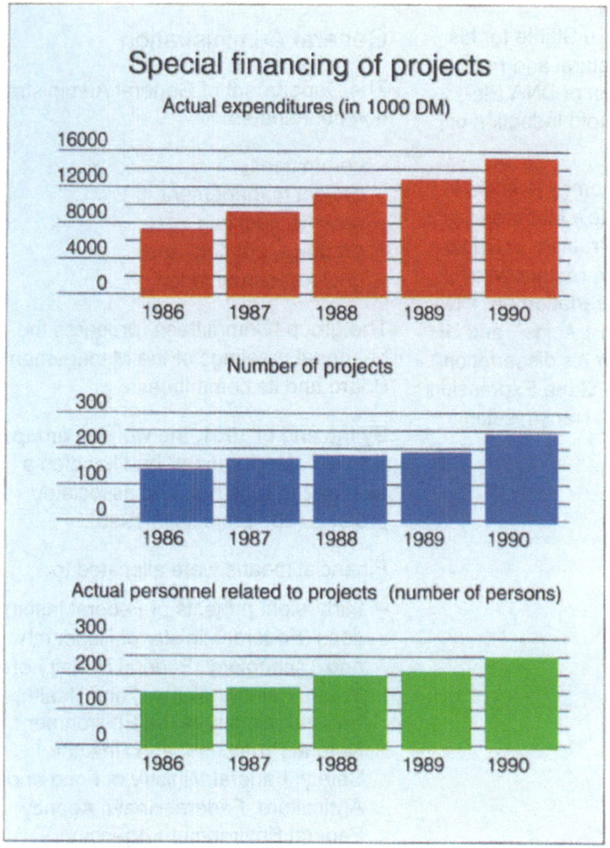

Fig. 156
General Administration. Special financing of research projects by external grants.

schungszentrum for the support of new research approaches.
The working group "Patents and Licenses" handles and applies for patents for inventions created at the Center.

The Deutsches Krebsforschungszentrum passes on its technological developments not primarily by licensing, as is done by more technological institutions, but rather by passing new techniques on to clinical practice and by industrial cooperations (such as for the development of new medical agents, computer software, or methods for the use of large-scale medical equipment). The Deutsches Krebsforschungszentrum plans to further extend the cooperation between the Center and industry.

Personnel and Social Matters

The Department of Personnel and Social Matters coordinates

- personnel matters,
- salary and wage accounting,
- ancillary personnel matters (travel expenses, financial aid),
- teaching, vocational training, postgraduate training,
- guest scientists, and the Center's guest houses.

By December 31, 1991, the Deutsches Krebsforschungszentrum employed a total of 1463 persons. Among these, 558 were scientists (including guest scientists, doctoral students, and scholars), 614 worked in the field of infrastructure, and 157 were wage-earning employees. In addition, the Center employed 49 diploma students and 85 apprentices in scientific, engineering, and administrative professions. The proportion of women varied greatly: 406 women worked in infrastructure (66%), 80 as wage earners (51%), and 155 as scientists (28%). There were also 22 female diploma students (45%) and 57 female apprentices (67%).

A total of 713, 729, and 739 permanent posts were funded by basic financing in 1989, 1990, and 1991, respectively. Funding for all other staff was mainly provided by projects that were sponsored by various organisations.

The fluctuation of employees is increasing: 26.3 and 24.3% of the Center's employees quit their jobs in 1990 and 1991, respectively. These high rates include auxiliary scientific staff, project staff, auxiliary staff, and guest scientists. Permanent posts had a fluctuation of only 6%. In 1991, the average age of the scientific staff was 40.1, of all other employees (including trainees) 35.8. In 1991, 63.8 percent of all employees were younger than 40, and 63.7 percent had been employed for less than 10 years.

In the annual average, the Center fully met with the Federal requirement on the employment of handicapped persons.

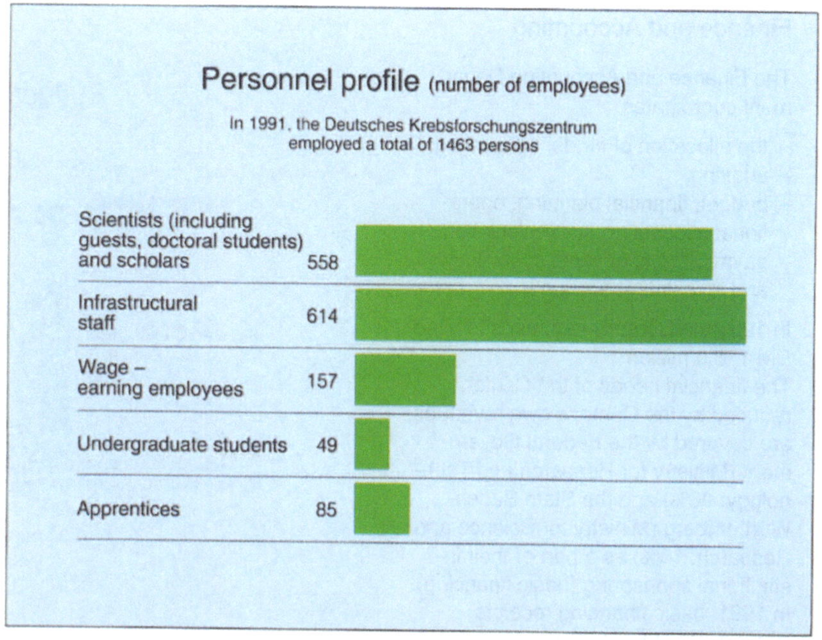

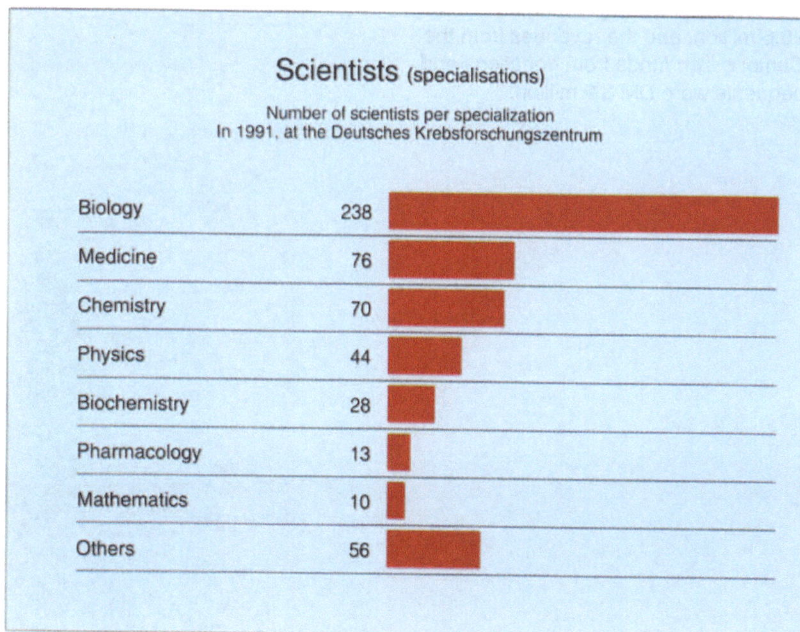

Figs. 157, 158

Finance and Accounting

The Finance and Accounting Department coordinates

- the allocation of funds, accounting,
- auditing,
- budget, financial planning, operational accounting, and calculation,
- payment transactions, special funds, and investment accounting.

In 1991 the Center's expenses totalled DM 178.9 million.
The financial needs of the Center, reduced by the Center's own revenues, are covered by the Federal Government (Ministry for Research and Technology: 90%) and the State Baden-Württemberg (Ministry for Science and Research: 10%) as a part of their institutional sponsoring (basic financing). In 1991, basic financing receipts totalled DM 155.1 million, whereas project-related financing amounted to DM 20.6 million, and the revenues from the Center's own funds from donations and bequests were DM 3.2 million.

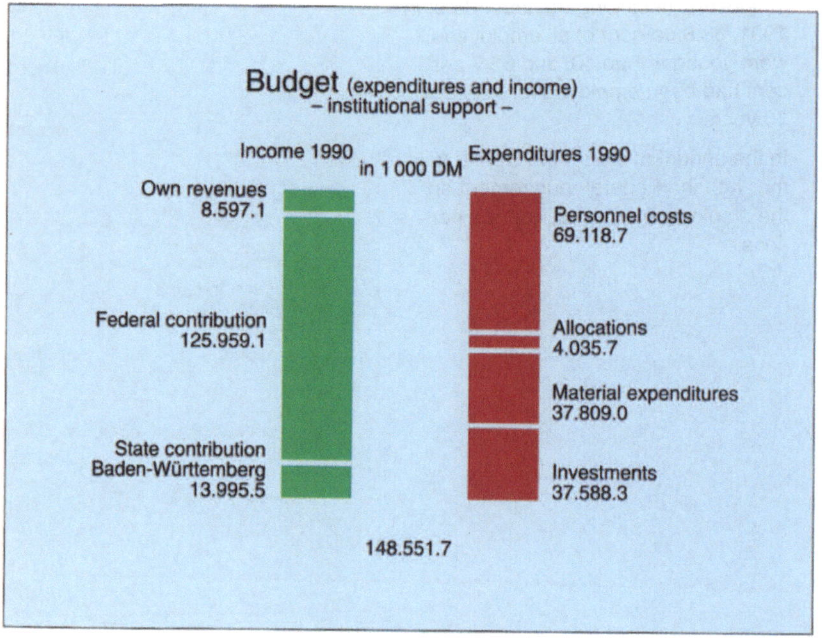

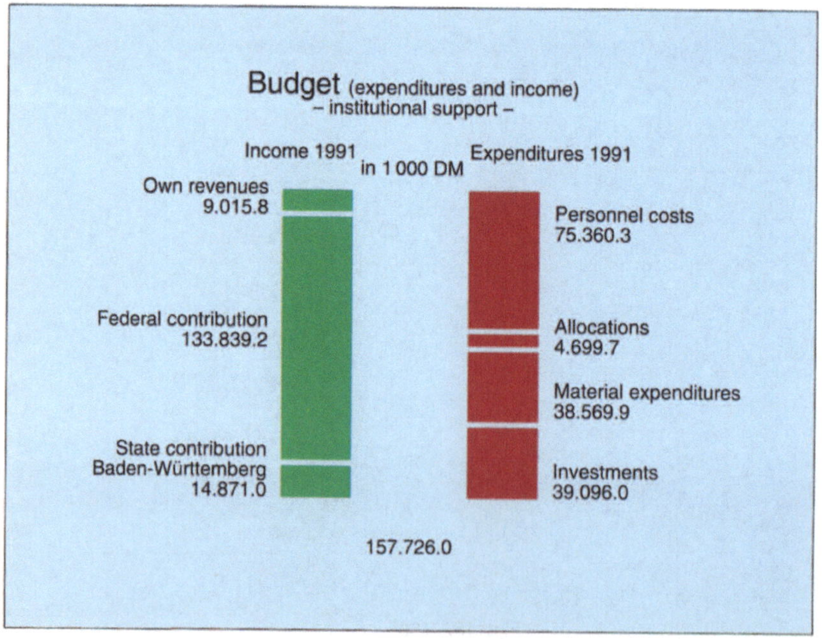

Figs. 159, 160

Procurement and Material Management

The tasks of the Department of Procurement and Material Management are

- acquisition,
- equipment management, and
- material management.

Acquisition

The group "Acquisition" purchases the equipment and the major part of the raw materials, process materials, and fuels needed by the Center. Outline agreements have been made with suppliers to fulfill these tasks economically and efficiently. The range of goods acquired reflects the broad demand research makes on acquisition, ranging from large computers to simple PCs, including all peripherals and software, from equipment for large laboratories to routine devices, from technical and office equipment to all kinds of materials. In 1991 the acquisition volume was DM 16 million for investments and DM 5 million for investment goods. In 1991, the goods department received 22000 deliveries.

Equipment Management

The group "Equipment Management" manages all investment goods of the Center and draws up an inventory. Currently, the Center handles approximately 32000 items. The management includes

- the conclusion of leasing and maintenance contracts,
- the collection and evaluation of repair costs, and
- the utilization or disposal of equipment taken out of service.

Material management

The group "Material Management" is responsible for

- chemicals and laboratory material,
- technical material, and
- office material.

It handles a total of approximately 10000 different items. The first step in realizing the Center's new storage concept was completed by the commissioning of the new central storage room for laboratory, technical, and office materials. The unification of formerly separate stocks is supplemented by a new computer system which allows the scientists to directly access the available stock and to order on-line. The new system also helps to improve supply planning.

Engineering and Construction

The Engineering Department is responsible for the Center's utilities and its energy supply. It also gives advice on the realization of research and development projects.

The department is divided into four subunits:

- electrics, communications, and supervision,
- heating, air conditioning, and sanitation,
- general and scientific machine shops, and
- constructions.

Special machine shops (such as for precision mechanics, glass-blowing, joinery, electric engineering) develop and manufacture devices and equipment not available on the market.
In 1991, 4035 (3946 in 1990) service contracts were handled for the institutes and central facilities, mainly in the maintenance and manufacture of scientific equipment. Construction and technical orders amounting to approximately DM 7 million were placed for small constructions, structural alterations, and the extension of existing buildings. These included

- the extension of the ventilation system of the Center's main building;
- the installation of fire doors;
- asbestos clearance;
- the renewal of the heat recovery system of the Center's main building;
- a new electric energy feed;
- the installation of energy-saving frequency-controlled drive motors into the central ventilation system;
- the installation of a 400 Hertz frequency converter for the central data department;

- the renewal of the elevators in the Center's main building including new drives and a digital control system; and
- the introduction of the HICOM communication system.

In 1991, an additional DM 19.9 million was spent on extensions and construction work such as
- the erection of the building for the Research Program Applied Tumor Virology; and
- the erection of a multi-storey car park.

General services

The General Services Department manages the property, the employees' dining hall, and the Center's bequests. Important tasks are the cleaning of the Center's building and the disposal of special waste (liquid and solid waste from the laboratories) in accordance with the German Waste Disposal Act.

Hazardous Goods Officer

In Germany, a large part of all hazardous goods are transported on the road. To ensure that all hazardous goods transports arrive safely at their destination, the legislature prescribed in the Hazardous Goods Act of October 1, 1991, that all companies and public institutions which pack, ship, load, or transport more than 50 metric tons of hazardous goods per calendar year must appoint a Hazardous Goods Officer.

The Deutsches Krebsforschungszentrum produces approximately 250 metric tons of hazardous goods per year which have to be disposed of safely.

All transports to special incineration plants are carried out either by officially licensed companies or by the Center's own special vehicles and highly qualified personnel.

On October 1, 1991, Hans-Joachim Buchholz was appointed as the Center's Hazardous Goods Officer. He ensures that the regulations on the transport of hazardous goods are followed. His main tasks are to examine all hazardous goods to be transported and to verify their classification, to check if they are marked as prescribed, to ensure that no goods are transported together with those which may not be, to check all transport precautions and the presence of the required accident instruction sheets.

The Hazardous Goods Officer documents his activities in protocols which may be inspected by the supervising environmental protection agencies at any time.

No defective vehicle will be allowed to transport hazardous goods until all defects have been remedied. To improve safety for the transport staff, the hazardous goods officer regularly offers courses on safety precautions or arranges training on the handling of hazardous goods through acknowledged external training institutes.

Teaching, Vocational Training, and Refresher Courses for Employees

Teaching

The scientists of the Deutsches Krebsforschungszentrum offer a wide range of seminars, colloquia, lectures, and laboratory courses for advanced students. All together, they teach more than 100 courses at the University of Heidelberg and, to a lesser degree, at the Universities of Karlsruhe, Tübingen, and Kaiserslautern, as well as at various professional colleges. From 1988 through 1990, 742 doctoral and diploma students participated in research work at the Center. During this period, they submitted 338 diploma, doctoral, and postdoctoral theses. The Center also organizes postgraduate training courses, refresher courses for staff members, and special courses for physicians, which are mainly held by the Division of Radiological Diagnostics and Therapy. Courses in ultrasound are offered regularly at three levels – introductory, intermediate, and advanced.

In order to promote highly qualified young researchers, five posts for young scientists and 10–15 posts within team-oriented project proposals are sponsored per year by the Center's special fund, i.e., by donations given to the Center. Within the framework of projects competitively proposed by the Center's scientists, young researchers are thus offered the possibility to do research work for up to 3 years. A trainee program is also devoted to the promotion of young scientists. Students of the Study Foundation of the German People (Studienstiftung des Deutschen Volkes) and of Stanford University (Krupp Foundation) are offered 8-week practicals.

The winners of the competition "Researching Youth" (Jugend forscht), held by the German Länder, are regularly invited to the Krebsforschungszentrum and may work for up to 2 weeks in a division of their choice. In addition, international courses for the introduction of scientists to new techniques and methods of research are organized by the Center on a regular basis.

The Center's colloquia are organized as an instrument for introducing new scientific ideas and for stimulating scientific discussion among researchers of the Center and of other institutions. From 1988 through 1990, scientists from more than 19 countries held more than 600 lectures. The Center's colloquia program is part of the program "bio-scientific lectures" of the University of Heidelberg, the Max Planck Institutes in Heidelberg, and the European Molecular Biology Laboratory. The lecture announcements of all of the above-mentioned institutions are compiled monthly by the Center's Department of Public Relations and mailed upon request.

Vocational Training

For the past 15 years, the Deutsches Krebsforschungszentrum has been offering vocational training according to the Vocational Training Law, which for the past 7 years was realized in cooperation with the professional colleges of Baden-Württemberg. Most of the young apprentices work in research laboratories. Vocational training has became an integral part of the Center's work and is held in high esteem by industrial companies of the Rhine-Neckar region.

In past years, the number of vocational training programs offered by the Center has increased significantly.

Laboratory professions:

- consulting-room assistant
- biology laboratory assistant
- chemistry laboratory assistant
- radiation protection assistant (diploma; Bachelor of Science [BS])
- animal keeper (care of domestic and experimental animals)

Technical professions:

- precision mechanics
- mechanics
- joiner

Administrative professions:

- business consultants (Bachelor of Science in economics)
- commercial clerk for office communication.

In view of the lack of apprenticeships in the region, the Deutsches Krebsforschungszentrum offers modern vocational training to many more apprentices than needed by the center. By the end of 1990, more than 500 apprentices had successfully passed their final examinations, despite the continuous high level of training. The young apprentices trained by the Center are generally offered good positions in and beyond the region. The high number of applicants demonstrates the attractiveness of the Center's vocational training programs.

Since the age groups with low birthrates are now leaving school, the number of applicants is decreasing considerably. In 1990, 452 school graduates applied for a total of 25 apprenticeships at the Center; in 1991 this number had dropped to 309. Demands on the quality of the apprenticeships will increase, however. The Center's apprentices are trained in the most sophisticated techniques that go far beyond current requirements both in administrative and in laboratory skills. During their training, the apprentices get to know various departments in order to become familiar with the ever-changing aspects of a research institution.

The practical training in the laboratories is deepened and completed by regular practical and theoretical courses held at the training laboratories, which thus guarantee a valuable synthesis of theory and praxis.

The Center's vocational training goes far beyond statutory requirements, which is demonstrated by the high number – almost 50% – of early final examinations. Last year, two of our apprentices ranked best within the area of our Chamber of Commerce and Industry in their examinations as biology laboratory assistants.

Three full-time instructors are responsible for the vocational training of the Deutsches Krebsforschungszentrum.

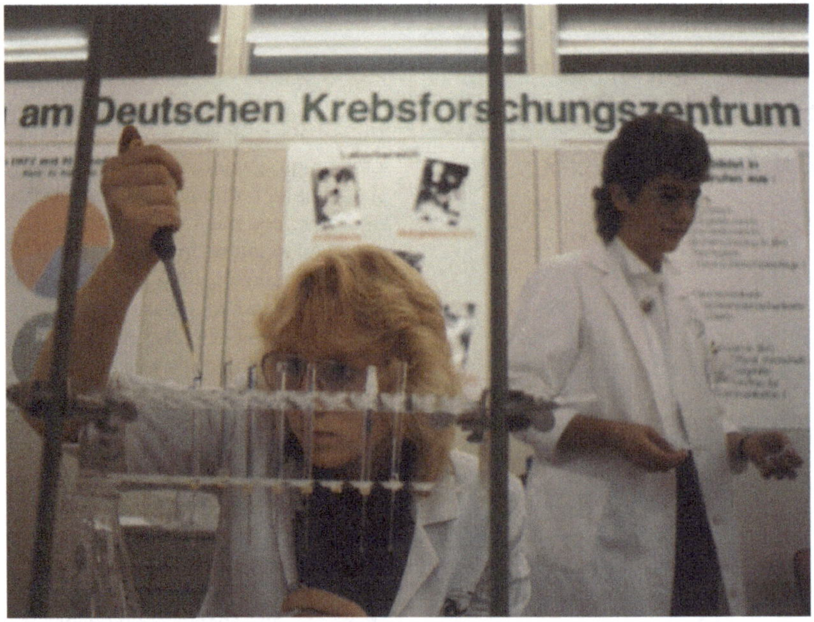

Fig. 161
Apprentices demonstrate their skills during the open house.

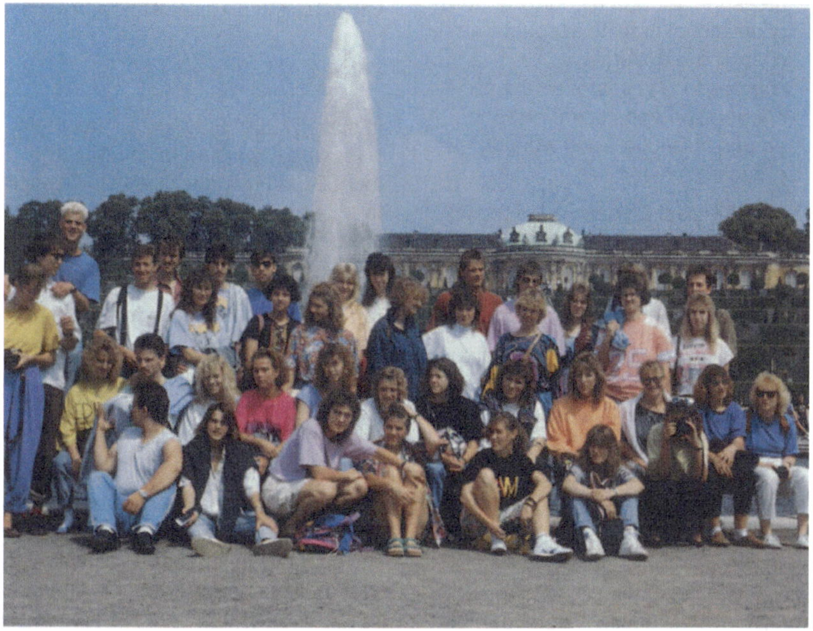

Fig. 162
The apprentices journey to Berlin.

Trainees

Apart from school classes visiting the Center to inform themselves about the focuses of work of our scientific laboratories, more than 70 high school students completed practicals offered by the Center's laboratories. Individual preferences of the trainees with regard to their field of work are taken into consideration. The practicals are an important aid for the professional orientation of young people; their duration may be between some days and several months.

More than 20 students of professional colleges majoring in biotechnology, computer sciences, electrical engineering, and industrial chemistry fulfilled their practical semester at the Krebsforschungszentrum.

Recently, the number of students in biology and medicine applying for practicals during the semester breaks has increased considerably. Preference is given to molecular biology, biochemistry, immunology, and genetics.

The large number of trainees (they are generally not paid) demonstrates the hopes and expectations that are placed on scientific laboratories for professional orientation.

Refresher Courses and Continuing Education for Employees

Since knowledge and know-how rapidly become obsolete nowadays, it is of vital interest for any company that its employees participate in refresher courses and in further training programs. During the past years, the spectrum of scientific work and its objectives have changed considerably; more complex and diverse tasks place great demands on all employees. The Center's success depends mainly on its staff. Learning is one form of work. Individual willingness to learn is also an expression of the commitment to the Deutsches Krebsforschungszentrum. Regular participation in refresher courses and further training programs are thus an important long-term investment for both the employees and the institution.

Based on a job agreement, the Center offers an extensive further training program to its staff. This program has been growing year by year. It includes successful courses from previous years and new courses selected from a multitude of general and specialized subjects on the basis of the divisions' needs and demands.

These considerations are reflected in the internal further training program, published annually, and in the decisions as to which employees should be released from work to attend courses. The Center's further training program includes

- specific measures to further the exchange of knowledge among individuals,
- measures for groups from various organizational units to account for changing requirements,
- courses for the improvement of cooperation and communication among individuals and working groups.

During the past 2 years, each participant spent a mean of 2.5 days on courses offered by the continuing education program. On average, each of the Center's employees thus spends 10 hours per year on further training. This figure, however, does not include scientific lectures, congresses organized by the divisions, or specific projects.

Since knowledge and know-how of the more than 250 diploma and doctoral students are considered vital for the efficacy of the Center's work and, thus, for its overall success, the department for continuing education has increasingly offered further training courses for these young scientists. Many participate both in the interdisciplinary 2- or 3-day seminars offered by the Graduates Promotion Program as well as in the lectures on general matters, e.g., writing scientific manuscripts or learning presentation techniques.

Graduate Student Adviser

In spring 1990 a graduate student adviser was appointed by the Management Board and the Scientific Council to support the about 300 graduates of the Center.

It is his task to help diploma and doctoral students to find an appropriate research project within the Center according to their own interests and abiblities, to establish a graduates promotion program and to help the graduates in delicate situations.

Many diploma and doctoral students have applied. Their number exceeds the capacity by three to five times. Most of the applicants come from Heidelberg, many from other German universities and some from abroad. The graduate student adviser's support is regarded as very helpful, because it is more personal and more efficient than the previous disorganized situation.

The graduate program is voluntary. It was in an experimental phase during its first year. Training courses for the improvement of communication or presentation skills were used very intensively. So were courses for methodological and theoretical know-how or for modern research techniques, which obviously are not sufficiently offered at the university.

These kinds of courses are to be offered continuously without disregarding general scientific and cancer related subjects. To foster contacts with the industry and to gain an insight into its recruitment policies in research, production, and management an information

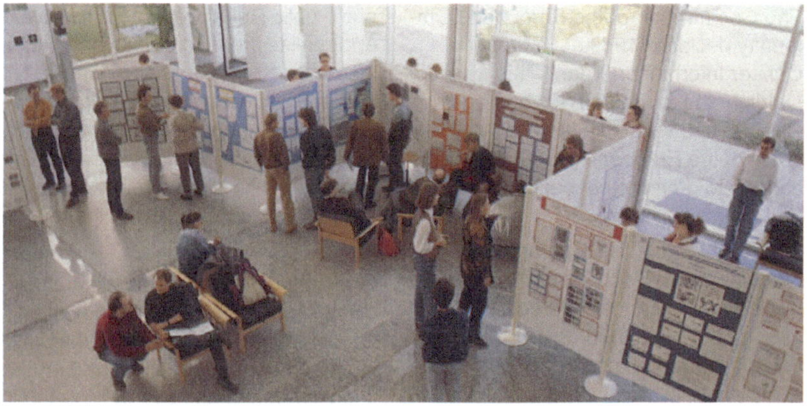

Fig. 163
Every year, a poster exhibition is organized in which the doctoral students demonstrate the results of their research work.

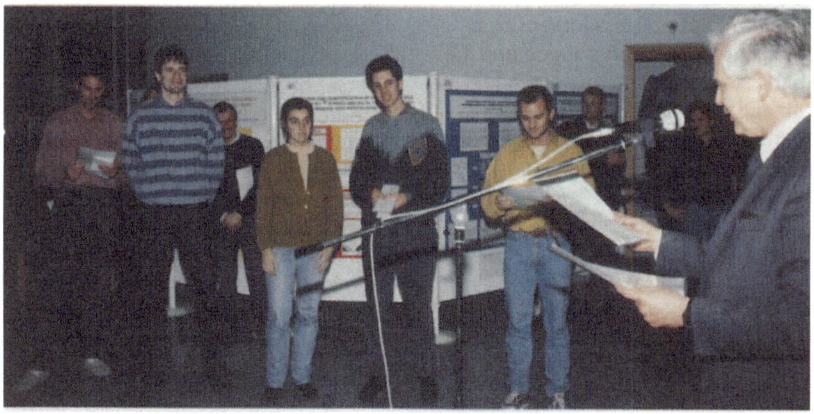

Fig. 164
Awards are presented for the best posters.

meeting was held to prepare the graduates for their careers.

Working together very intensively sometimes leads to problems; often, graduates feel at a disadvantage in a complicated situation. In such cases the active support by a neutral person has proven to be very helpful.

The experiences of the first year have confirmed that the appointment of a graduate student adviser has been very helpful.

Graduate student adviser:
Prof. Dr. Eberhard Spiess

17

Press and Public Relations

The Commission of the European Community declared 1989 as "European Cancer Information Year." This was to highlight the campaign "Europe against Cancer" and to realize the essential goals of the European program to fight cancer, to promote cancer prevention and health education.

The main goal of the program "Europe against Cancer" is to lower the expected rate of cancer-related deaths by 15% by the year 2000. By addressing various interested social groups, or likely to be interested in cancer and cancer research by use of different media, the Deutsches Krebsforschungszentrum wanted to establish a form of communication between science and the public that might serve as a model for the future. At the same time, the Department of Press and Public Relations devoted much of its attention to the preparation of the celebration of the 25th anniversary of the Deutsches Krebsforschungszentrum. The activities in the field of press and public relations were to document the Center's contribution to international cancer research and particularly the improvement of the fight against cancer in Germany.

By continuously presenting to the public results of the various research programs' and their relevance to cancer prevention, early diagnosis, and therapy of cancer diseases, the Deutsches Krebsforschungszentrum has assumed a key role in the fight against cancer in Germany. Since it is a "neutral" Federal institution, people expect it to produce "first hand" and authoritative information about the state of research on, and the fight against, cancer.

The concept of the Center's program of activities was worked out at the beginning of 1988. The Department of Press and Public Relations set out to develop and realize ideas to employ the various instruments of information effectively and productively. The goal was to open the Center along with its programs and research results to the general public and to specific target groups and to elucidate its contribution to the fight against cancer.

One cannot inform the public about cancer research in the same way as about high energy physics. When talking about cancer, irrational and emotional components have to be taken into consideration, taboos, psychological and mental barriers, suffering and grief, high expectations and desperation because of the perceived restrictedness of diagnostical and therapeutical possibilites. In addition, the messages about the possibility of preventing certain types of cancer such as lung cancer have only a limited effect, since they have to compete with, for example, the smoker's "cognitive dissonance" and the unavoidable abstractness of the information that in general cannot take account of the specific social environment and the individual situation.

1. The Region

As a national institution, the Krebsforschungszentrum is part of a tight network of international, European and non-European, research activities. At the same time it has to justify its expenses to the German tax payer and should thus involve the local community in such a way that it understands and supports the Center as "its" institution.

Series of popular-science lectures

A concept of popular-science lectures was elaborated in intensive discussions with the Center's scientists; its realization began in the spring of 1989. The local community is thus given the advantage of obtaining comprehensible "first-hand information" from cancer experts and of discussing with the researchers in person.

Topics of the lecture series "Cancer Research News," held between May 1989 and May 1990

Medication against Cancer (the late Prof. Dr. Dietrich Schmähl)

Immunotherapy – an Additional Strategy in Cancer Treatment? (Prof. Dr. Volker Schirrmacher)

Cancer Diagnosis with new Methods – Insights into the Human Body (Prof. Dr. Gerhard van Kaick)

Viruses as a Cause of Cancer? (Prof. Dr. Harald zur Hausen)

Environment and Cancer – Strategies for Cancer Prevention (Prof. Dr. Rudolf Preußmann)

Cancer – Disturbed Intracellular Communication (Prof. Dr. Friedrich Marks)

With the Arms of the Immune System – New Approaches for Diagnostics and Therapy (Prof. Dr. Peter Krammer)

Cancer Diseases in the General Population – Frequency, Regional Variations, and Possible Causes (Prof. Dr. Jürgen Wahrendorf)

Cancer – a Genetic Accident? (Prof. Dr. Manfred Schwab)

Defense of Cancer – Directly Changing the Immune System (Prof. Dr. Stefan Meuer)

Open house

On Saturday, September 23, 1989, the Deutsches Krebsforschungszentrum invited the general public to an open house. In a building of more than twelve floors, narrow hallways, eight institutes, and a number of central installations, the planning of and the preparations for such an undertaking take many months, thus reducing the research capacity of the Center.

An open house offers the general public an immediate insight into research and an opportunity to contact and to talk to scientists. In addition, almost all the life and natural sciences that are working on cancer research are present in the Deutsches Krebsforschungszentrum. As a contribution to the Cancer Information Year, the open house thus seemed to be the best way to offer up-to-date information. About 9000 visitors were introduced to problems of cancer research, its methods and working conditions, and its latest results between 10 a. m. and the official closing at 5 p.m., which in fact was extended to 8 p.m. The public was informed about the event on billboards and by supporting prereports in the regional media. The underlying idea was to open the Center without any restriction. Problems related to the use of animals in cancer research were also discussed. For this purpose a closed sta-

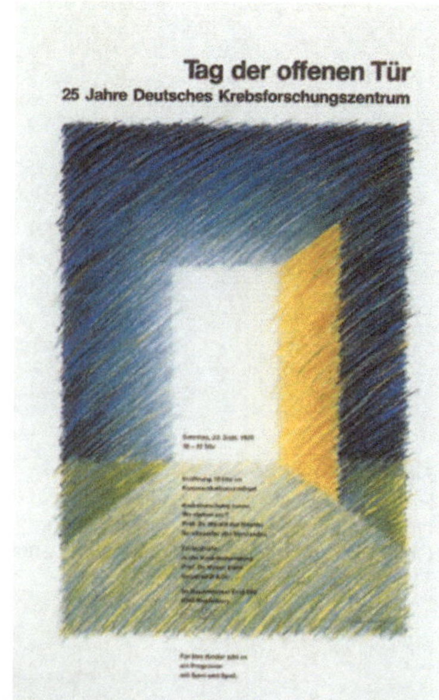

Fig. 165
An open house was organized on the occasion of the 25th anniversary of the Deutsches Krebsforschungszentrum.

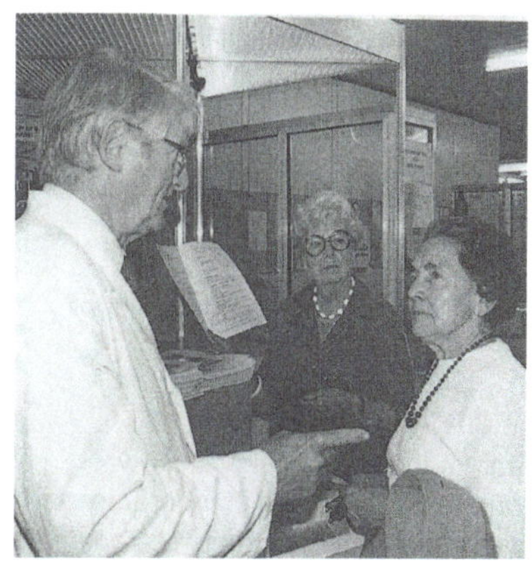

Fig. 166
Prof. Dr. Klaus Munk talking to visitors.

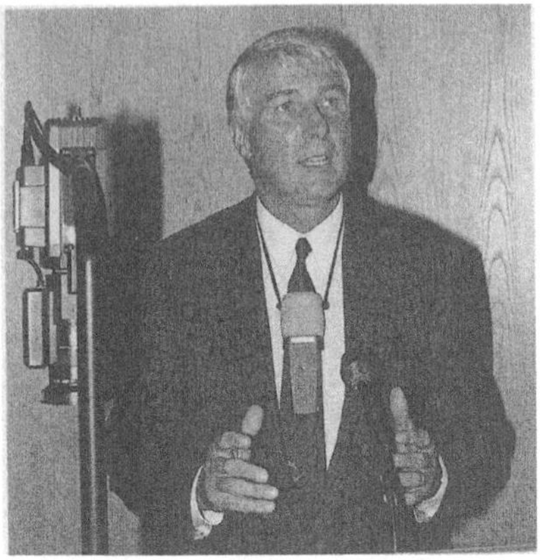

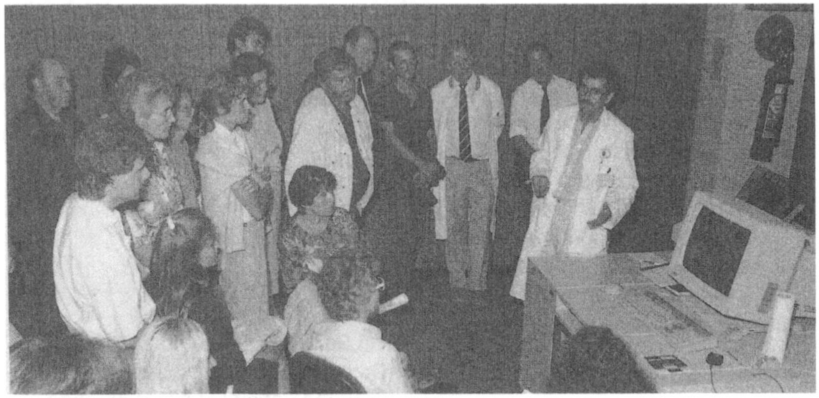

Fig. 167
Prof. Dr. Volker Diehl, director of the University Clinics of Internal Medicine, Cologne, lectured on "Advances in Cancer Therapy".

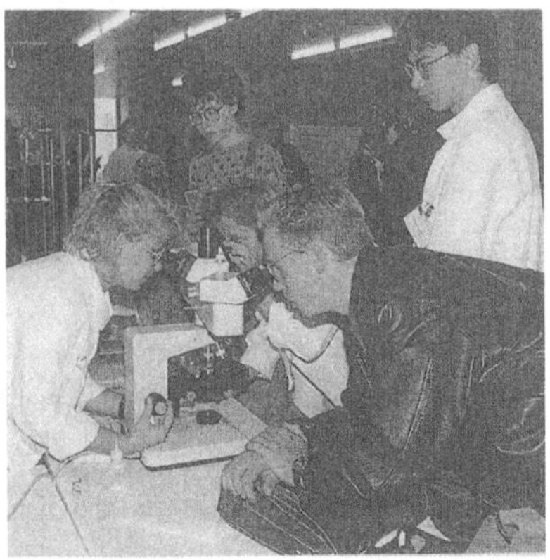

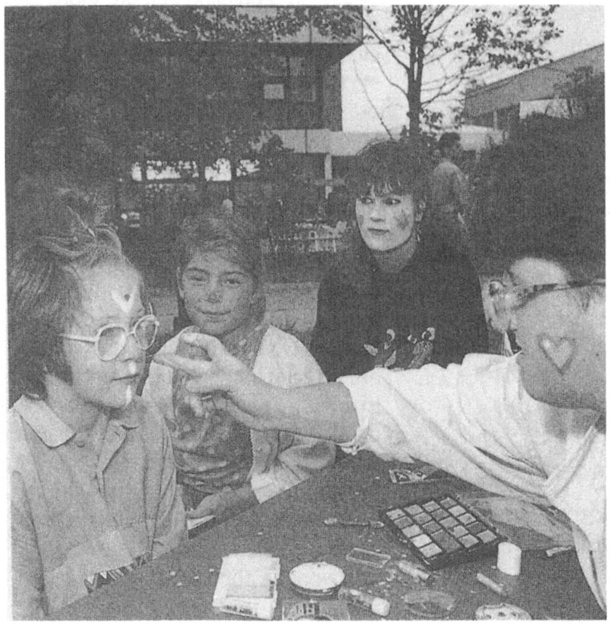

Figs. 168–170
Communication with various groups of visitors.

tion of the animal laboratory was opened. All species of laboratory animals held in the Center were presented and the investigations done with them or on them were explained to the interested public.

Besides information booths from each of the Center's sections, the central information booth provided publications and descriptions on all of the Center's divisions open to the public. Written by scientists, this background information served to deepen the understanding of the facts presented. The visitors to the Center's open house were integrated into the campaign "Europe Against Cancer" with the help of a booklet that the Center had published for the first time. "Die zehn Regeln zur Bekämpfung des Krebses und ihre wissenschaftlichen Grundlagen" (The Ten Rules for Cancer Prevention and Their Scientific Background) contains the European codex against cancer and integrates the scientific background of worldwide research results.

Individual questions were answered at the booth of the Cancer Information Service (KID), from which a free, anonymous telephone hotline was installed to the Center's KID office.

2. The General Public

It was decided that, in addition to informing the local population, all members of the general public interested in the results, and problem areas, of cancer research should be targeted. Not only patients and relatives, but all those afraid of possibly falling ill with cancer were to be clearly informed about the progress made in cancer research, the application of which in the clinical practice is not usually immediately possible. Currently available diagnostic and therapeutic options were to be shown in order to demonstrate how the individual can benefit from today's knowledge.

A. Special edition of the magazine "einblick"

Since the importance of this step-by-step progress becomes clearer if seen in the historical context, the Deutsches

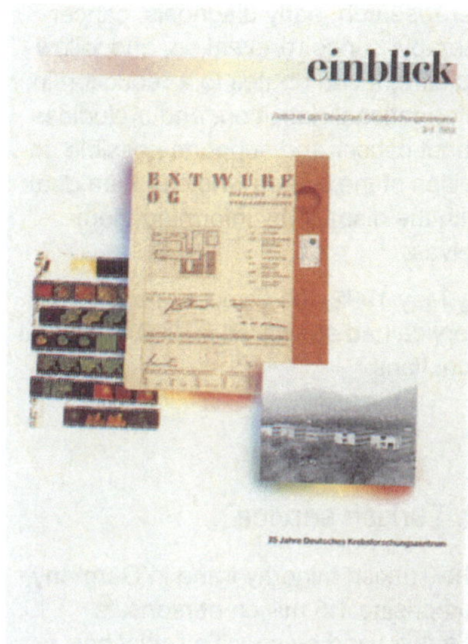

Fig. 171

Krebsforschungszentrum has published a double issue of the magazine "einblick," dedicated to the history of the Center, its institutes, research programs, and projects. This issue also contains an historical overview of the scientific and health-political background that led to the foundation of the Center and have determined its structural development.

Texts that are easy to understand, descriptive pictures, a stimulating layout, these are the tools "einblick" has used since 1987 to publicize science.

The key concepts behind the idea of "einblick" are transparency, information, and communication. The reader is given an insight into the many scientific disciplines which work together on solving the cancer problem. "Einblick" also wants to provide the reader with ready criteria that will help him to assess the importance of scientific results. Freelance journalists, who assist the editorial staff, write from a critical and unbiased "outside point of view".

The constantly growing number of subscribers – presently there are 6000 – indicate the public's great interest in cancer research.

B. Current Cancer Research – Reports from the Deutsches Krebsforschungszentrum

On the occasion of the 25th anniversary of the Deutsches Krebsforschungszentrum, a commemorative volume was published, which extensively reviewed the research program.

Springer-Verlag Heidelberg, New York, Paris, Tokyo and Steinkopff-Verlag Darmstadt published a first English edition in 1989. It had fostered the communication with scientists and science journalists from abroad.

C. Cancer Information Service for the public

Even the best publication cannot hide the fact that immediate personal contact is the most successful mediator of facts. Only in a face-to-face conversation is it possible to consider the personal situation of our vis-à-vis, his individual problem and his level of language. It is possible to clarify misunderstandings, to hold back unrequested facts, and follow an associative line of talk.

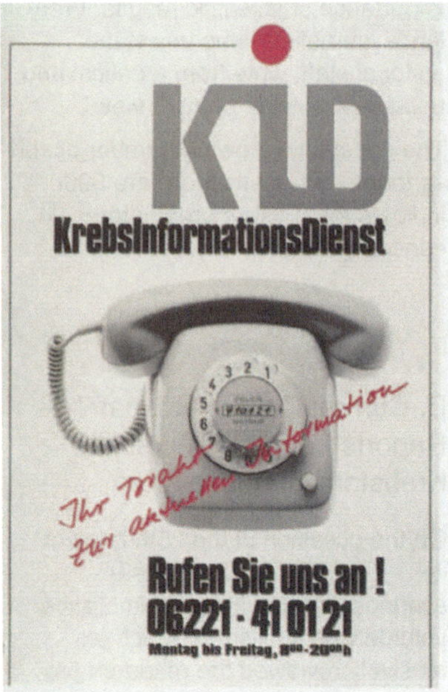

Fig. 172

All this was the basis for the creation of the telephone Cancer Information Service (KID), which was established as a model program in 1988. This service, which addresses the general public, is supported by the Deutsches Krebsforschungszentrum and the Tumor Center Heidelberg/Mannheim and is financed by the Federal Ministry of Health. The Ministry of Labor, Health, Family, and Women of the State of Baden-Württemberg also provides considerable financial support for the project.

The Cancer Information Service is a bridge in cancer information and corrects problems in the communication of scientific results to the public. Its task is to promote or to establish fast access to the latest information on cancer, cancer research, early diagnosis, cancer therapy, cancer prevention, and follow-up care. It contributes to a reduction in informational deficit on, and prejudices about cancer and supports possible activities of the callers who can then deal with the disease by informing themselves.

By May 1992, the Cancer Information Service had answered 60 000 individual questions.

D. Turkish service

The Turkish minority living in Germany, comprising 1.5 million persons, is characterized by specific social barriers, language problems, and cultural isolation, and will no longer be excluded from an often vital, easily accessible information service on cancer.

E. The "Ten Rules for Fighting Cancer"

"Einblick," "Current Cancer Research," the "Cancer Information Service," the series of lectures "News from Cancer Research," and the open house were supplemented by the brochure "Die zehn Regeln zur Bekämpfung des Krebses und ihre wissenschaftlichen Grundlagen" (The Ten Rules for Fighting Cancer and Their Scientific Background), which was published, on the basis of the Center's research results, for the European "Cancer Information Year".

The concept behind this publication was to explain the basic message of the program "Europe against Cancer" – which, as is described in the "European codex against cancer," illustrates the importance of cancer prevention and its early diagnosis – and to prove its relevance by presenting research results in such a way that even a critical citizen is willing to consider the facts.

The brochure was compiled on the basis of scientific publications that support or discuss the message of the codex. With the support of the Commision of the European Community, 20 000 copies were printed and published in 1989.

F. Health education in schools

The measures mentioned also address two important subgroups of the general public, namely school children and teachers. Young persons, being open for information and capable of reorienting their lives, are a particularly important audience for information on health and research, as are their teachers, who are better multiplicators than most other professionals.

In the region of Heidelberg, students and teachers were thus important target groups for information on the Center's series of lectures and its open house. Many school classes used the open house to find out about cancer research. During 1989, the Department of Press and Public Relations organized guided tours for 25 school classes with 446 students, explaining projects and methods of cancer research. (In the same year, a total of 880 visitors participated in guided tours through the Center.) Groups of students came from all parts of Germany.

3. Journalists and the "Cancer Information Year"

In our modern society, journalists of the print and broadcast media play a decisive role in spreading information about cancer. The Department of Press and Public Relations is thus in continuous and close contact with journalists from Germany and abroad, especially with scientific and medical journalists.

There was a particularly high number of press reports during 1989, which was due to initiatives taken by the Commission of the European Community and supported by the German Federal Government's "National Coordinating Cancer Control Program." Television teams from private and public TV stations produced reports for well over 50 telecasts. One hundred and fifty interviews and background talks with the Center's scientists were arranged by the Department of Press and Public Relations. The visitors were offered, among other things, discussion programs, documentations, and preparative talks.

A total of 38 press releases were the basis for press reports on current research topics. As a consequence, about 500 newspaper articles, with a total circulation of well over 80 million copies, reported on the Deutsches Krebsforschungszentrum.

In collaboration with the heads of the specialized and press departments of the Federal Ministry of Research and Technology a press symposium was organized in Bonn. The aim was to discuss cancer research in the context of the Federal government's research promotion program "Health for Everybody" and the government's science policy. Addressees of this seminary were the correspondents and science journalists living in the area of Bonn; they were given specialized information, supplemented by current political evaluation through the Federal Secretary of Research and Technology.

A special edition of the British magazine "Interdisciplinary Science Reviews" (Vol 14, No. 3), London, on the Center's role in the international research network featured articles written by the Center's scientists. The special edition was published on the occasion of the Center's 25th anniversary. Mailed out to European and non-European science and medical journalists, this issue was an important basis for reports on the state of cancer research in the Federal Republic of Germany.

4. Internal Communication

The increased efforts to inform the public about the current state of cancer research and about the contribution of the Center has required a motivated staff, especially highly motivated researchers who accept this task as an integral part of their work. They are needed for establishing and furthering internal and external contacts, as authors of reports and articles, as

Fig. 173
Opening of the art exhibition of Maria-Luise Krapp (right): Beate Weber, at the time a member of the European Parliament, today chief mayor of the city of Heidelberg, and Dr. Reinhard Grunwald, administrative member of the Board of Trustees.

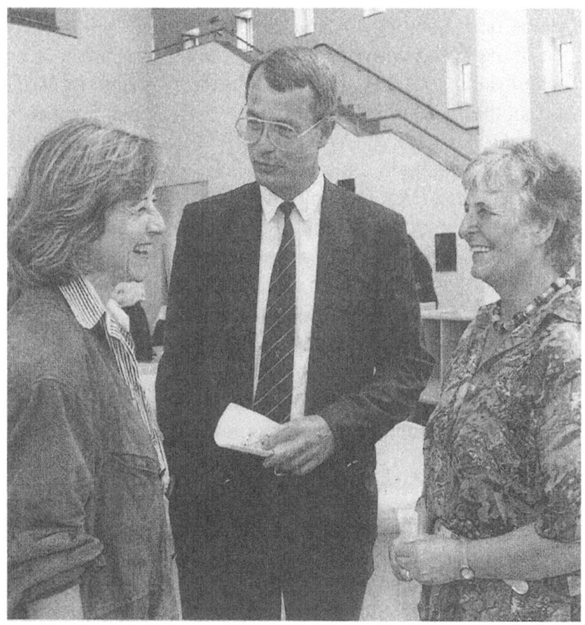

referees, as interview partners, and as speakers.

Ways and methods had to be found to get the scientists to participate – in the sense of corporate identity – in activities that they perceived either as a pleasure or which gave them access to new scientific information. As a special offer to both established and young researchers of the Center, a symposium "Concepts in Oncology" was conceived by the Management Board. This symposium brought together researchers from the United States, Israel, the United Kingdom, Sweden, and Germany. It was accompanied by a guided tour through the Center, which also helped to deepen the contacts.

Commemoration of the Center's 25th anniversary

On the occasion of the commemoration of the 25th anniversary of the Center on October 31, 1989, the President of the Federal Republic of Germany, Dr. Richard von Weizsäcker, Baden-Württemberg's Minister of Science and Arts, Prof. Dr. Helmut Englert, and the undersecretary in the Federal Ministry of Research and Technology, Dr. Gebhard Ziller used the opportunity for extensive discussions with scientists of the Center and to acquire information about their research results. The festivities summarized the contribution of the Center to the continuous development of cancer research and to its part in improving the fight against cancer.

A book titled "Krebsforschung in Deutschland – Vorgeschichte und Geschichte des Deutschen Krebsforschungszentrums" (Cancer Research in Germany – A History of the Deutsches Krebsforschungszentrum) was presented to document the historic context of this ceremony. It was edited by Prof. Dr. Gustav Wagner, emeritus and director of the former Institute of Epidemiology, Biometry, and Statistics, and by Andrea Mauerberger, doctoral student at the Institute of Recent History of the Ludwig Maximilian University in Munich (Springer Verlag Heidelberg, 1989).

Also on this occasion, the Deutsches Krebsforschungszentrum, together with the Springer Verlag, edited a facsimile reprint of a seminal work of the founder of the Center, Prof. Dr. Karl-Heinrich Bauer's "Mutationstheorie der Geschwulstenstehung" (Theory of the Mutation of Tumor Development), published for the first time in 1928 by Julius Springer Verlag Berlin.

The new communications center, which consists of a 290-seat lecture hall, two connecting conference rooms, and – in addition to a spacious entrance hall – rooms for teaching laboratories, had been finished just in time for celebrating the 25th anniversary and were inaugurated in a separate ceremony.

Current activities

In addition to the activities centured around the Center's 25th anniversary and the European "Cancer Information Year," the Deutsches Krebsforschungszentrum and its visitors' service have tried to offer each visiting group an individual guided tour through the Center. During 1989/1990, a total of 200 groups consisting of 3500 persons toured the Center's laboratories and were introduced to its tasks and structure. In addition, the Press Department has organized more than 80 congresses and workshops and given advice for a number of lectures organized by the university or other research institutions.

Press symposia were held on the occasion of the international symposium of the Section Experimental Cancer Research of the German Cancer Society on April 12, 1989, and of the annual meeting of the Association of Major Research Institutions, which took place for the first time on November 7, 1990, in Heidelberg under the chairmanship of Prof. Dr. Harald zur Hausen. Other press symposia discussed the current state of Papilloma research (May 15, 1990), the state of the collaboration of the European cancer information services (October 19, 1990, on the occasion of the meeting of the European working group of the cancer information services, which was organized by the Center's Cancer Information Service), and the annual report of the Tumor Center Heidelberg/Mannheim (November 27, 1990).

In 1990, about 90 journalists and teams took part in background talks, interviews and film productions. Thirty press releases, among these, two on the Tumor Center Heidelberg/Mannheim, supplemented the spectrum of information.

The working programs of 1989 and 1990, as well as the preparations for the Center's 25th anniversary in 1988, were greatly supported by trainees working in the press department. In the past, the Center made genuine efforts to promote young science journalists. Science journalism and public relations are still dominated by persons of the first generation, which has lead to a deficit in well-trained young journalists and public relations specialists. Trainees, who are often fellows of the Robert Bosch Foundation or of the Study Foundation of the German People, are given independent editorial work to teach them the organizational processes and coordinating mechanisms necessary in the public relations work of a research center.

Three, seven, and nine trainees worked in the Department for Press and Public Relations in 1988, 1989, and 1990, respectively. They were graduate biologists, natural sciences teachers, graduate students of biology, students of ecotrophology, journalism, and public relations. From 1986 to May 1992, a total of 41 trainees worked in the press department. For some, their writing for the Center's magazine "einblick" was the starting point of a career as a freelance science journalist, which has led them to jobs on the editorial staff of large newspapers, magazines, or science programs on television. Without the editorial and organizational work of the department's trainees it would have been hardly possible to carry out all of the public relations measures described above.

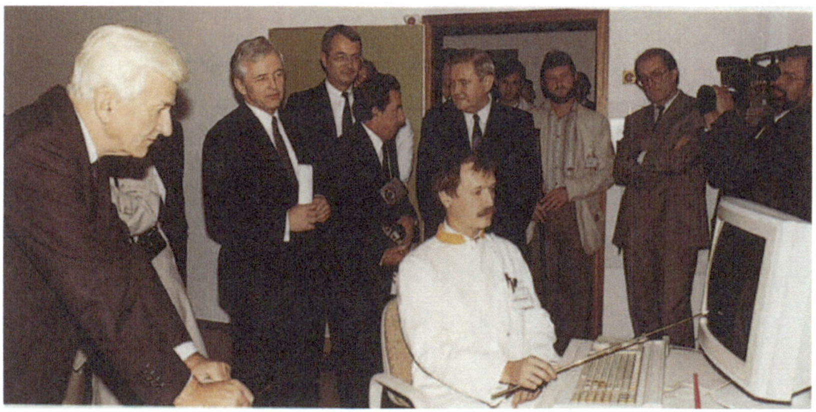

Fig. 174
Prof. Dr. Gerhard van Kaick explains details of the positron emission tomography to the President of Germany Dr. Richard von Weizsäcker.

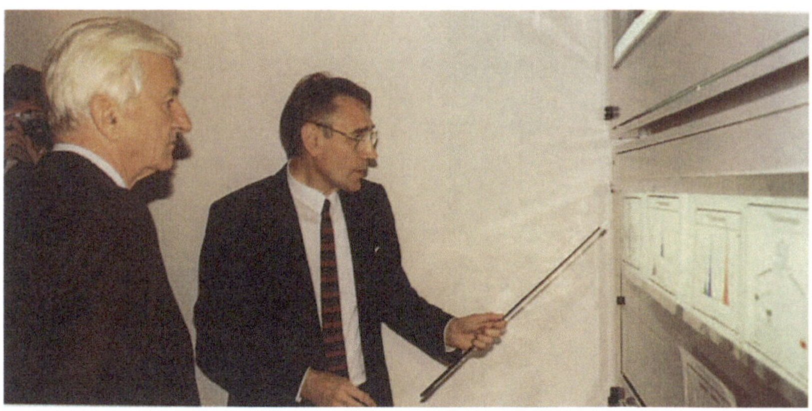

Fig. 175
Priv.-Doz. Dr. Wolfhard Semmler demonstrates an examination with the magnetic resonance tomographer.

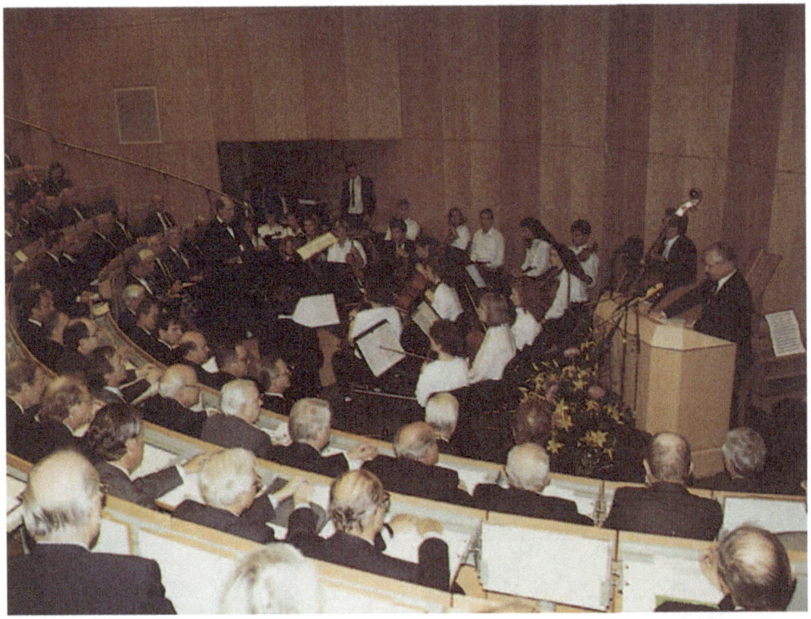

Fig. 176
Celebration of the inauguration of the newly built communication center on October, 31, 1989.

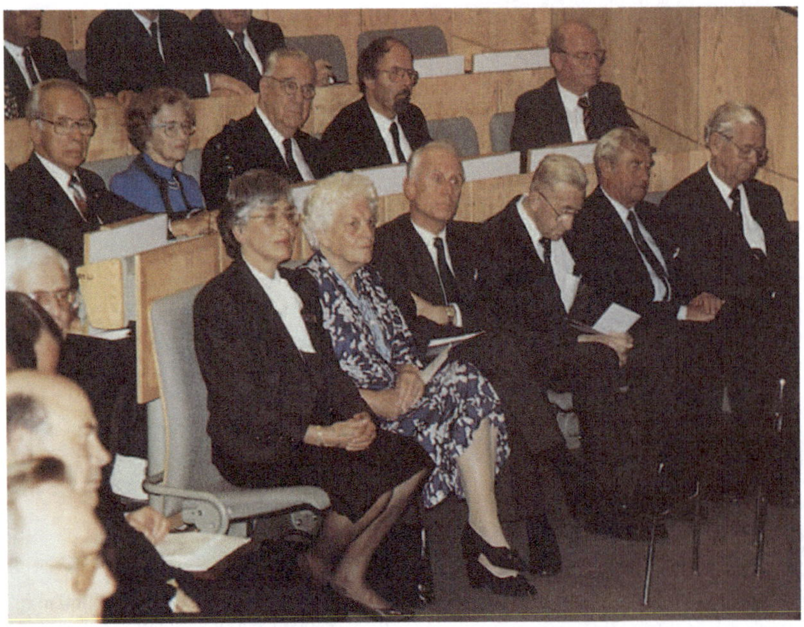

Fig. 177
From left to right: First row: Ingeborg Bauer and her daughter, Dr. Monika Gottstein, Prof. Dr. Ulrich Gottstein, Prof. Dr. Bernhard Timm, Prof. Dr. Gotthard Schettler, Prof. Dr. Fritz Linder. Second row: Prof. Hans Neurath and Susanne Neurath, Prof. Dr. Wilhelm Doerr.

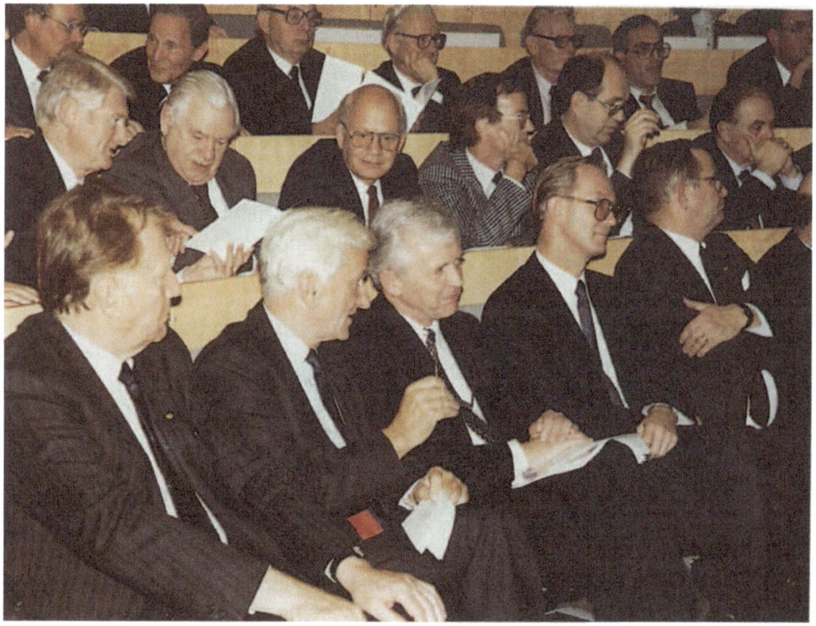

Fig. 178
From left to right: First row: The Minister for Sciences of the State Baden-Württemberg Dr. Kurt Engler, the President of Germany Dr. Richard von Weizsäcker, Prof. Dr. Harald zur Hausen, Prof. Dr. Hubert Markl, President of the German Research Association (Deutsche Forschungsgemeinschaft), undersecretary Dr. Gebhard Ziller of the Federal Ministry for Research and Technology. Second row: Prof. Dr. Klaus Munk, Prof. Dr. Gustav Wagner, Prof. Dr. Erich Hecker, Prof. Dr. Günter Hämmerling, Prof. Dr. Werner Franke, chairman of the Scientific Council, Prof. Petre Tautu – former and managing directors of the Center. Last row: Dr. Ernst-Lüder Solte and Prof. Dr. Otto Westphal, former members of the Board of Trustees of the Deutsches Krebsforschungszentrum.

Fig. 179
The German President talks to the chairman of the coordinating committee of the Tumor Center Heidelberg/Mannheim, Prof. Dr. Christian Herfarth (center), and to Prof. Dr. Walter Lorenz.

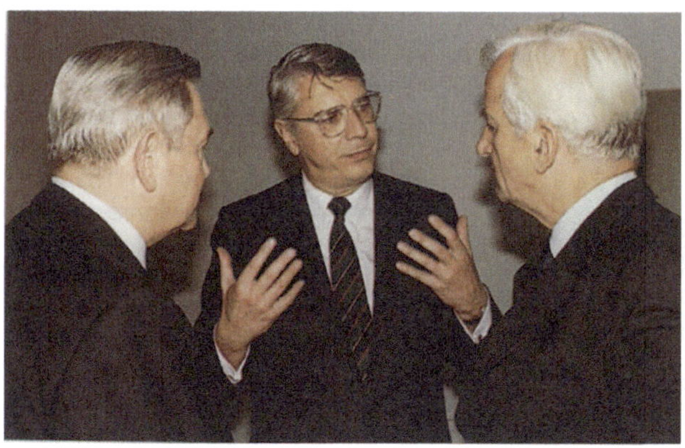

Fig. 180
Prof. Dr. Bernard Mechler explains a microscope preparation of drosophila to the President Dr. Richard von Weizsäcker. Drosophila is used to investigate the genetic causes of the development of cancers.

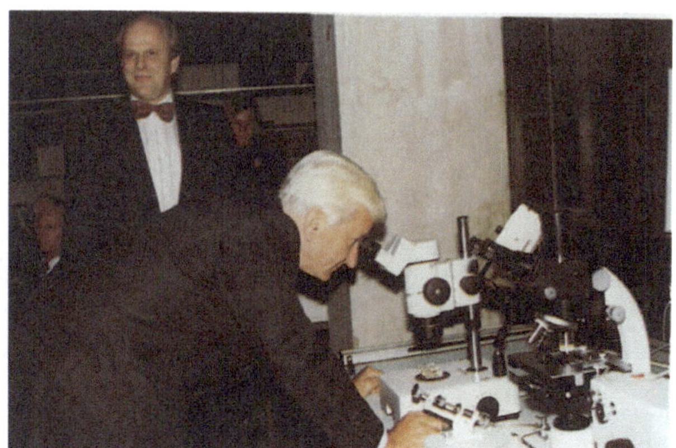

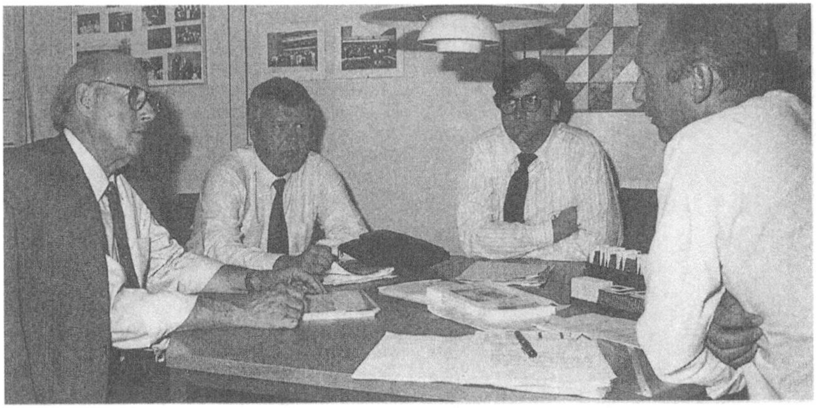

Fig. 181
Visiting the Deutsches Krebsforschungszentrum. Members of parliament Christian Lenzer (left) and Erich Maas (second to left), and Wilfrid Kraus (second to right), secretary of the research and technology working group of the Christian Democratic Union of Germany (CDU), talking to the epidemiologist Prof. Dr. Jürgen Wahrendorf.

Fig. 182
The chairman of the Board of Trustees, undersecretary Dr. Josef Rembser (second to right) and the vice-chairman, assistant secretary Dr. Heribert Knorr (third to right) inquire about activities in the areas of diagnostics and therapy research. Talking to them (from right to left): Prof. Dr. Walter Lorenz, Dr. Wolfgang Maier-Borst, Prof. Dr. Gerhard van Kaick. In the back: Hans Hietzker.

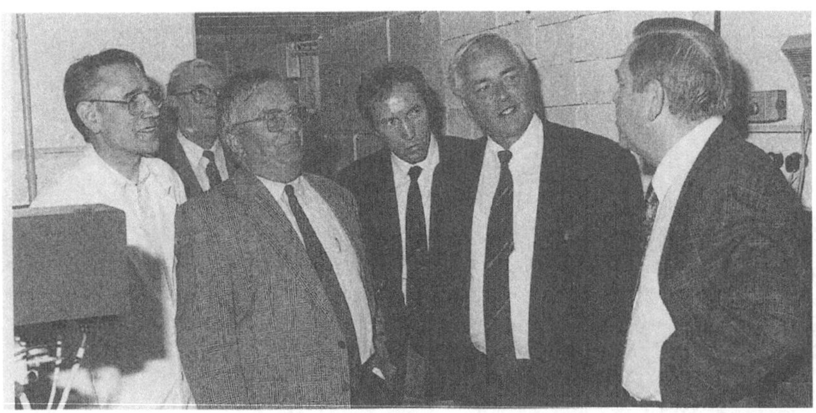

The Cancer Information Service - Mediator between Science and the Public

Since 1986, the Deutsches Krebsforschungszentrum has offered a telephone Cancer Information Service (KID). From Monday through Friday, 8 a.m. to 8 p.m., anybody can call – anonymously, if so desired – to obtain free information on all cancer-related questions. The telephone service is sponsored by the German Cancer Research Center and integrated in the Tumor Center Heidelberg/Mannheim. Initially financed as a model program by the Federal Ministry for Youth, Family, Women, and Health, the public's increasing interest demonstrates that KID has become a successful mediator between research and the public. Since 1991, KID has been funded on a long-term basis by the Federal Ministry of Health. Annual financial support is also given by the Ministry of Labor, Health, Family, and Women of the Land of Baden-Württemberg.

This service is based on the public's strong interest in cancer research and cancer therapy, and the host of inquiries directed to the Deutsches Krebsforschungszentrum indicate that there is a great demand for information in oncology, a field which is extremely complex and confusing for a layman. Though cancer is a potential vital threat to many people, not enough factual information on the subject is, in general, available. Experience shows that physicians and medical specialists often cannot meet the needs and expectations of patients and their families once the primary treatment has been carried out. When it comes to questions regarding personal details of the treatment, or the significance of various diagnostic methods, or the future life, especially concerning the appropriate diet, the patient and his family often feel left alone. The mass media, as a possible source of information, tend to confuse the patient with unrelated news rather than to help him with useful information. Experience, however, has shown that factual information can be of substantial help in dealing with problems that arrive and in promoting the patient's own activities.

The Cancer Information Service thus set itself the task of compensating for the lack of reliable information about the causes, prevention, early diagnosis, and therapy of cancer, as well as about social matters and matters in the field of social legislation. KID attempts to reduce fears by promoting factual information. The results of national and international research have been incorporated into a new concept of cancer information geared to the interested public, cancer patients, their families and friends. KID was inspired by and based on the National Cancer Institute's Cancer Information Service in the USA., which has been working successfully since 1975. The telephone offers the possibility to answer questions individually and to open up active access to current knowledge in oncology to the caller (who may remain anonymous).

It is the primary goal of the Cancer Information Service to provide rapid access to up-to-date information on cancer, cancer research, prevention, diagnosis, therapy, follow-up, as well as to provide addresses of health institutions working on cancer problems. Also, KID promotes the public's awareness of cancer prevention by offering information on prevention and early diagnosis. KID informs both healthy persons who ask for information on methods of prevention or the current state of cancer research, as well as cancer patients, their families and friends, who need information in order to be able to deal with their own or a patient's situation.

A multidisciplinary team of 27 employees and freelance cancer communicators works toward achieving this goal. The task of giving telephone information is undertaken by 20 free-lance cancer communicators who operate KID's four telephone lines each Monday through Friday between 8 a.m. and 8 p.m. They are the heart of the Cancer Information Service and embody its basic idea; to provide clear, well-founded, and topical information on cancer, tailored to the individual caller. All of them are health professionals: physicians, pharmacists, chemists, nurses, psychologists, or medical-technical assistants. However, none are specially trained oncologists, so the use of technical language is reduced to a minimum. Once a year, all staff members participate in a basic training program on oncology, during which clinical and research specialists teach new trends in medicine and methodology as well as conversational techniques. This teaching course is supplemented by continuous information on various matters and on current events in oncology.

The necessary support information is compiled by the team of full-time staff members who are KID's organizational backbone. Here, the Deutsches Krebsforschungszentrum and the Tumor Center Heidelberg/Mannheim are valuable sources of information for KID, without which the staff members would not be able to answer the sometimes very complex questions. Most information is obtained by personal contact or by telephone from scientists of the Krebsforschungszentrum, oncologists at clinics of the Tumor Center Heidelberg/ Mannheim, clinicians and researchers of other research institutions throughout Germany and abroad, and from administrations of German public health organizations. The staff consults the Center's central library which comprises more than 63000 volumes, as well as the international biomedical online literature data bases, which are available in the department of scientific information. The information is then translated into comprehensible language and given to the telephone staff, who use it to answer incoming questions. The scientific staff prepares text based on frequently asked questions or matters of particular interest, this guarantee that standardized responses are given to relevant inquiries, and these texts are updated on a regular basis.

As a consequence of the continuous compilation of information, KID's database has increased considerably over the years. The information is structured, organized, and made accessible to the telephone staff through the aid of a special database (PARADISE) installed PC network. KID's database contains and organizes two main data sets:
1) text information of basic topics in oncology, accessible through key words, and 2) about 1700 addresses of tumor centers, oncologic and research institutions, aftercare clinics, psycho-social cancer counselling services, self-help groups, and other organizations that the caller may be referred to if necessary, as well as specialists at various medical centers who can be contacted by the scientific staff for specialized infor-

mation. KID carried out surveys to obtain current information on aftercare clinics and psycho-social counselling services. Important abstracts, publications in non-scientific periodicals, manuscripts of lectures in oncology, summaries and announcements of the American National Cancer Institute, and other papers are compiled in a retrieval system which presently contains 3000 entries. This system allows KID to rapidly and easily access the stored data. KID's database, its reference library containing the most important oncologic manuals, and – if printed material is asked for – its collection of brochures on cancer (offered by various German publishers), make it possible to immediately answer about 75% of all questions. The remaining questions are new or so complex that they require further investigation. The caller may call again later to obtain the results of the investigation or, upon request, is called back by KID.

Continuous exchange of information with clinicians and scientists of the Tumor Center, who may also refer to colleagues of other institutions, ensures that all information given is well-founded and up-to-date. Continuous staff training and periodical training by an experienced psychologist that includes in-depth discussions of individual cases, ensures that all information given is of high quality. The scientific council of the Cancer Information Service, composed of clinicians of the Tumor Center and scientists of the Deutsches Krebsforschungszentrum, is responsible for basic decisions with regard to content.

A call record form for continuous statistical evaluation has been developed to analyze all incoming calls. It contains – anonymously and coded – the most important aspects of each call. This makes it possible to respond to the callers' needs and to continuously evaluate, develop, and improve KID. For example, KID tries to define and to remove specific information deficits among certain population groups. The Turkish service, for example, is available three times a week in order to serve the largest ethnic minority in Germany. Another example is the need for information in eastern Germany. The latter poses new challenges to the Cancer Information Service, not only with regard to the number of calls and hence the number of investigations, but above all because of the particular medical care infrastructure and attitude towards cancer, and thus new contents of communication. In 1991, these additional requirements were accounted for by increasing the capacity for investigations and enlarging the telephone service. Deficiencies of telecommunications between eastern and western Germany have meant that people in eastern Germany have been obliged to write letters, as a result of which KID has established a special letter service for answering these written inquiries.

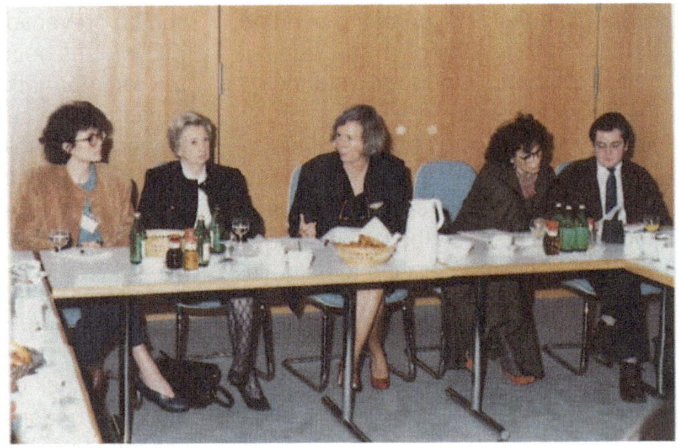

Fig. 183
Press conference at the meeting of the European cancer information services in Heidelberg. From left to right: Representatives of the British, French, German, Israeli, and Spanish cancer information services.

The population in western Germany makes extensive use of KID by telephone; 41.2% of the callers are patients, 36.6% relatives of patients, 9.4% interested citizens, who are affected neither directly nor indirectly and who are a prime target with regard to cancer prevention, and 7% are professionals from various health institutions, mostly physicians and nursing staff. Approximately two thirds of the callers are women, and the majority of the inquiries are on breast cancer. Male callers mostly inquire about cancers of the colon, prostate, and lung. Inquiries about treatment account for 69.2% of the questions, which corresponds to the large number of patients among the callers. Most of the callers are between

40 and 59 years of age. Most of the calls referring to a specific disease are made after the first treatment, i.e., after primary medical care. This seems to indicate that most patients and their families are frequently left without proper information. KID focuses on providing support and information. Callers that are interested but not affected mainly inquire about symptoms, followed by risk factors, diagnostical methods, and early diagnosis.

Beyond these statistical analyses, KID's experience has revealed a host of new questions which have been investigated since 1987 in accompanying studies. One project being carried out in cooperation with the Research Institute of Social Developments of the University of Mannheim, deals with the "investigation of the public's point of view on cancer related issues". The data is compiled by surveying approximately 300 randomly selected callers who consented to a telephone interview. One section of the investigation tries to elucidate attitudes, opinions, hopes, and knowledge with regard to cancer, cancer medicine, and prevention. In this context, too, one focus is to determine the primary and secondary prevention behaviors and the acceptance of early diagnosis examinations as provided by law. The purpose of this study is to establish if there is a correlation between ideas and expectations on the one hand, and scientific and personal realities on the other hand. The study also tries to elucidate the role of the print media in developing people's ideas and feelings of insecurity about cancer. It is the goal of the study to contribute to the future development of communication and user-oriented information in the field of public health with regard to cancer problems, based on a definition of its present state.

KID represents and evaluates a new concept of cancer information and is part of the Federal government's cancer control program. Within the past years, cancer telephone information services and helplines have been established all over Europe and beyond. A first international workshop was initiated and organized by KID in 1987, followed by annual meetings, at which staff from information services and helplines discussed aspects of their work and evaluated options for coordination and cooperation.

Present user data shows that in Germany the establishment of the cancer information service has proven successful. KID fulfilled the goal of the initial pilot phase to evaluate and to meet the assumed public's demand for information on cancer. The number of calls is a measure of KID's success. During the 6 years since its establishment, more than 65 000 calls were answered by KID. KID is accepted both by scientists and clinicians, who supported KID from the beginning. The experiences during the initial pilot phase (ending in 1990) were used to constantly improve the service, its structure, and its expansion in order to serve populations who previously had no access to information on cancer. The results also mark the beginning of a new stage of work, which started in 1991 with the financing of KID as a permanent project of the Deutsches Krebsforschungszentrum.

KID – the public cancer information service can be reached by calling +6221/410121.

Meetings, Workshops, and Symposia

Since its inauguration, the Deutsches Krebsforschungszentrum has been concerned with intensifying and promoting the exchange of information between scientists at home and abroad, both by events in the field of their own program-related research work and in other scientific topics.

In particular, the following events which took place during recent years, should be mentioned:

Fifth Symposium of the Section Experimental Cancer Research (SEK) of the German Cancer Association on "Current Problems and Results of Experimental Cancer Research" on the occasion of the 10th anniversary of the SEK, German Cancer Association and Deutsches Krebsforschungszentrum:
April 10–12, 1989.

Project-Symposium "Radiotherapy with Heavy Ions" of the Gesellschaft für Schwerionenforschung, Darmstadt, organized jointly with the Deutsches Krebsforschungszentrum:
May 12, 1989.

Symposium "Computer Assisted Molecular Modeling":
June 1–3, 1989.

Second Flow Cytometry Symposium Heidelberg:
October 19–20, 1989.

International Symposium "Concepts in Oncology" on the occasion of the 25th anniversary of the Deutsches Krebsforschungszentrum:
October 30, 1989.

Second International Symposium on "Improvement of Antitumor Drugs Therapeutic Index by Toxicity Reduction"; organized jointly by the Imperial Cancer Research Fund, London, and by the Deutsches Krebsforschungszentrum:
November 6–7, 1989.

Symposium "Cancer and Genes":
November 23–25, 1989.

Symposium on Genetic Epidemiology of Cancer:
January 22–23, 1990.

Symposium "Cytokines: From the Gene to Therapy"; Research Center for Environment and Health, Munich, organized jointly with the Deutsches Krebsforschungszentrum:
Februar 15, 1990.

Meeting of the Expert-Committee of the European Association for Cancer Research (EACR):
March 10, 1990.

Eighth Annual Meeting of the European Organization for Cooperation in Cancer Convention Studies (ECP), organized jointly with the Deutsches Krebsforschungszentrum:
April 2–3, 1990.

International Workshop "Papilloma Viruses":
May 13–17, 1990.

Symposium "De Novo Cancers in Organ Transplant Patients"; University of Cincinnatti, USA, Medical Center College of Medicine, Department of Surgery, organized jointly with the Deutsches Krebsforschungszentrum:
May 28–29, 1990.

Workshop "On Modeling of Cell Replacement in the Gut":
June 7–10, 1990.

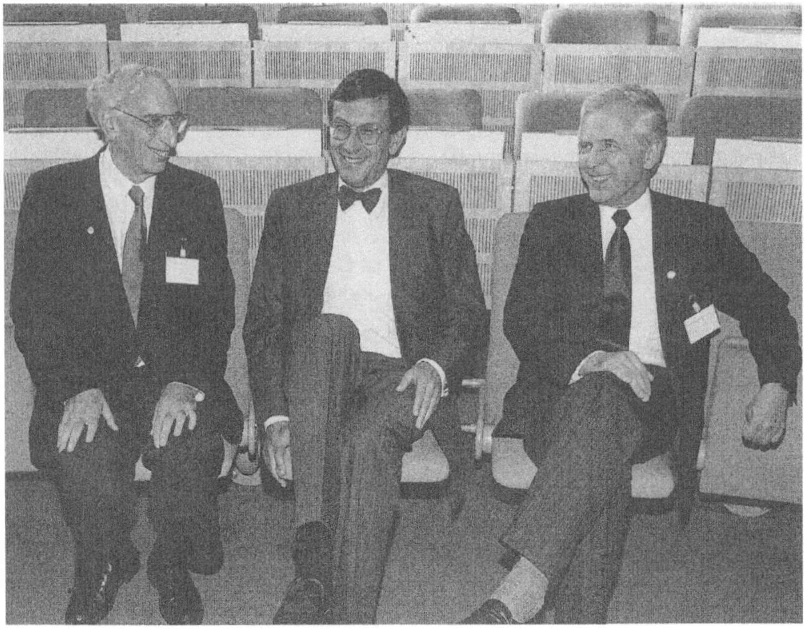

Fig. 184
In November 1991, the annual meeting of the Academia Europaea took place in the Deutsches Krebsforschungszentrum. *From left to right:* Sir Arnold Burgen, president of the Academia Europaea, Dr. Heinz Riesenhuber, Federal Minister for Research and Technology, and Prof. Dr. Harald zur Hausen.

European Workshop on Fluor Dexyglucose (FDG) in Oncology:
June 15–16, 1990.

Meeting of the German Saudi-Arabian Joint Committee for Cooperation in Science and Technology:
September 4–5, 1990.

Scientific Colloquium on "Biometrical Methods in Cancer Research":
September 17, 1990.

Symposium on the occasion of the 100th anniversary of K. H. Bauer; Surgical University Clinic Heidelberg, German Association of Surgery, Association of the Promotion of Cancer Research in Germany and Deutsches Krebsforschungszentrum:
September 26, 1990.

First German-Czech Workshop "Organizational Structures of the German Science in Biomedical Research" of the Czechoslovakian Committee of the Academy of Sciences and Universities of the CSFR, organized jointly with the Deutsches Krebsforschungszentrum:
October 1–4, 1990.

Conference "The Management Problems of Biomedical Research":
October 7–10, 1990.

Fourth International Workshop of the European Task Force of Cancer Information Services, Heidelberg:
October 18–19, 1990.

Third Flow Cytometry Symposium Heidelberg:
October 18–20, 1990.

Twentieth Annual Meeting of the Association of the Large Research Institutions, organized jointly with the Deutsches Krebsforschungszentrum:
November 6–7, 1990.

International Workshop "Epidemiological Methods" of the German Region of the Biometric Society, jointly with the Deutsches Krebsforschungszentrum
November 9–10, 1990.

Presentation of posters by diploma and doctoral students:
January 28–February 1, 1991.

Workshop "Biostatistical Analysis of the Micronucleus Mutagenicity Assay", German Region of the International Bibliometric Society, Working Group "Chemical Pharmaceutical Research", and Deutsches Krebsforschungszentrum:
February 6, 1991.

Sixth Symposium of the Section Experimental Cancer Research, Division for Experimental Cancer Research of the German Cancer Society and Deutsches Krebsforschungszentrum:
April 10–12, 1991.

Workshop "Bioinformatics Aspects of the European Human Genome Project":
April 26, 1991.

Workshop “Genes Controlling Cell Growth and Tumorigenesis in Drosophila”, Human Frontier Science Program and Deutsches Krebsforschungszentrum:
September 7–10, 1991.

Plenary Meeting of the Academia Europaea:
September 18–21, 1991.

Forth Cytometry Symposium Heidelberg, Cytometry Society and Deutsches Krebsforschungszentrum:
October 17–19, 1991.

Symposium “Skin Carcinogenesis in Man and Experimental Models”, University of Heidelberg jointly with Deutsches Krebsforschungszentrum:
October 29, 1991.

Meeting of the Executive Committee of the European Association for Cancer Research (EACR):
November 3–6, 1991.

Second European Workshop on FDG in Oncology, European Communities' concerted action “PET in Oncology” and Deutsches Krebsforschungszentrum:
December 9–11, 1991

Workshop “Molecular Biology of Aging”
December 13–14, 1991.

Presentation of posters of diploma and doctoral students:
February 3–6, 1992.

International Symposium “Human Tumor Viruses”:
May 3–6, 1992.

International Symposium on “Computational Methods in Genome Research”, European Data Resource for Human Genome Analysis and Deutsches Krebsforschungszentrum:
July 1–4, 1992.

Conference “New Methods in the Biochemistry of Proteins and Nucleic Acids, Study Group for Analytics of Proteins and Nucleic Acids of the Society of Biological Chemistry and Deutsches Krebsforschungszentrum:
September 10–12, 1992.

First Meeting of the Working Group “Molecular and Cytogenetics” of the German Cancer Society:
September 24–25, 1992.

Third Indo-German Workshop on Recent Results in Cooperative Cancer Research, Coordinating Committee for Cancer Research in the Arbeitsgemeinschaft für Großforschungseinrichtungen and Deutsches Krebsforschungszentrum:
October 4–7, 1992.

German-Japanese Workshop on “Host Defence Mechanisms and Molecular Basis of Cancer”:
October 18–21, 1992.

Fifth Cytometry Symposium Heidelberg, Cytometry Society and Deutsches Krebsforschungszentrum:
October 22–24, 1992.

Europe Against Cancer, Workshop for Journalists on “New Aspects in Cancer Research – A Network of European Cooperation in Science”:
November 29–December 1, 1992.

19

Statutes and Articles of the Foundation Deutsches Krebsforschungszentrum

in the version according to the resolution passed by the Board of Trustees dated 21 June 1991, published in the Legal Gazette Baden-Württemberg on 9 August 1991

I. General Provisions

Section 1
Legal Form, Seat

The Deutsches Krebsforschungszentrum, a foundation under public law of the Land Baden-Württemberg, has its seat in Heidelberg.

Section 2
Purpose of the Foundation

(1) It is the purpose of the Foundation to engage in cancer research.
(2) The Foundation may undertake other tasks in this connection, inter alia further education and advanced training, and especially the promotion of young scientists.
(3) The research results are to be published.

Section 3
Non-Profit Institution

(1) As a non-profit institution the Foundation shall exclusively and directly serve the public interest, in particular scientific interests according to fiscal regulations.
(2) Any profits made may only be used for the purposes laid down in the Statutes and Articles. The Foundation may not grant benefits to any person by expenditures which run counter to the purposes of the Foundation or by disproportionately high awards.

Section 4
Assets of the Foundation

The assets of the Foundation shall consist of the goods and titles which have been or are being created or acquired with the aid of the funds placed at its disposal by the Federal Republic of Germany, hereinafter referred to as the Federal Republic, the German Land Baden-Württemberg, hereinafter referred to as the Land, or by third parties. The assets of the Foundation shall be used for the purposes laid down in section 2.

Section 5
Financing of the Foundation

(1) The Federal Republic and the Land will provide for the necessary expenditures of the Foundation in as far as this is not covered by income from other sources or by own or foreign means – with the exception of donations and investment returns therefrom – by allowances according to further agreement.
(2) The means to be provided according to paragraph 1 will be allocated to the Foundation according to the provisions of the budgetary law within the framework of the approved budgets of the Foundation and the budgets of the Federal Republic and the Land.

Section 6
Budget of the Foundation

(1) The budget of the Foundation must contain any receipts to be expected in the fiscal year, any probable expenses, and any probable authorizations to incur liabilities. Receipts and expenditures must be balanced.
(2) The budget will have to be approved by the authority controlling the Foundation.
(3) Grants made to the Foundation are to be recorded in an appendix to the Foundation's accounts.

II. Organs of the Foundation

Section 7
Executive Organs

The organs of the Foundation are:
a) the Board of Trustees,
b) the Management Board,
c) the Scientific Council.

Section 8
Tasks of the Board of Trustees

(1) The Board of Trustees will supervise the legality, expediency, and economy of the conduct of the Foundation's transactions. It will decide on the aims of research and important research policy and financial affairs of the Foundation. It will determine the principles of management and those governing result control. It may give directives to the Management Board in special matters of research policy and finance as well as for the implementation of result control.
(2) The Board of Trustees sets up the annual budgets and the long- term financial plans including the programs for development and investment. It will decide on changes in the Statutes and Articles and on the dissolution of the Foundation as well as on other matters laid down in these Statutes.
(3) The following matters must be previously approved by the Board of Trustees:
a) the annual and long-term research programs;
b) taking up further tasks and discontinuing previous tasks;
c) the foundation, dissolution, and amalgamation of research programs, divisions, and central facilities, the start and termination of projects, and the extension of research programs and projects;
d) the appointment and recall of the heads of divisions, of the administrative director as well as of the directors of central facilities and projects, as well as the appointment of the coordinators of the research programs;
e) the regulations for research programs and projects;
f) the regulations for elections and the rules of procedure;
g) the regulations governing appointments;
h) principles governing the utilization of the research results of the Foundation;
i) extraordinary legal transactions and measures exceeding the framework of current business operations which may exert considerable influence upon the position and activity of the Foundation; significant agreements concerning cooperation with other German undertakings and institutions, and agreements concerning cooperation with foreign undertakings and institutions; entering into contracts which impose upon the Foundation obligations exceeding a period of one year, inasfar as they are not within the scope of normal business or provided for in the approved budget;
k) drawing up, changing or terminating employment contracts in excess of or outside the tariff, granting other benefits in excess of or outside the tariff, as well as entering into contracts exceeding an amount fixed by the Board of Trustees;
l) measures of collective tariff commitments or formation and general

regulations concerning remuneration and social benefits, as well as setting up directives governing the granting of reimbursement of travel and moving costs, of separation allowances, and of expenses for the use of motor vehicles.

(4) For particular types of legal transactions and measures, the Board of Trustees may give its agreement in general.

(5) In urgent cases it is sufficient to have the prior written consent of the President and the Deputy President of the Board of Trustees. The other members of the Board of Trustees are to be immediately informed by the President about the action.

Section 9
Composition of the Board of Trustees

(1) The Board of Trustees consists of, at most, eighteen honorary members.

(2) Out of these

a) four members – one of them being the President – will be delegated and removed from office by the Federal Republic,

b) two members – one of them being the Deputy President – will be delegated and removed from office by the Land,

c) three scientists working for the Foundation and without a seat on the Management Board – at least one of them being head of a division – will be appointed by the Land in agreement with the Federal Republic from a list of six nominees drawn up by all members of the scientific staff. Further details will be settled by election regulations to be issued by the Management Board in consultation with the Scientific Council and with the consent of the Board of Trustees. If those appointed have seats on the Scientific Council, their membership in the Scientific Council will be terminated upon acceptance of their appointment to the Board of Trustees,

d) seven external members (mainly specialists) will be appointed by the Land in agreement with the Federation upon consultation with the Management Board and the Scientific Council,

e) two members as the representatives of the University of Heidelberg, i.e. one proposed jointly by the Faculties of Medicine and Natural Sciences as well as the Rector (President) during his term of office or a professor charged by the latter, will be appointed by the Land in agreement with the Federal Republic.

(3) The members referred to in paragraph 2, items c, d and e will be appointed for a maximum period of three years. Re-appointment is permitted. After expiration of their term of office they will remain in office until the new appointments have been made according to paragraph 2, items c, d and e. Members may be removed from office for important reasons. Members leaving before their terms of office have expired must immediately be replaced from among the non-appointed applicants from the list of nominees according to paragraph 2, item c or by a new appointment according to paragraph 2, item d. Should the list of suggestions be exhausted, the procedure according to paragraph 2, item c shall be applied. Suggestion and appointment will be valid for the remaining term of office.

Section 10
Scientific Committee of the Board of Trustees

(1) The Scientific Committee prepares the decisions of the Board of Trustees in all scientific matters within the framework of section 8.

(2) The Scientific Committee bears the responsibility for the timely evaluation of the results of research programs, divisions and projects based on scientific expertise. As a rule, they set up ad hoc commissions manned by external scientists for this purpose.

(3) The Scientific Committee of the Board of Trustees consists of the external scientific members of the latter according to section 9, paragraph 2, item d. From among its members a chairman and a deputy chairman are elected. The President and the Deputy President of the Board of Trustees may take part in the sessions as guests. The Scientific Committee may set up standing rules which also determine the competence and procedures of the ad hoc commissions in greater detail.

Section 11
Standing Rules of The Board of Trustees and its Committees

(1) The Board of Trustees may set up standing rules which also determine the competence and procedure of the Committees in greater detail. Persons who are not members of the Board of Trustees may also hold a seat on the Committees; they will not take part in passing resolutions in Committees granted jurisdiction. A representative of the Federal Republic will assume the chair.

(2) The Board of Trustees may set up Committees to prepare its decisions as well as for certain matters to be decided by the Committee itself. At least one member each according to section 9, paragraph 2, items a through d must hold a seat on each Committee.

Section 12
Meetings of the Board of Trustees and its Committees

(1) The Board of Trustees will be convened by the President once in six months as a rule, but at least once every calendar year.
(2) The members of the Management Board as well as the chairman of the Scientific Council and the chairman of the staff representation or their deputies are entitled to attend the meetings of the Board of Trustees and its Committees in a consulting capacity, inasfar as the Board of Trustees or the Committee do not decide otherwise.

Section 13
Resolutions of the Board of Trustees and its Committees

(1) The Board of Trustees will constitute a quorum if two-thirds of its members are present or are represented in compliance with paragraph 2. The President or his deputy must be present. Committees holding power of decision will constitute a quorum if one member each according to section 9, paragraph 2, items a through c is present or represented.
(2) If unable to attend, the members of the Board of Trustees delegated by the Federal Republic and the Land may arrange to be represented by members of their administration, other members may be represented by a member of the Board of Trustees provided with a written limited power of attorney valid for the individual contingency.
(3) Resolutions of the Board of Trustees are passed with a majority of the valid votes cast. The President and the Deputy President have a double, transferable vote. In case of parity, the President shall have the casting vote. With important questions of research policy, in financial matters, in matters according to section 8, paragraphs 2 and 3, as well as with the appointment of the members and the release of the Management Board, resolutions may not be passed counter to the votes of members of the Board of Trustees delegated by the Federal Republic or the Land.
(4) Paragraphs 2 and 3 apply to the Committees correspondingly.
(5) In individual cases, the President, or if he is prevented, his deputy may cause resolutions to be passed in writing, by telex or by cable, insofar as no member of the Board of Trustees registers his immediate protest.

Section 14
Functions of the Management Board

(1) The Management Board directs the Foundation.
(2) The Management Board seeks the prior approval of the Scientific Council on the matters set down in section 8, paragraph 3, items a through g, as well as on

- the annual budget and long-term financial plans including the programs for development and investment;
- measures for the implementation of efficiency control of scientific work;
- measures to promote the flow of scientific information within the Foundation (work reports, colloquia, hearings);
- the co-operation with universities, other research institutions and international establishments;
- the submission of the scientific progress report to the Board of Trustees.

(3) Insofar as the Scientific Council's proposals in these matters should deviate, the Management Board will initiate a renewed joint discussion with the Scientific Council. If agreement cannot be reached, the Management Board will decide. If the Management Board makes a decision which deviates from the recommendations of the Scientific Council, it will have to supply an explanation in writing to the Scientific Council and the Board of Trustees.

Section 15
Composition of the Management Board, Scope of Authority

(1) The Management Board consists of at least one scientific and one administrative member. The administrative member shall be qualified for employment in the higher administrative service. The term of office for the members of the Management Board is limited and will, as a rule, amount to five years. Re-appointment is permitted. Appointments may be revoked at any time.

(2) The chairman of the Management Board and the other members will be appointed and recalled by the Board of Trustees after consultation with the Scientific Council. The Scientific Council has the right of nomination for scientific members and for the chairman.
The members of the Management Board may not at the same time be coordinators of research programs or be members of the Scientific Council. The President of the Board of Trustees, who in this capacity represents the Foundation, will enter into, change or terminate contracts with the members of the Management Board.
(3) The chairman of the Management Board will be the scientific representative of the Foundation. Together with the administrative member he will represent the Foundation judicially and extrajudicially. In matters of current administration the administrative member may represent the Foundation on his own.
(4) The Management Board will set up standing rules which require the approval of the Board of Trustees. The standing rules will also regulate the authority according to paragraph 3, sentences 2 and 3 in the event the authorized representatives are prevented from fulfilling their function.
(5) The administrative member of the Management Board will be in charge of budget affairs in the sense of section 9 of the budget regulations of the Land Baden-Württemberg.

Section 16
Tasks of the Scientific Council

(1) The Scientific Council advises the Board of Trustees and the Management Board in all significant matters of a scientific nature. In particular, it will offer advice concerning

a) the annual and long-term research programs;
b) appointment procedures, in particular the drawing up of appointment lists;
c) the appointment and recall of the heads of divisions as well as the directors of central facilities and projects;
d) taking up further functions and discontinuing previous functions;
e) founding, dissolving and amalgamating research programs, divisions and central facilities, starting and terminating projects, as well as extending research programs and projects;
f) issuing regulations for research programs and projects;
g) the appointments procedure;
h) principles for the utilization of the research results of the Foundation;
i) the annual budget and long-term financial plans including programs for development and investment;
k) measures for the implementation of result control of scientific work;
l) measures for the promotion of the flow of scientific information within the Foundation (work reports, colloquia, hearings);
m) the co-operation with universities, other research institutions and international establishments;
n) the scientific progress report.

In these matters the scientific Council, insofar as this is necessary according to section 14, paragraph 2, will pass resolutions about its consent with the intended decisions of the Management Board. If agreement cannot be reached, the procedure according to section 14, paragraph 3 will be applied.
(2) The Scientific Council may demand information from the Management Board on scientific matters and matters of research policy.

Section 17
Composition and Resolutions of the Scientific Council

(1) The Scientific Council consists of
a) the coordinators of research programs,
b) an equal number of representatives of the scientific staff.

(2) The members according to paragraph 1, letter b will be elected for a period of three years by the scientific staff of the Foundation in compliance with an election order. The election order is laid down by the Management Board in consultation with the Scientific Council and with the consent of the Board of Trustees.
(3) The Scientific Council elects from its midst a chairman and a deputy chairman.
(4) The members of the Management Board, the President of the Board of Trustees or a member of the Board of Trustees to be determined by the latter and a member of the staff representation may attend the meetings of the Scientific Council in a consultative capacity insofar as the Scientific Council does not decide otherwise in any individual instance.
(5) The Scientific Council will constitute a quorum if two thirds of its members including the chairman or the deputy chairman are present. Resolutions require a majority of the valid votes cast.
(6) The Scientific Council in consultation with the Management Board and with the consent of the Board of Trustees will set up standing rules governing the representation of the members.

III. Research Programs, Divisions, Projects and Central Facilities

Section 18 Research Programs and Divisions

(1) Research programs are the thematically defined and temporary collaboration of divisions.
(2) Divisions are scientifically independent research units co-operating within research programs. There are temporally limited and unlimited divisions. They are headed by heads of divisions who are appointed for an unlimited or limited period of time.
Being organizational units, the divisions serve the purpose of the Foundation. Within the divisions, working groups may be organized.
(3) The management of a research program consists of the heads of the divisions of that research program. It coordinates the scientific work of the divisions of that research program and makes all necessary decisions.
(4) The management of the research program nominates, with the consent of the Scientific Council and the Management Board, a coordinator from among its members. After approval from the Board of Trustees, the coordinator will be appointed by the Management Board. The term of office will amount to three years; re-appointment is possible. The tasks of the coordinators of the research programs are laid down in the standing order of the research programs, which also provides a research program committee and a research program assembly.
(5) The Management Board sets up standing rules for the divisions and the research programs after approval by the Scientific Council and the Board of Trustees.

Section 19 Projects

(1) The Foundation may carry out part of the research program in the form of projects. A project is understood to be a research activity largely structured in detail which is temporally and financially limited, bound towards a certain aim, and which exceeds the framework of a research program and which, due to its size and scientific importance, requires an independent organizational structure.
(2) The organization and implementation of projects are laid down in a project order which the Management Board will issue with the approval of the Scientific Council and the Board of Trustees.

Section 20 Central Facilities

(1) Central facilities shall serve to fulfill tasks of the entire Deutsches Krebsforschungszentrum or of several research programs and projects. They are reporting directly to the Management Board.
(2) The participation of the scientific staff in the elections to the Scientific Council and the Board of Trustees is regulated by the Management Board in the respective election orders with the approval of the Board of Trustees and the Scientific Council.

IV. Administration and Personnel Affairs

Section 21 Accounting, Auditing and Acceptance of the Accounts

(1) Accounts must be rendered annually by the Management Board concerning the income and expenditure as well as the assets and liabilities of the Foundation. Notwithstanding the legal auditing rights of the Federal Audit Office and the Audit Office of Baden-Württemberg, the annual accounts must be audited by a chartered accountant or auditing establishment. The Board of Trustees will decide who is to be entrusted with this task.
(2) At the end of the calendar year a business report and a statement of account is to be submitted to the Board of Trustees, the authority in control of the Foundation and the auditing authorities.
(3) Section 109, paragraph 3 of the budget regulations of Baden-Württemberg is applicable to the release. Organ for decision making is the Board of Trustees.

Section 22 Scientific Staff

The scientific staff as defined in these Statutes and Articles consists of all employees of the Foundation who are either university graduates or who carry out corresponding activities in the scientific field on the basis of equivalent abilities and experience and who have entered into an employment contract with the Foundation.

Section 23
Personnel Affairs

(1) Prior to the appointment of heads of divisions and the employment of scientific staff according to section 8, paragraph 3, item d, an appointment procedure is to be carried through pursuant to further regulations laid down in an appointment order to be issued by the Management Board in consultation with the Scientific Council and with the consent of the Board of Trustees.
(2) Decisions concerning the legal status of civil servants employed by the Foundation will be made by the competent authorities according to the legal regulations of the Land on the basis of applications which are decided upon by the competent organs of the Foundation.

Section 24
Changes Affecting the Statutes and Articles and Dissolution of the Foundation

Resolutions concerning changes affecting the Statutes and Articles and the dissolution of the Foundation may not be passed without the votes of the members of the Board of Trustees delegated by the Federal Republic and the Land who have a double vote in such matters. The Management Board and the Scientific Council are to be previously consulted. The resolutions will not take effect until they have been approved by the authority in control of the Foundation.

Section 25
Accumulation of Assets

(1) In the event of the dissolution of the Foundation, the Foundation's assets will pass to the Federal Republic and the Land in proportion to the value of the grants made by each of them, insofar as these assets do not exceed the value of the grants awarded and any contributions made in kind at the time of dissolution. Any balance then remaining will, in agreement with the Federal Republic, be used on a non-profit basis in the sense of the paragraph titled "tax-privileged purposes" of the tax code.

Section 26
Effective Date and Transitional Provisions

(1) These Statutes and Articles will go into effect on the day following their announcement in the Law Gazette of Baden-Württemberg.
(2) With the enactment of these Statutes and Articles, the Statutes and Articles of February 7, 1983 (Law Gazette, p. 86) and July 9, 1986 (Law Gazette, p. 278) become ineffective.
(3) The membership of the acting directors of the institutes and the scientific staff members of the Scientific Council continues in the framework of their term of office until the coordinators of the research programs are appointed and new scientific staff members have been elected.
(4) The terms of office of the acting directors of the institutes will be terminated upon the enactment of these Statutes and Articles.

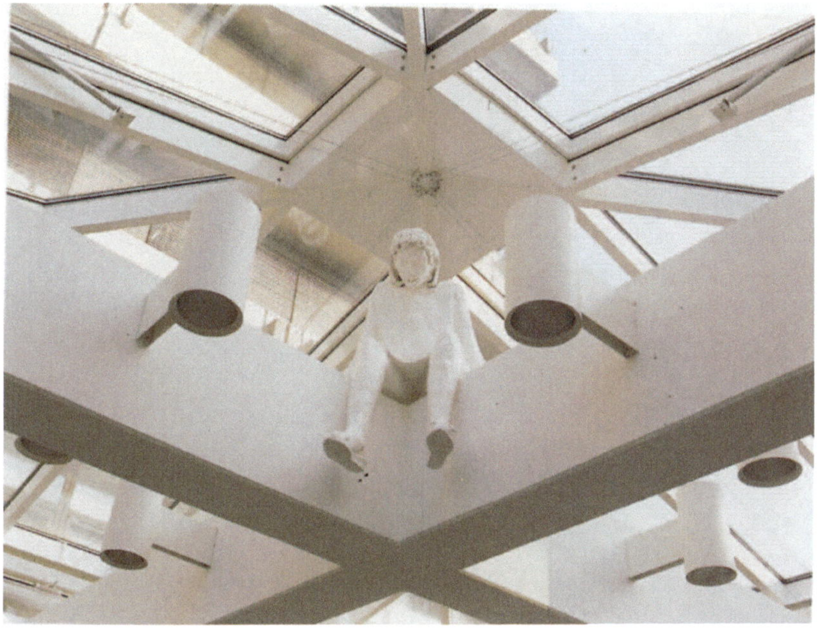

Fig. 185
Life-sized figures decorate the hall connecting the main building to the new communication center. The figures were made by students of the Tack painting school in Saarbrücken.

20

Index

Additional information of this book

(*Das Asbestzement-Druckrohr*, *978-3-798-50898*-9) is provided:

EXTRA
MATERIALS
extras.springer.com

http://Extras.Springer.com

GPSR Compliance

The European Union's (EU) General Product Safety Regulation (GPSR) is a set of rules that requires consumer products to be safe and our obligations to ensure this.

If you have any concerns about our products, you can contact us on ProductSafety@springernature.com

In case Publisher is established outside the EU, the EU authorized representative is:

Springer Nature Customer Service Center GmbH
Europaplatz 3
69115 Heidelberg, Germany

Batch number: 10578399

Printed by Printforce, the Netherlands